SURVIVING

CANCER

COVID-19, & DISEASE:

The Repurposed Drug

Revolution

by

Justus Robert Hope, M.D.

Published by Hope Pressworks International, LLC, Redding, California.

First Edition

Library of Congress Cataloging-in-Publication Data has been applied for.

ISBN: 978-0-9980554-2-8

The information presented in this book is the result of years of practice, experience, and clinical research by the author. However, it is not a substitute for evaluation and treatment by a medical doctor. The information contained herein is for educational purposes only. It is not intended to be a substitute for professional medical advice. The reader should always consult with his or her physician to determine the appropriateness of the information for his or her own medical situation and treatment plan. No prescription medication should be obtained or taken without a personal physician's prescription, care, and supervision. Reading this book does not constitute a physician-patient relationship. The stories in this book are true. The names and circumstances of the stories have been changed at times to preserve privacy.

Cover design by Daniel Ojedokun

By George Fareed, M.D.

2015 California Rural Physician of the Year
Former Assistant Professor, Harvard Medical School
University of California School of Medicine
Team Physician, United States Davis Cup Tennis Team
1991-2001

"This is a monumental treatise which should educate, inform, and impact medical care, public health, public policy and our world positively and also be of immense benefit to patients with cancer, infectious diseases and in particular those directly or indirectly affected by the Covid-19 pandemic. Dr. Justus Hope has assembled and explained critical facts and research on repurposed drugs in the most scholarly manner."

By Roger Seheult, M.D.

Associate Clinical Professor
University of California Riverside School of Medicine
Assistant Clinical Professor
Loma Linda University School of Medicine.
MedCram Co-Founder & Instructor

"The only thing necessary for the triumph of evil is for good men
to do nothing"
-Edmund Burke

*"This quote from Edmund Burke is true of Dr. Hope. He turned
his anger at his friend being diagnosed with Glioblastoma into
the book you are holding.
We must always be ready to admit that we do not understand
everything and have the humbleness of heart to change our
practices if the evidence confirms."*

FOREWORD by Dr. Ben Williams

When I was diagnosed with a glioblastoma multiforme brain tumor in 1995, I was told that the standard treatments of surgery, radiation and chemotherapy were ineffective and that no one survived my diagnosis. Fortunately, this was when the success of the HIV cocktail was in prominent focus, which raised the prospect that the cocktail approach applied more generally, including to the treatment of cancer. At least conceptually, the evolutionary dynamics that produce treatment resistance for AIDS applies to cancer cells as well as to viruses, so targeting the cancer cell with multiple treatment agents at the same time would produce more effective treatment with longer-lasting efficacy.

Having a philosophy of treatment is one thing. Implementing the philosophy is another. Identifying drugs that can be combined with other drugs, without excess toxicity, is a daunting task that must be addressed with caution. It is also extremely difficult given that the standard practices of our medical system has been to actively discourage the use of drug combinations outside of clinical trials.

At the same time the cocktail approach to treatment was gaining traction, the revolution in cellular biology was increasingly successful in understanding the dynamics of cell division, and provided the framework for understanding how many widely used drugs could be adapted for cancer treatment. Because many of these drugs have been used for decades, their toxicities are well understood, as are their interactions with other drugs, thus ideal candidates for use in drug cocktails.

This book is an important resource for all cancer patients. It identifies many commonly used drugs that have shown efficacy against multiple types of cancer. Because of their toxicities are well known, they can be added easily to standard treatment. Several different cocktail protocols are explicitly discussed, including clinical outcomes from different types of clinical trials. Hopefully, the wealth of evidence that is discussed will overcome the resistance to cocktail treatment plans so often encountered by patients from their oncologists.

August 2020   -Ben Williams, PhD
                     Professor Emeritus of Psychology
                     University of California at San Diego

                     Author of *Surviving Terminal Cancer: Clinical Trials, Drug Cocktails, and Other Treatments Your Oncologist Won't Tell You About*

FOREWORD by Dr. M.-E. Halatsch and Dr. R.E. Kast

In the shadow of the SARS-CoV-2 pandemic, which has claimed an acute death toll and critically challenged healthcare systems, societies and economies worldwide, many oncological diseases, including glioblastoma at a prominent position, remain notoriously difficult to treat. The traditional clinical research architecture of drug (target) discovery and validation in subsequent clinical trial phases is hampered by long time periods needed, high financial costs involved, and, in case of diseases with low prevalence, unfavorable return-of investment for drug-developing pharmaceutical companies, to name just a few points. On a different level, ethical issues with traditional randomized clinical trial designs continue to be raised by patient advocate groups, if such trials are available at all.

Against this background, the concept of individual drug repurposing has drawn significant attention from both patients and physicians. This concept hypothesizes that drugs able to yield better treatment results than today's first-line therapies for life-threatening, incurable diseases are already available and marketed, yet often unidentified or unproven for their "repurposes" by traditional standards; are comparatively cheap due to off-patent status; are relatively well-tolerable based on long clinical post-marketing experience with many patients; and last not least, can be legally prescribed for off-label use.

In addition, the drug repurposing concept is attractive to patients as it implies enhanced participation in the treatment effort, similar to dietary interventions, although there are more differences than similarities in this comparison. The broad availability of drugs for rational repurposing may provide a "democratic" element in that previous sense.

From a clinical science perspective, the positive theoretical considerations cited above must not substitute for the proof of effectivity and tolerability provided by randomized clinical trials. From the patient perspective, however, one persisting dilemma is that especially enrolling in confirmatory (vs. adaptive) clinical trials may serve future patients more than the actual trial participants themselves. This may hold true despite the non-disputed fact of clinical benefit for trial participants in general, even in control arms. The second dilemma stems from the irresolvable task to weigh a potential benefit of unknown magnitude associated with randomized clinical trial participation against the sometimes more or less theoretical – albeit often elaborate and plausible - concepts that constitute the basis of drug repurposing by individual patients.

Despite the availability of large knowledge bases regarding side effects of many repurposed drugs in their original indication, off-label use will be experimental in many cases. "Experimental" is not a precluding or judgmental term but reminds us that estimating the risk-benefit ratio of drug repurposing must be done responsibly. Responsibility is also mandatory in the face of broad drug availability. It is conceivable that this availability may affect the conduct of clinical research in the future.

One pressing, giant need is to rationally score drugs according to their evidence base , be it theoretical, molecular, cell culture-based, preclinical, case-based or derived from early-phase clinical trials, and to balance these scores with single-drug tolerabilities and drug-drug interactions, allowing the synthesis of optimized multi-drug regimens. It seems obvious that artificial intelligence is likely to play a major role in this effort. Whether or not drug scoring should also consider drug target molecule expression levels and drug target signaling pathway activations, among others, in individual diseased tissue may remain a matter of debate. Apart from potentially misleading sampling errors, so-called targeted therapy may lead to clonal selection and development of cellular resistance by signaling pathway cross-activation and other mechanisms. Time will tell if a consciously "non-targeted", broad, balanced combination of multiple repurposed non-oncological drugs may favorably modulate postoperative glioblastoma re-evolution during adjuvant medical treatment.

In the realms of this complexity, which has only been touched above, the current book by Dr. Justus Robert Hope represents a formidable attempt to provide guidance to patients and physicians wishing to consider the use of repurposed drugs.

August 2020   -Marc-Eric Halatsch, M.D., Ph.D.
                   Professor of Neurosurgery
                   Chief Consultant and Vice Chair,
                   Department of Neurosurgery
                   Ulm University Hospital
                   Ulm, Germany

                   Richard E. Kast, M.D.
                   IIAIGC Study Center
                   Burlington, Vermont, USA

CONTENTS

Foreword By Dr. Ben Williams 5

Foreword By Dr. M.-E. Halatsch and Dr. R.E. Kast 7

Dedication 13

Acknowledgements 15

Introduction 19

SECTION I: REPURPOSING DRUGS TO FIGHT CANCER 25

    Chapter 1 Can Doctors Prescribe Off-Label? 27

    Chapter 2 Treating Cancer with Repurposed Drugs............................ 33

    Chapter 3 My Own Repurposed Drug Regimen: The S.A.M. Cocktail... 47

    Chapter 4 The Redo Project: The Revolution Begins 55

SECTION II: THE SCIENCE BEHIND REPURPOSED DRUGS...........65

    Chapter 5 Pleiotropy.. 67

    Chapter 6 The Warburg Effect 79

    Chapter 7 Tumor Resistance, EMT and Autophagy 99

SECTION III: PERSONALIZING YOUR CANCER TREATMENT 117

    Chapter 8 Choosing the Right Plan for You............................. 119

    Chapter 9 The Coming Revolution in Cancer Care............................157

SECTION IV: REPURPOSING DRUGS AGAINST CORONAVIRUS .. 175

    Chapter 10 Repurposing Drugs Against Coronavirus 177

    Chapter 11 Human Trials Against Covid-19... 187

    Chapter 12 White Coats vs Blue Coats 195

SECTION V: THE SCIENCE OF CORONAVIRUS 199

    Chapter 13 Zoonotic Transfer 201

    Chapter 14 The Cytokine Storm 223

SECTION VI: THE POLITICS OF THE CORONAVIRUS 231

    Chapter 15 The Demonization of Hydroxychloroquine....................... 233

    Chapter 16 Getting to the Truth 241

Afterword.. 255

Epilogue.. 259

References 269

Appendix A: Myths and Misconceptions.. 299

Appendix B: Frequently Asked Questions...303

Appendix C: Informed Consent for Repurposed Drugs 307

Appendix D: Abbreviations Glossary 309

Appendix E: Redo Data Base of Repurposed Drugs 322

Appendix F: The Physicians' Position: 100 Points of View 323

Appendix G : Open Letter to Dr. Anthony Fauci 377

Appendix H : The Miracle of the Imperial Valley 393

Appendix I : YouTube Censors the Senate and Bans Dr. Pierre Kory 399

Postscript 407

DEDICATION

I was angry. Evan, my friend and colleague of 30 years, who was almost exactly my age, was diagnosed with glioblastoma. Several months prior, he was a healthy, successful professional with an adoring family.

My patients raved about how he treated them after their Medicare stopped paying. They marveled at his compassion, his concern for their pain, their lives, and their well-being.

Evan didn't deserve glioblastoma. But he also didn't deserve the standard treatment protocol of surgery, chemotherapy, and radiation treatments. As I used my background as a trained physician and researched every stitch of up-to-date technology, I grew angry—angry at the deception, angry at the bureaucracy, and angry at the system.

What I discovered in my research would make anyone angry. Dominic Hill, the producer of the film *Surviving Terminal Cancer*, said it best, "If you make enough people angry, the system will change." Evan deserved better. Every terminal cancer patient deserves better. Our current and outdated cancer treatment system needs reform, and now.

To Evan and everyone who suffers from terminal cancer, I dedicate this book.

Justus R. Hope, M.D.
Redding, California
May 2020

By Congressman John Lewis
1940-2020

Co-Organizer of the 1963 March on Washington
Co-Leader of the 1965 March on Selma
Presidential Medal of Freedom Award
Robert F. Kennedy Book Award
John F. Kennedy Profile in Courage Award

"When you see something that isn't right – isn't fair, that isn't just – you have a moral obligation to say something, to do something."

***

By Albert Schweitzer, M.D., Ph.D.
1875-1965

Priest, Physician, Humanitarian and Concert Musician
Medical Missionary
Founder of the Schweitzer Hospital of Lambaréné, Gabon
Goethe Prize Award
Nobel Peace Prize 1952

"The purpose of human life is to serve and to show compassion and the will to help others."

ACKNOWLEDGEMENTS

This book has given me hope for both cancer prevention and treatment. It has allowed me to find my friend Evan some realistic encouragement and, at least in some small way, has added one more brick to the repurposed drug revolution. This book would not have been possible without my eye-opening experience in reading Jane McLelland's work, *How to Starve Cancer without Starving Yourself*. Her book inspired me to discover the Care Oncology Clinic's impressive efforts, the Anti-Cancer Fund, and the Metronomic Movement. Jane's work proved to be the tip of a massive iceberg in this revolution.

First and foremost, I owe a debt of gratitude and appreciation to an icon, Dr. Ben Williams, the humble individual that started the repurposed drug revolution back in 1995. Ben's true story is retold herein and remains the stuff of legend. He cured himself of glioblastoma with a cocktail of repurposed drugs despite the refusals of his oncologists to prescribe them. Inspired by the AIDS cocktails, he single-handedly ignited a paradigm shift in cancer care that has today become a world-wide movement.

Ben returned my telephone call on a Saturday morning, answered my questions, and candidly relayed his personal experiences. As Dominic Hill said about Ben, "But he could have kept that to himself and gone to the mall or watched a ball game, but he didn't — he wrote a book, and he shared that information, and there are patients alive today, probably as a direct result of him choosing to write that book." It was one of the great honors of my life to speak with Ben.

I must thank Dr. Gregory Riggins, whose mice led to the chance discovery of the wonder drug, Mebendazole and its anticancer effects. Thanks to Dr. Pan Pantziarka for getting the world and *New York Times* to notice the topic of repurposed drugs. And a personal thanks to Dr. Pantziarka for never being too busy to answer a flood of e-mails from a frustrated physiatrist and aspiring writer with a confusing pen name, Justus R. Hope. Thanks to Dr. Pantziarka's research team, including Dr. Gauthier Bousche, Dr. Lydie Meheus, Dr. Vidula Sukhatme, and Dr. P. Vikas.

A heartfelt thanks to a great man, a man of fortitude, honor and compassion, to Dr. George Fareed, the pride of the Imperial Valley. George rejuvenated me when I felt alone in this fight. To the Harvard trained 2015 California Physician of the Year, who has set a glowing example for other doctors on what it means to crusade for patient care.

A patriotic thank you to Dr. Brian Tyson, whose message was censored by YouTube, but now lives on forever in the pages of this book. To Dr. Fareed's courageous young associate, the man behind the unbelievably true account of "The Miracle of the Imperial Valley," the energetic physician who achieved a 100% cure rate in his 1900 COVID-19 patients. To the El Centro family doctor who changed the world.

A sincere thanks to Dr. Roger Seheult, the young Loma Linda Intensivist who co-founded the MedCram review courses, and who was far ahead of the curve in proposing the HCQ/Zinc combination for COVID-19. To the gifted physician who gave the world the Seheult Supplement Cocktail.

Thank you to Dr. Samir Agrawal, a world-renowned hematologist/oncologist and the authority on aspergillosis. He took the time to review my manuscript when I was low on hope and could not reach other scientists. Dr. Agrawal proved to be a kind, down-to-earth, and incredibly patient gentleman who was always available to answer questions. I thank Dr. Agrawal for his generosity in time and spirit and his associates who co-founded the Care Oncology Clinics. The Care Oncology Clinic has been a beacon of hope and light in a dark world.

Thanks to the teams at the Care Oncology Clinics in both the United States and Europe including Dr. Zoraida Mendez, Dr. Paul Zhang, and Dr. Charles Meakin. Thanks also to the Care Oncology Team in the United Kingdom, including Dr. Agrawal, Dr. Vamadevan, Dr. Mazibuko, Dr. Robin Bannister, Dr. Ralph Swery, Dr. Wilson, and Dr. Edwards.

A special thanks to the Care Oncology Clinic for being there for my friend, Evan, and inspiring Jane McLelland. Without the Care Oncology Clinic, Jane would likely not have written her book, and you would not be reading this one.

Let me extend a personal thank you to Dr. Marc-Eric Halatsch, the German Neuro-Oncologist who introduced me to the extraordinary mind of Dr. Richard Kast, a massive force in the repurposed drug revolution and the inventor of the CUSP9 drug cocktail. I appreciated Dr. Halatsch's dedication, scientific accuracy, and willingness to help a fellow doctor he had never met.

Dr. Kast led me to discover the Metronomic Chemotherapy Movement, which is also a worldwide force to change the way chemotherapy is delivered, especially to pediatric and third-world patients.

My faith in organized medicine and human nature had been crippled by the politics of the worldwide pandemic, but has now been restored by people like Dr. Kast, Dr. Halatsch, and Dr. Agrawal. We are all in this together, rich or poor, educated or not, modern or third-world, and we all deserve the best chance to survive cancer and viruses. I am indebted to the support groups and charities that continue to support cancer research and funding.

I appreciate the trail-blazing efforts of Dr. Mark Moyad, a brave physician who is perhaps the world's foremost authority on the subject of dietary supplements, as well as the inventor of the S.A.M. cocktail for prostate cancer prevention. Thanks to Dr. Moyad for allowing me to adopt S.A.M. in this book. Thanks to Matt DeSilva for taking time away from his company, Notable Labs, to indulge the questions of an aging country doctor.

Allow me to apologize in advance to any individual I may have slighted in this book. There are many fine oncologists, fine regulators, and fine organizations seeking beneficial change and seeking to add repurposed drug cocktails and change outdated chemotherapy paradigms. Allow me to thank Dr. Jeffrey Fudin, who generously gave his time and wisdom to review this manuscript and who told me not what I wanted to hear but what I needed to know.

Allow me to apologize to any pharmacists I may have offended. Pharmacists and physicians work together as part of a team approach to ensure the best interests are met for each patient, including safety and efficacy. Pharmacists are an indispensable part of the treatment team, and I never meant to marginalize them in any way.

Thanks to my longsuffering wife, April, who supported this project every step of the way and without whose support I would not have completed it. Thanks to my transcriptionists, Candice Barner and Della Bowman who were a consistent hardworking force of nature.

Thanks to my editors Dan Crissman for reviewing the first half of the book and Dr. Andrew Diamond for the last half. Thanks to my artists for the cover and illustration work. Daniel Ojedokun did the cover and is also known as Danny_Media at FIVERR. The Cancer Tree illustration is by Rani.D (http://www.instagram.com/dewaranii/). Thanks also to Dr. Gregory White who helped me find my way through a very challenging journey.

Finally, thanks to Dr. Harvey Risch, who granted me approval to use his quote on the back cover. Dr. Risch is perhaps the most crucial voice in this book, the man who answered my email in less than five minutes on a Saturday evening. Dr. Risch is the distinguished Yale epidemiologist who would not be silenced. He is the man who will be remembered as the ultimate voice of reason in this great pandemic, the soul who stood tall to save lives with a repurposed drug. Dr. Risch's words will stand the test of time.

INTRODUCTION

Dr. Gregory Riggins, a neurosurgeon at Johns Hopkins University, had given his mice cancer. By carefully implanting malignant cells from a live tumor into each of their brains, they would now all grow brain medulloblastomas. New drugs and human cancer treatments could be tested.

But before the experiment could begin, his mice came down with a bad case of worms. Dr. Riggins did what any good scientist would: He treated them with a pinworm drug. Following the deworming treatment, the mice were once again healthy and worm-free, but quite inexplicably they were also cancer-free.[1]

After the mice got the pinworm drug, Dr. Riggins reported, "Our medulloblastomas stopped growing."

Riggins began studying the pinworm drug he gave them, mebendazole (or MBZ, for short) as an anticancer treatment. Mebendazole has been used safely for 40 years to treat parasites. Preliminary results showed MBZ to be effective at treating a large variety of cancers, including leukemia, lymphoma, lung cancer, colon cancer, and brain cancers such as glioblastoma and medulloblastoma.[2]

Compared to vincristine, the current standard treatment for pediatric brain tumors, MBZ is relatively safe, and nontoxic.[3] Vincristine is old school chemo, replete with side effects such as nausea, vomiting, hair loss, and immune suppression. Both vincristine and mebendazole work by blocking microtubule assembly in cells. If MBZ has been shown to be similarly (and perhaps) effective at fighting cancer, why would anyone not prefer a treatment with fewer side effects?

The answer, unfortunately, is money. The average cost to bring a drug to market in 2020 is approximately 1.8 billion dollars. Only a large pharmaceutical corporation with a good chance to make a profit would make such an investment. For old drugs to be used for new purposes, such as MBZ, the studies would simply not be cost effective. There would be no monetary incentive for a drug company to develop these along the traditional route. And because these billion-dollar Phase II and Phase III clinical trials have not yet been done, if a physician were to prescribe a pinworm medication like MBZ to treat cancer, he could risk his license. Unlike general practitioners, cancer specialists and oncologists are bound by a stricter set of guidelines, and any use of non-approved drugs or off-label use for cancer could mean being ostracized, losing hospital privileges, lawsuits, and license discipline.

As Jane McLelland's remarkable story shows, getting a prescription for off-label MBZ can be next to impossible. McLelland is a physical therapist who developed stage 4 cervical cancer with lung metastasis at barely age 30. She was given months to live along with recommendations for traditional surgery, radiation, and chemotherapy. Her primary chemotherapy drug, which almost killed her, was 5-FU, also known as 5-fluorouracil. Among oncologists, the drug was nicknamed "5 Feet Under."

STANDARD TOXIC CHEMO

Drug	Side Effects
• 5-FU aka 5 Feet Under	* Hair Loss, Inflammation
	* Low Blood Cell Count
	* Nausea, Vomiting
• Vincristine	* Hair Loss, Lung Damage
	* Low White Cells
	* Immune Suppression
	* Mouth Sores, Nerve Damage
	*Nausea, Vomiting

As a doctor, this kind of passive acceptance of dangerous medicine bothers me. No one should die from the treatments they receive from their physician. But somehow, this is acceptable in cancer care. Jane McLelland, however, refused to play by the rules. She did her own research and designed a combination of off-label drugs used for non-cancer purposes to treat her cancer. She almost single-handedly started the movement of repurposing old drugs for cancer treatment. Her book, *How to Starve Cancer without Starving Yourself*, has been an inspiration to many around the world.[4] She has survived her terminal cancer now for over 20 years.

There is a reason that cancer rates are rising to become the number one cause of death in developed and Western countries. Our current cancer system works well if one has an early disease. The cure rates and survival are generally excellent. The lesion is removed, and so long as the tumor has not spread, that may be the end of it. The problem comes with advanced disease. When dealing with stage 4 cancer, those that have spread and seeded distant locations, the chances of cure drop. The chances of toxicity rise. At this point, the patient often dies, either from cancer itself or from complications of the treatment.

Why do we accept this reality? Why have we not adopted less toxic therapy that is known to prevent tumor resistance, and metastatic spread, as it exists in the form of repurposed drugs? Perhaps it is because, in the early days of treating cancer, there was no alternative other than death. Our cancer care treatment protocols have not kept pace with technology.

Today, we have targeted immunotherapy. We have precise radiation beams. Most importantly, through our genetic knowledge of tumors, we have existing drugs that can prevent resistance by targeting key cancer stem cell pathways.

We have sequenced the genome. But we have not yet applied this knowledge in treating terminal cancer. We still treat terminal cancer patients with the old protocols of 50 years ago—surgery, chemotherapy, and radiation.

Take the case of a five-year-old with a brain tumor, medulloblastoma. When other effective nontoxic drugs exist, like MBZ, why does this five-year-old receive outdated chemotherapy so toxic, that he will be left with permanent brain damage and lifelong loss of pituitary growth function? Which one would you want your child to receive, if God forbid, they had a medulloblastoma?

By now, you may be seeing exactly why I am so passionate about reforming our current barbaric cancer care system. If drugs like mebendazole are available now, and most of us do not know about them, why is that? I can tell you after having done the research, and as an experienced physician, that it is not because they do not work. Consider this: mebendazole used to cost around $4.00 per pill and was widely available. After its cancer-killing properties were discovered, its price rose to around $400 per pill. Inexplicably, the price stayed low outside the United States. Today my friend with GBM cannot obtain it unless it is shipped from overseas.

Cancer chemotherapy, however, remains big business. One month of standard American chemotherapy can cost a healthy $10,000. The average cancer patient's total treatment cost is between $100,000 and $150,000. Eleven of the last 12 cancer drugs the FDA approved in 2012 were priced at more than $100,000 per year.

And Big Pharma's profits and monopoly are not just limited to cancer drugs. Consider this: hydroxychloroquine (HCQ) costs pennies. It has been used for decades by millions around the world for lupus and rheumatoid arthritis. It is used against cancer today. It was considered so safe that it was available over-the-counter in the UK and India. Like Mebendazole, once its antiviral effects against COVID-19 were discovered, it suddenly became scarce. Now a prescription is required to obtain it overseas. In the US, even with a prescription, most pharmacists refuse to fill it for COVID-19 despite a physician's order.

The time has come to make repurposed drugs widely available for everyone.

Existing and nontoxic medications that are FDA-approved for other treatments can and will turn the tide on our war against cancer. They can save you and your loved ones untold misery, but only if you can gain access to them. In the pages that follow, allow me to tell you about the repurposed drug movement and how that will translate into lifesaving treatment for terminal cancer and other conditions.

I will identify nontoxic and common medications that can be employed for maximum cancer preventative effect. I will also show you how common prescription medications in your medicine cabinet might just save your life if you already have terminal cancer. Drawing from my background as a physician, I will teach you which studies to show your doctor to convince him to prescribe these drugs off-label for you.

SECTION I:
REPURPOSING DRUGS TO FIGHT CANCER

Chapter 1

CAN DOCTORS PRESCRIBE OFF-LABEL?

While most of this book will explore the benefits of repurposed drugs for treating cancer, it is important to begin with a practical question: Is it legal for doctors to prescribe drugs for treating disease beyond their approved purposes?

The answer is yes. In fact, it happens all the time. As a pain specialist, I frequently prescribe lidocaine patches for my patients with nerve pain. The patch numbs the skin and reduces pain. However, the labeled use or the approved FDA indication for a Lidoderm patch is for post-herpetic neuralgia, a type of pain that can develop after a patient has developed shingles.

Ninety-nine percent of the time, my pain patient does not carry a diagnosis for the indication post-herpetic neuralgia or zoster. However, as a physician, I am legally allowed to prescribe the drug if there is a valid scientific basis that it will work, so long as it does not have a likelihood of causing harm. Similarly, a physician can prescribe metformin to a nondiabetic patient if there are published studies and good science to support a reasonable use.

With that said, most oncologists I know will not prescribe off-label drugs to treat or prevent cancer. I suppose it is because they might lose standing or be ridiculed by their colleagues. But this hesitance has consequences. To get a label use for a drug requires passing Phase I, Phase II, and Phase III clinical trials. A Phase I trial is to establish drug safety in humans, which all FDA-approved drugs pass. To test a new drug use for an old medication, however, Phase II and Phase III trials can cost many hundreds of millions of dollars. Traditionally, only the financial backing of a large pharmaceutical company could accomplish this. Without the incentive of billions in profits and a patentable drug, there would be no reason to invest this money. The necessary trials would not get done. Therefore, off-label use is currently the only practical option.

Why Won't Oncologists Cooperate?

Jane McLelland, an inspiration for this book, was met with anger and indignation when she asked the UK oncologist to prescribe off-label drugs for her cancer. My hope is that, as a physician, I can bolster the pioneering work Jane has already accomplished.

Her book *How to Starve Cancer without Starving Yourself* inspired me to research this further and led me to discover the Care Oncology Clinic in the UK, which is now doing clinical trials on glioblastoma. Their work has already produced impressive results in many cancers. Earlier this year, my friend and colleague Evan was diagnosed with glioblastoma, a malignant brain tumor with an average survival of 15 months, and I advised him to enroll in the Care Oncology Clinic's study. The preliminary data they've released about the combination standard treatment and repurposed drugs is encouraging. Simply adding metformin, doxycycline, atorvastatin, and mebendazole can increase GBM average survival from 15 to 27 months, almost a doubling.[6]

GLIOBLASTOMA AVERAGE SURVIVAL

Type of Treatment:	Survival Time in Months:
• Standard Rx	15 months
• COC Protocol + Standard Rx	27 months

In my opinion, the COC four-drug protocol should be offered to all GBM patients in light of the METRICS study results at Care Oncology Clinic.

Everyone in the world with GBM should know about the potential benefits of repurposed drugs and the Care Oncology Clinic. Why is it that we don't? If I had not stumbled across this information to help my friend, you would not be reading this book today.

My friend and his family do not have the time to wait for official approval and further clinical trials. Still, he certainly can legally join the existing trial at the Care Oncology Clinic. I find myself wondering, what if my friend had started taking these four drugs years ago not to treat the glioma, but to prevent it? Would he still be coming down with GBM today?

This brings us back to mebendazole (MBZ), the deworming drug that Dr. Riggins discovered that could make his mice's brain tumor stop growing. Since 2011, when Dr. Riggins stumbled across the unintended benefits of the MBZ, more than 100 additional studies have been conducted that confirm the suspected anticancer effect.

Mice with glioma survived an average of 30 days in a control group. Mice treated with MBZ survived an average of 49 days, an increase of some 16.3%.[7] Dr. Riggins reported in 2015 that MBZ works by preventing the tumor's microtubule formation. It also has anti-angiogenesis mechanisms that interfere with tumor blood vessel growth.[8] MBZ, when combined with chemotherapy, can strongly suppress melanoma growth as well.[9]

When combined with radiation, MBZ prevents triple-negative breast cancer from forming radiation-sensitive tumor cells, thereby greatly enhancing tumor control.[10] MBZ and Sulindac can prevent tumor initiation, the starting point of colon cancer formation. MBZ, in combination with Sulindac, reduces 90% of precancerous polyps seen in the worst case familial adenomatous polyposis.[11] MBZ is nontoxic.

MEBENDAZOLE INHIBITS CANCER

- Colon
- Leukemia
- Melanoma
- Ovarian
- Lung
- Brain
- Kidney

Additionally, it was found to decrease the activity in the Hedgehog (Hh) pathway that is common to gliomas, melanomas, lung cancers, ovarian cancers, and colorectal cancers.[12] But MBZ targets mainly cancer stem cells (CSC). It promotes apoptosis or death of cancer cells and has little to no effect on normal cells. This explains its major effectiveness against a broad collection of tumors and its lack of toxicity at normal doses. In testing in the lab, MBZ had high activity against leukemia, colon cancer, and melanoma with lesser activity against ovarian, renal, and non-small cell lung cancers.[13] In colon cancer, 80% of cell lines were sensitive to MBZ.

The use of MBZ has been proposed for treating dozens of cancers. Approvals are coming, but not nearly soon enough. I have not yet personally prescribed it or taken it, but I believe it may be reasonable to have a course of MBZ twice per year for prevention purposes in certain high-risk groups. Obviously, more studies are needed to fine-tune these recommendations. But the research so far is encouraging, to say the least.

A Word About Science

Physicians rely on science because supposition, hunches, conventional wisdom, and so-called miracle cures are the province of quackery. Scientific studies provide the foundation of modern medicine, and the best studies remain prospective randomized placebo-controlled double-blind trials. Retrospective reviews, however, those with proper matching and large numbers can provide good associations. Determining cause and effect requires multiple such studies.

We are protected from charlatans and snake oil salesmen by insisting on science before recommending that desperate souls buy into unproven treatments. However, the science in favor of using repurposed drugs to treat cancer has been building for many years. Today, the evidence has reached the persuasive level.

But hiding behind science today, in the face of the hundreds of promising studies, to attempt to deny the effectiveness of repurposed drug use in cancer is neither scientific nor humane. Today, our problem with modern cancer care is neither quackery nor junk science. It is rising cancer mortality and a dearth of new research and development.

Pharmaceutical companies are bringing fewer and fewer new cancer treatments to market. With an R & D price tag of billions for each new molecule and a 70% failure rate, it is seldom worth the risk, at least for cancer drugs. Meanwhile, in 2018, the world saw 18 million new cancer cases and 9.6 million related deaths. We already have some 2,000 FDA-approved drugs that have passed the phase I trials certifying their safety in humans.

Why not use this massive, immediately available resource to solve our cancer care dilemma? Why not use old drugs as anticancer treatments? Due to financial and regulatory constraints, not scientific roadblocks, the public, and most physicians simply are not aware that better and more efficient cancer treatment options are currently available. This is tragic, as many millions worldwide continue to suffer and die when better alternatives now exist.

The movement to license repurposed drugs will open the door to marketing them. With luck, the pharmaceutical companies will be allowed to advertise their uses. Under current laws, any informing of the public by drug companies about off-label use could result in criminal prosecution and penalties.

Fortunately, we live in the age of social media. The word is slowly getting out that even cancer does not have to be fatal if people use repurposed drug combinations. Long-term survivors of glioblastomas and other terminal cancers, once rare, are becoming more commonplace with the use of these drugs. With every long-term survivor who employs repurposed drugs, it becomes more and more difficult for the old guard to pass them off as another statistical freak. There is a clear pattern emerging that cannot be ignored.

A world-renowned Glioblastoma expert, who asked to remain anonymous, has stated that physicians are ethically obligated to investigate these long-term survivor case histories to determine the factors that contributed to their survival. They should not continue to be simply disregarded, but instead responsibly studied. In Belgium, The Anticancer Fund supports further widespread clinical trials of repurposed drugs.[14] Licensing and regulation reform could take years and maybe even decades. But these repurposed drugs are available today from your GP or family physician, legally and scientifically based upon off-label use.

ANTICANCER POTENTIAL OF REPURPOSED DRUGS

- Number of New Cancers Yearly   18 Million
- Number of Cancer Deaths Yearly   9.6 Million
- Number of FDA Approved Drugs   2,000
- Approved Drugs with Anticancer Activity   310

Today's greatest barrier is lack of awareness. Most people have never even heard about repurposed drugs for cancer. I aim to change that with this book. Now is the time for grassroots efforts by everyone to join the repurposed drug revolution. You, your loved ones, or anyone affected by cancer or who is at risk should know as much about these as they already know about common cancer screening tests. The best time for people to learn about repurposed drugs' potential health benefits is before cancer strikes, not after.

BARRIERS TO USE OF REPURPOSED DRUGS

- Big Pharma   * Cheap off-patent Drugs not Profitable
- Regulators   * Regulators are Cozy with Big Pharma
- Lack of Public Awareness
- Lack of Physician Awareness

Chapter 2

TREATING CANCER WITH REPURPOSED DRUGS

So what should you do if, God forbid, you are diagnosed with cancer? Let us look briefly at a few true stories.

Dr. David Jennings and Barry Downs

Dr. David Jennings, a New Zealand GP physician with 40 years of experience, encountered cancer and repurposed drugs up close and personal.[15] A close friend, Barry Downs, was diagnosed with terminal gallbladder cancer. Barry had found out late in the disease after the cancer had spread to his lungs and beyond. He was given three weeks to live. His pain was so severe he needed morphine 60 mg twice a day to cope. Barry's wife, Adrian, did not feel that he would make it through the week.

"Davey," she said, "I think we have a dead man walking. He is really, really bad. We have an appointment for an MRI on Thursday, but I don't think we're going to get there."

The oncologist's appointment to discuss chemotherapy was six weeks away, and there was a good chance that Barry would not make that either.

Dr. David Jennings did what any good friend would do. He researched the cancer and everything that could be done to help his friend. The good doctor discovered five repurposed drugs: metformin, atorvastatin, mebendazole, loratadine, and cimetidine that had scientifically proven anticancer effects. The medications were approved for other treatments like diabetes or ulcers, but Dr. Jennings felt Barry had nothing to lose as they were nontoxic.

"We immediately felt that this was worth a shot. There was nothing else on the table. Nobody was offering anything else," said Adrian.

Very quickly, Barry responded. The tumors shrank, and Barry started to gain weight. The crushing pain let up, and he dropped his morphine dose from 120 to 20 mg per day. Barry eventually received chemotherapy down the line, but Adrian and Dr. Jennings were convinced that the repurposed drugs had made all the difference.

Barry had a birthday, and Adrian had a birthday. He attended birthdays for his two grandchildren, and he enjoyed quality time with his wife and family. He survived almost six more months, far more than the few weeks predicted.

Although the cancer ultimately claimed Barry's life, Dr. David Jennings was forever changed. He became a believer in the use of repurposed drugs in cancer treatment.

Dr. Ben Williams

Dr. Ben Williams was a psychology professor who had earned a PhD from Harvard. At the age of 50, he was diagnosed with glioblastoma (a brain tumor).[16] This was not just any glioblastoma; it was glioblastoma multiforme, the nastiest most aggressive form. This is the same tumor my friend Evan developed. It is typically fatal within a year and is known in medical circles as "The Terminator."

Dr. Ben Williams did what Dr. Jennings did. He researched the tumor and studied all the ways to slow its growth or kill it, especially by using prescription drugs off-label.

He read about clinical trials and soon discovered that the drug Accutane, commonly used to treat acne, could fight it. He found that tamoxifen, a drug used to treat breast cancer, was also effective. He learned that the tumor could shield itself from chemotherapy by calcium channels. So, he decided to add the calcium channel drug, verapamil, to thwart this. Verapamil is usually used blood pressure.

He asked his cancer doctor if he could add these and about a dozen other "repurposed drugs" to his treatment plan.

"He just out and out refused to allow the tamoxifen, he was unwilling to bend, and we had a major altercation over the phone," Ben recalls. "It is a big mystery to me how you can just deny something that has credible evidence." The two parted ways, and not so politely.[17]

Ben persisted. He found a mushroom extract used in Japan routinely in almost all cancer treatment protocols. Ben states, "It is never mentioned in the United States. It is nontoxic. It has been used by millions of Japanese for years to treat cancer." Ben was flabbergasted that the United States physicians did not even recognize supplements and medications that had strong proven anticancer effects.

Eventually, Ben re-established care with his neuro-oncologist, after his neurosurgeon backed Ben up. "Going against the advice of my doctor was initially an act of desperation, but I was not concerned about offending him. I was concerned about staying alive. So, I was going to use anything I could get my hands on, and if that made them angry, then that was too bad."

With that strategy, Ben designed a prescription drug cocktail that would attack the cancer from as many angles as he could. Within six months and the first chemotherapy regimen, the tumor began shrinking. Encouraged, Ben redoubled his efforts and added even more supplements and drugs. His tumor withered after the third round, and by the completion of the fourth, it was gone. He received a clean MRI of his brain.

At that point, in hindsight, his oncologist suggested he was a rare case with an excellent response to chemo. He suspected the additional supplements and repurposed drugs Ben added did nothing, and that his cancer remission was a statistical fluke. Perhaps just a lucky patient who found himself among the 3% of GBM patients who survive more than five years.

"The irony is that almost every oncologist will agree that multiple agent approaches are going to be necessary to cure cancer. No one disagrees with that. The question is, what goes into the cocktail and what kind of criteria or evidence you have to have for putting those cocktails together?"

Dr. Ben Williams has since gone on to continue his cocktail and now, with over 25 years of survival, has become a staunch advocate for reform of the current US cancer care treatment system. "We will never know for sure why I am still alive."

Jane McLelland

Jane McLelland wrote a remarkably similar story in her book, *How to Starve Cancer without Starving Yourself.* Jane contracted cancer at the age of 30 and was eventually informed that it had spread to her lungs, making it stage IV and terminal.

Jane embarked on a research program similar to Ben's. In 1996, the internet was a very basic instrument compared to the Google monster that we have today. Nevertheless, Jane found some helpful information. There were a few success stories by people who had adopted a radical change in diet. She discovered that glucose and insulin fueled most cancers.

Jane began cutting out sugar and refined carbohydrates in her diet. She advised her mother to do the same as her mother had ironically been diagnosed with terminal breast cancer at the same time Jane was diagnosed with her own disease. However, her mother's oncologists were not nutritionally-minded and told her (mistakenly) that diet really did not matter.

Jane reports that her mother obediently followed the oncologist's advice to eat cake and biscuits "for energy." Jane watched as her mother lost weight and grew battered from chemotherapy. After she passed away, Jane became alienated and distrustful of modern medicine. Eventually, Jane rebounded with renewed optimism about researching and battling her own cancer.

Soon Jane was researching prescription drugs effective against cancer pathways. More specifically, she realized that combinations of drugs were effective in saving the lives of AIDS patients, and she asked why these might also help slow the disease of cancer patients? She felt that the right combination of repurposed drugs and supplements could keep cancer in remission permanently.

Jane, like me, became a PubMed explorer. She took advantage of the free National Library of Medicine search engine to look up all studies under a given topic. It was sort of like Google for doctors or healthcare professionals with one major exception. Regular Google often results in misinformation. But the studies on PubMed are scientific, not the product of social media. They are peer-reviewed and evidenced-based.

Jane's systematic research led her to the truth. In particular, Jane's research supported that she take an aspirin, both before and after surgery, as surgery can cause inflammation. Her oncologist disputed this and told her that there was not enough evidence to support aspirin's use. He was worried about stomach bleeds. Despite his advice, she made the decision—the correct one based on today's new evidence—to take low dose aspirin prior to surgery. Jane's reasoning was, "if only I had known the risk of GI bleeding with aspirin was a mere 2% compared to my 100% risk of dying in stage IV cancer. It would have made my decision easier."

"My developing theory was that anything that might make the tumor less had to be a good thing." Jane went on, "attack it from every angle. That was my mantra. This was war. No question, I was going to take aspirin."

Eventually, Jane discovered that old drugs like dipyridamole (usually used to prevent heart attacks) also had a strong anticancer effect. Dipyridamole had also been used in conjunction with AZT to treat AIDS (off-label) because of its antiviral properties.

Jane recognized that statins, in combination with anti-inflammatory agents, could increase cancer cell death by fivefold.[18] This is termed apoptosis. With her doctor's permission, she added aspirin, a statin, and dipyridamole for several months and saw her cancer biomarkers drop. She was succeeding in suppressing her cancer, and soon her cancer biomarkers dropped from 397 to 21.5. A level of 15 was considered normal.

As Jane approached her 40th birthday, she loosened up on her diet. Having been in remission for almost five years, and defying all odds in surviving stage IV cancer, she became lax with her cocktail. She took aspirin only infrequently. She celebrated her 40th birthday and soon noticed symptoms like leg swelling and coughing up of blood. When she retested her tumor markers, she was horrified to see the levels back up to 200, levels similar to when the tumor was active.

She immediately resumed her statin/dipyridamole combination. Within weeks, her biomarkers returned back to near normal. She is now committed to continuing her repurposed cocktail permanently.

Eventually, Jane became a staunch advocate for cancer treatment reform. She helped her friend with malignant melanoma by accompanying her to her oncology visit. The oncologist berated the patient's decision to cut out sugar from her diet. "I have already explained to you that changing your diet is a waste of time," the doctor proclaimed.[19]

Jane spoke up on her friend's behalf, asking about dipyridamole and statins. Without answering, the oncologist scowled and left the room. Her friend did not get the two repurposed drugs, although based on the science, they would likely have helped. Jane's friend passed away some six months later. Jane's use of repurposed drugs saved her life. She has now survived over 20 years with a disease that typically kills in a year with standard care.

Dr. Angela Chapman

Dr. Angela Chapman, PhD, is an ornithologist and second author of the publication, *Breast Cancer with Brain Metastasis Prospects from a Long-Term Survivor.*[20]

She was also the patient. Dr. Chapman developed her HER2+ positive cancer at age 61 in November 2012. It quickly spread to her liver, and at stage IV, she was given just a 23% chance of surviving five years. Both she and her partner began furiously researching the available medical literature. Her partner, Dr. Christopher Kofron, worked as a biologist specializing in endangered species. Both had extensive experience in scientific research.

Angela received the standard treatment of chemotherapy and monoclonal antibodies at UCLA, to which her body responded quickly, with a complete remission within six months. She suffered severe nausea and vomiting, fatigue, and loss of hair and nails.

She enjoyed nearly 18 months of full remission with a return to normal life and function. By June 2014, her speech suddenly became garbled, and the cancer was found to have spread to her brain. An MRI of the brain showed some 20 tumors, the largest being three-quarters of an inch (the size of a large marble). The prognosis for survival suddenly changed to months, with an 8% chance for five-year survival.

In 2014, she was started on capecitabine and lapatinib, the only options according to the medical standard of care. The side effects were severe and left her debilitated. Since the patient and her partner were both PhD educated biologists, they continued to extensively review the available scientific literature. Since the patient and her partner were both PhD educated biologists, they continued to extensively review the available scientific literature.

At the patient's request, off-label trastuzumab was infused. The two felt that these large molecules could cross the damaged blood-brain barrier. In addition, Dr. Chapman supplemented with off-label drugs and supplements such as artemisinin, aspirin, chloroquine, doxycycline, hydroxychloroquine, as well as melatonin, nanocurmin, Omega III fish oil, pterostilbene, and quercetin, and resveratrol. She also utilized turkey tail mushroom (trametes versicolor) and vitamin D3.

Since March 2013, there has been no evidence of cancer recurrence outside the brain or central nervous system. Angela was forced to abandon capecitabine and lapatinib due to their intolerable side effects, but, like Jane, Angela has continued her cocktail of aspirin, melatonin, nanocurcumin, Omega III fish oil, pterostilbene, and vitamin D3.

Her cancer has not returned, as shown on the recent chest, abdominal, and pelvic MRI scans. Her recent brain MRI of 2019 showed no further recurrence. Her estrogen receptor status, combined with her HER2+ status, is reported to make her long-term survival unlikely, even with the standard medical care.

Both Dr. Kofron and Dr. Chapman credit her survival to three things:

- An excellent oncologist with whom they developed a partnership

- Informed exploration of the available scientific literature

- The use of numerous substances, supplements, and repurposed drugs in concert with the standard of care treatment.

The two doctors pointed out that Angela's recovery was directly due to not only standard of care, but to the repurposed drugs. All patients should take an active part in their treatment, research available treatment options, suggest them to their physicians, and work with them to negotiate an optimal treatment plan.

The authors write, "It seems likely that the patient's supplementation with numerous repurposed drugs and other substances, reported to have antitumor properties have been a key factor in her long-term survival."

Do Your Own Research

What do Ben Williams, Jane McLelland, and Angela Chapman have in common? For one, they are all doctorate level, highly educated individuals with backgrounds in the biological sciences. More importantly, they all availed themselves of the latest medical research on their tumor's biology and discovered a wealth of anticancer substances ranging from supplements to prescription drugs.

What should an average patient do? What can a person who lacks a Harvard PhD accomplish to save themselves from terminal cancer? First, enlist the help of a trusted GP or family doctor who is willing to work with you. Second, you or an educated family member or friend should conduct a computer search on PubMed, or simply go to Google and type in your tumor type + PubMed + repurposed drugs.

Print out the five best articles on repurposed drugs with low toxicity and take them to your family physician. Family physicians are much more open to prescribing repurposed drugs for cancer than oncologists. However, most physicians will not suggest these to you on their own. If you come prepared with excellent articles and evidence, though, many will prescribe them feeling that it could not hurt.

You must partner with an oncologist who is willing to work with you and your family doctor. Perhaps because they were fellow scientists, Dr. Chapman and Dr. Kofron were able to convince their oncologist to work with them. Dr. Kofron was kind enough to grant me an interview and insight into this process.

Although Jane McLelland and I utilize PubMed, the free search engine of the National Library of Medicine, Dr. Kofron used Google Scholar as he was familiar with its use in everyday work as a biologist. I tried both, and they are each simple and easy to use. Just search "Google Scholar" and click on the site. Dr. Kofron said he first searched for "mushrooms + breast cancer" and "polysaccharide K + breast cancer" as the literature suggested beneficial effects.

PUBMED: GOOGLE FOR DOCTORS

• Free Search Engine	* Anyone Can Use
• Scientific Papers	* Peer Reviewed Studies
• International	* Avoids Bias
• Search by Cancer	* Search by Drug or Supplement
• Search Author	* Last name and first initial

I replicated the search for breast cancer and mushrooms. Noticing that Dr.'s Kofron and Chapman had included turkey tail (trametes versicolor) mushroom in her cocktail, I searched trametes versicolor + breast cancer + mushroom. I read about Krestin, otherwise known as PSK or polysaccharide K. The substance was first identified in the 1970s and originally tested in Japan. In the United States, more recent studies have shown that PSK, combined with chemotherapy, improves survival and treatment response.[21]

Why would someone not take this nontoxic mushroom supplement? Because they aren't aware of it. That is the problem. If you have stage IV HER2+ breast cancer, you will get advice to use standard toxic chemotherapy and radiation. Still, I can assure you that your oncologist will not breathe a word about turkey tail mushroom.

Like Jane McLelland, Dr. Kofron read life extension publications. Dr. Kofron recommends a book entitled *"Disease Prevention and Treatment"* edited by Blake Gossard.[22] He read the Fifth Edition, but the sixth is already in print. It is a "must reference" for any family, and I would include it as a good starting point in your research.

It reports on recent evidence-based studies, fresh out of PubMed, that combat many diseases including Alzheimer's, atherosclerosis, and all major cancers. There are sections on glioblastoma, pancreatic cancer, and breast cancer.

By itself, it would provide anyone with an easy to understand foundation of knowledge. In addition to turkey tail mushroom, nanocurcumin was added due to the research showing intense antitumor activity. This is not the common over-the-counter curcumin. The over-the-counter version does not absorb well. Nanocurcumin, by contrast, is micronized and easily absorbed. The two requested off-label use of pegfilgrastim to help Angela with radiation brain injury.

This brings me to the next part of off-label drug use. Although it is legal for a physician to prescribe a drug for off-label use, it may not be covered by insurance. Insurance generally only covers the drug if it is used for an FDA-approved indication.

Although Dr. Kofron found competent evidence to support the use of pegfilgrastim, the coverage was denied, and the two had to come up with the $6,000 price tag for a year. After a lengthy appeals process including a 90-page scientifically based letter authored by Dr. Kofron, the drug was retroactively covered, and they were reimbursed.

Angela is currently cancer-free but continues to suffer from complications of whole-brain radiation. She is unable to walk and suffers from neurologic decline, including loss of short-term memory and technical skills. In the article they published, Dr. Kofron strongly recommends that preventative follow-up MRIs be routinely performed to detect brain metastasis. Had this been done with Angela, her tumors could have been picked up earlier where they would have been smaller, and less radiation would have been required. There would have been less brain damage.

Angela's story is all too common. The traditional standard of care treatment is now as follows:

Blast the cancer with the latest, greatest, and most expensive debulking agent, have a party when the patient goes into remission, and do absolutely nothing while the remaining tumor cells dust themselves off and like transformer automatons, reassemble into a much more deadly version that now may be radiation resistant and impervious to all known chemotherapeutic agents.

Instead, how about this? Research PubMed and find the latest supplements with anticancer effects, whether it be turkey tail mushroom or nanocurmin, in Angela's case, or berberine in Jane's case. Take the best five low dose anticancer drugs like chloroquine or doxycycline in Angela's case, like Accutane in Ben Williams' case, dipyridamole or lovastatin in Jane's case and then allow the chemotherapy at a reduced dose.

Jane wrote that she had to beg and plead with her oncologist to reduce her dose. She is convinced that if she had been given the full standard dosage treatment, she would not have survived. Remember what Dr. Ben Williams said, "I did not care about offending my oncologist. I was interested in saving my life." You need to draw the line at too toxic a dose of chemotherapy or radiation treatment.

ADD YOUR REPURPOSED DRUGS

- First research your cancer and your standard care
- Search PubMed for Repurposed Drugs that show effectiveness
- Print out the articles
- Negotiate with Your Oncologist
- If your Oncologist refuses, ask your family doctor

The treatment you agree upon with your oncologist must be an informed negotiation. I would also advise you to decide on your cocktail regimen in advance with your family doctor. Be sure it is based on good science, and there are no drug-to-drug interactions or toxicities. Run this by another physician first, your family doctor or trusted GP for 20 years, for example. Gain his approval that your decision is reasonable.

Bring your printed out studies from your Google Scholar or PubMed and negotiate with him on as many drugs as he will allow. Generally, the more, the better, and that applies to supplements as well. If you are a pushover, bring your bulldog partner, sibling, or relative to the oncology appointment. Argue for the drugs that show synergy with either radiation therapy or chemotherapy. They will give you the most benefit.

Angela and Chris mastered this part. They insisted on adding chloroquine to the trastuzumab during the initial chemotherapy that included monoclonal antibodies. They found the 2013 study by Dr. Cufi and colleagues published in "*Science Reports*" that showed that chloroquine reversed 90% of the trastuzumab resistance.[23]

With very little arm twisting, their oncologist added both chloroquine and hydroxychloroquine to the chemotherapy regimen. Flaxseed oil also enhanced the effectiveness of trastuzumab.[24] Also added was doxycycline that killed cancer stem cells, the roots of cancer.[25] As shown earlier, aspirin also improves breast cancer survival.[26] Angela and Chris employed all of these.

ADJUST YOUR DIET & LIFESTYLE

- Lower High Glycemic Foods [Lowers IGF]

- Add Time Restricted Eating [Fasting up to 16 hours overnight]

- Lose Weight if Obese

It bears repeating that diet does matter, as Jane's story shows. A low-glycemic, low animal fat diet is safest as it keeps the insulin growth factor (IGF) and insulin levels low. If you are overweight or carry belly fat, then, by all means, do everything possible to get healthy. Lose weight, even five to ten pounds can make a huge difference. Engage in time-restricted eating with overnight fasts of

16 hours four or five days a week. Avoid concentrated sugar, whether it is natural or not. It does not matter if the sugar comes from fruits or honey; it will still spike your sugar and insulin levels and "feed the cancer."

Above all, take a page from Dr. Chapman's playbook. Do you believe the criticism of many oncologists that her long-term survival against all the odds was a fluke of chance and unrelated to her repurposed drug cocktail? I think not. She continues to take pterostilbene, which has been shown to suppress brain cancer metastasis. She takes it every day to this day.

Why would she not? If you or I were in her shoes, why would we not? The only reason might be because we did not know. After you read this book, you will always know, or at least know how to find out. Hopefully, you will pass this knowledge along to others, too. Spread the word that terminal cancer doesn't have to be a death sentence anymore if one adds repurposed drugs.

Chapter 3

MY OWN REPURPOSED DRUG REGIMEN: THE S.A.M. COCKTAIL

As I'm forced to watch my friend Evan struggle with this terrible disease, I am even more shocked at our current cancer treatment system. We are not just ignoring the first dictum of medicine "Do no harm"; we are trampling all over it. Out of one side of our mouths we teach, "Do not use off-label drugs for fear of toxicity." At the same time, we teach the use of toxic chemo and radiation regimens.

With cancer, studies are beginning to clearly show that multiple nontoxic repurposed agents have a multiplied or synergistic effect. There is a huge advantage in effectiveness with much less toxicity in using a multi-drug cocktail, compared to using one drug at a toxic dose. If a cocktail of multiple anticancer drugs is added to chemotherapy from the beginning, the tumor is hamstrung from rewiring itself and can be prevented from returning later on. I believe this is why we hear so many success stories of terminal cancer survivors who swore by their cocktails, as we saw in the previous chapter.

Physicians use combination approaches all the time in treating diabetes and blood pressure. They work in the same way. At low doses, three blood pressure agents do a much better job than a single agent at a toxic dose. I've seen this in my practice countless times. It wasn't until I read Jane McLelland's book that I began looking for a repurposed cocktail of my own—not for treatment, but prevention.

Inflammation

As a pain specialist, I have done many thousands of therapeutic injections to help patients. As a result, my injection thumb developed arthritis about 20 years ago, and the pain was terrible.

Compounding matters was that I also used my right thumb for handwriting; I take notes at every patient visit.

Between injections and handwriting, my thumb hurt 24/7. It kept me awake at night. It let me know when the weather was going to change. I could predict the rain. I booked an appointment with my orthopedic surgeon believing I would need an operation. I could feel the bone spur at the base of my thumb. At first, I thought the growth might be bone cancer, but then I saw the x-ray.

"Just mild arthritis," the orthopedist told me. "Take some Celebrex." So I did.

Celebrex 200 mg once a day worked like a charm. My pain went down from a seven to a one. That was in early 2000 before I reversed my insulin resistance. I had a lot of inflammation in my thumb. For that matter, I had a lot of inflammation everywhere—in my joints, my arteries, and my brain. Little did I know then that by reversing my inflammation, I would turn around my health.

That was before I started drinking coffee, before I developed my muscles, before I got healthy. It was before I lost my belly fat. (See my previous book, *The Coffee Cure Diet*, for more about that.) With Celebrex, I did not need to do any of that. I could remain fat, out of shape, and inflamed. The Celebrex magically removed my inflammation for one day, and I was good as long as I took it each and every day.

Soon, I recommended Celebrex for half of my patients. It seemed that inflammation was a very common problem. How correct I was. Today, one-half of all Americans now have either prediabetes or diabetes, both of which lead to chronic inflammation. Like many Americans, I had four of the factors that characterize the metabolic syndrome that often accompanies diabetes—the thick waist, high blood pressure, high triglycerides, and borderline high blood sugar.[27] Being a physician, I knew that I was headed for a heart attack or possible cancer.

Imagine my relief when I came across a preliminary study that suggested that consistent use of Celebrex reduced the risks of colon cancer by up to 60%. I proudly informed my patients that in addition to helping their inflammation, Celebrex could also help prevent cancer. However, the study was quickly halted when a bombshell came down in the medical community: NSAIDs can cause heart attacks.[28] A cousin of Celebrex, Bextra was so risky the FDA took it off of the market. Soon studies came out linking other NSAID medications like Celebrex and Vioxx to the risk for heart attacks. Doctors became reluctant to recommend NSAID medication for anyone.

Aspirin

NSAIDs are only one way to control inflammation. Aspirin is another. Aspirin does not cause heart attacks. It actually helps prevent them. Studies show aspirin use to be associated with reduced risk for a number of cancers including prostate, pancreatic, and rectal. Dr. Harvey Risch of the Yale School of Public Health noted a nearly 50% reduction in aspirin users' rate of pancreatic cancer.[322] Studies on aspirin preventing colon cancer show between a 30% and 50% reduction in the risk of colon cancer. Like NSAIDs, aspirin can cause bleeding in a small percentage, around 1%. With baby aspirin, the chances are much less. A 2017 study in the United Kingdom looked at 340,000 cancer patients for over 12 years, with one-half taking baby aspirin, and the other half not.[29] There was a 34% reduction in the development of colon cancer.

The U.S. Preventative Services Task Force advocates a policy of low dose aspirin for the prevention of colorectal cancer and cardiovascular disease in certain high-risk groups.[30] I take baby aspirin daily. I would advise you to clear it with your physician first and possibly add an antacid to lower GI bleeding risk. Or take enteric-coated baby aspirin. Cimetidine, as we shall later see, is a good antacid that also has anticancer activity.

Metformin

The second piece of my cocktail might be the most important. In 2002 when I first began to take metformin, it was not because I had the condition of type II diabetes mellitus, its main use. It was because I had the condition of prediabetes, a fasting blood sugar of 102. Normal fasting blood sugar is under 100. Diabetes is diagnosed with two fasting readings on two separate occasions greater than 125. I took metformin off-label for prediabetes, which is also known as insulin resistance. I had researched the scientific studies on PubMed, and I noticed that patients who took metformin were less likely to progress to full-blown diabetes.

I wish I could say I was smart enough 18 years ago to take metformin to prevent cancer, but I cannot.

Today we know that metformin is a safe and nontoxic treatment for insulin resistance, but we have hundreds of scientific studies showing that the longer one takes it and the higher the dose, the lower the risk for many cancers. In 2005, Dr. Josie M. Evans published a study that examined 314,000 people in Tayside, Scotland.[31] Some 11,000 were diagnosed with type II diabetes. Some were treated with metformin, and others were not. Nine hundred twenty-three were later diagnosed with malignant cancer. The chance of getting cancer for those taking metformin was roughly 40% less than non-metformin users. This was a pilot study and triggered hundreds of further studies, which have since confirmed cause and effect with metformin and cancer. It turns out I was lucky, not smart, as the saying goes.

Why is it that we do not read about metformin and cancer prevention on the cover of *Time* magazine or the lead story in AARP or in Dr. Oz's columns? Why is it that 1.8 million people a year and rising continue to develop cancer with another 600,000 deaths each year?

We could all be taking the pill with our doctor's approval (and prescription, of course) that could realistically drop these numbers by up to one-third. Never in my career have I been more sobered by a statistic.

Aspirin and metformin are two of three medications of the trinity that I take and advise for those with insulin resistance. We know insulin resistance (IR) causes inflammation and high levels of blood sugar and insulin, both of which are fuel for cancer. Thus, there is a very low-risk and a huge benefit to taking these two medications together.

Statin

The third member of my preferred cocktail is a statin, preferably a lipophilic one. Statins, dervied from fermented fungus, have gotten a bad rap. Red Rice Yeast extract is chemically similar to lovastatin and not a prescription, but has the same action. Contrary to popular belief, they are not dangerous, they do not cause Alzheimer's, and they not only prevent heart disease, but they also help prevent cancer in a big way.

Like metformin, the longer one takes the lipophilic statin, the lower the death rate from cancer if it develops. Statins increase survival if cancer forms.[32] They both block sterol synthesis through the HMGCR pathway. Certain statins, the lipophilic ones like atorvastatin and lovastatin, can induce cancer cell apoptosis or cell death. The hydrophilic (water soluble) statins, like pravastatin, have minimal to no anticancer effects. I take atorvastatin every day. Why? Because statin use, like aspirin and metformin, decreases the chance of death from all causes.

A 2012 study looked at almost 300,000 Danes between 1995 and 2007 aged 40 or more.[33] Compared to patients who never used statins, the statin users had a 15% reduction of death from any cause and a 15% reduction of death specifically due to cancer. The New England Journal of Medicine reported on this study, and the authors saw that a drop in cholesterol resulted in a decrease in cancer cell division and multiplication. This was due to the blocking of the mevalonate pathway.[34] Statins make the cancer cell weaker and more vulnerable to death from radiation therapy.

The conclusion is that statins are effective both before and after cancer diagnosis and should ultimately reduce cancer-related death. This hypothesis was tested in the Danish community, and the results confirmed it. Statins help people die 15% less and live longer by reducing both cancer mortality and death from all causes.[35]

The S.A.M. Cancer Prevention Cocktail

Dr. Mark Moyad, a professor at the University of Michigan Medical Center, calls this holy trinity simply by the name S.A.M. which stands for statin, aspirin, and metformin.[36] Dr. Moyad believes that the S.A.M. combination is particularly effective against prostate cancer, especially in light of the USA's insulin resistance epidemic. He believes people should be taking this every day to prevent it.[37] He believes insulin resistance is due to our Western diet of high sugar, high fat combined with lack of exercise. My feeling is the same.

Jane McLelland found that merely adding a cocktail of off-label medications was not enough to cure her stage IV cervical cancer; she also had to practice very diligent control of her diet and lifestyle. Jane found that when she strayed from her diet with indulgences in sugar, fat, or alcohol, she immediately noted pain in her arthritic knee.

I had a similar experience with my insulin resistance. Even today, when I stray from my Coffee Cure Diet or exercise program, I also notice that my thumb pain returns. It is a useful reminder that helps me stay on track.

So, do I believe that off-labeled use of medication can help prevent and treat cancer? Absolutely. But do I think that taking pills alone will protect me? No. Remember Jane McLelland's mother, who was diagnosed with advanced breast cancer at the same time as her daughter, but followed the standard advice of many oncologists at the time. "Eat anything you want because diet will not affect your cancer treatment." Jane's mom passed away within months. By contrast, Jane continued to follow her strict diet of no sugar, low carbohydrate, low fat, and daily exercise. She ate lots of fresh vegetables and limited her fruit due to its sugar content. Armed with her repurposed drugs and dietary changes and against all the odds, she beat stage IV cancer and is still alive 20 years later.

Diet alone isn't sufficient, either. Exercise, especially resistive, lowers blood sugar by driving glucose into the muscle. I prefer it over simply walking. These lifestyle practices must be done daily.

The worst behavior is to do nothing and remain insulin-resistant. You become a sitting duck for cancer and heart disease. My advice is to reverse your insulin resistance with the diet and lifestyle changes while at the same time taking your daily regimen of S.A.M. This is the best cancer prevention strategy that I have found.

Chapter 4

THE ReDO PROJECT: THE REVOLUTION BEGINS

Stories like the ones you've read about so far may have remained anecdotal, were it not for the actions of Dr. Pan Pantziarka, a mathematician and computer scientist who had lost both his son and wife to cancer. He possessed both the ambition and the intellect to lead the charge. In 2014, Dr. Pantziarka and a bold group of distinguished researchers launched the Repurposing Drugs in Oncology (ReDO) Project. His goal was to drive the fast track research and approval process of existing drugs to treat cancer.

In memory of his son, Dr. Pan Pantziarka also established the George Pantziarka TP53 Trust, a charitable foundation designed to help families with Li Fraumeni syndrome and related conditions.[38] The description of the trust further describes the kind of man its founder is:

> "He is a scientist working at the Anticancer Fund (ACF) in Belgium, where he is coordinator of the Repurposing Drugs in Oncology Project. In addition to researching the re-use of existing non-cancer drugs, as new sources of cancer treatment, the project looks at the social and institutional factors influencing cancer policy."[39]

After the skirmishes of Dr. Ben Williams and Jane McLelland with their oncologists, Dr. Pan Pantziarka took up the mantle and declared war. He criticized the current cancer treatment paradigms as expensive, toxic, and ineffective, and vowed to revolutionize them. In a 2014 article announcing the purpose and goals of the ReDO project, Pantziarka and colleagues threw down the gauntlet to the old guard:

> "The authors of this (project) are a diverse group of researchers, clinicians, and patient advocates all working in the non-for

profit sector. We seek new (cancer) treatments that meet the needs of existing patients in as short of time frame as possible and at a cost that is affordable, both in developed and developing countries. Most of all, we seek treatments that are at least as effective as existing standard of care treatment, including the newer targeted therapies which are emerging into clinical practice but with lower toxicity and offering an improved quality of life to patients.

There are numerous hurdles to overcome to make drug repurposing a reality, but perhaps the first of them is convincing clinicians and patients alike that there really are old drugs contained in the pharmacist's cabinet, which can provide some value to cancer patients in fighting their disease. We hope in this (project) and those papers that accompany it to focus on individual drugs that can provide the scientific rationale and the evidence that is the case."[40]

The selection process for repurposed drugs was identified:

- They are well-known drugs, with many years of widespread clinical use, rather than newer agents recently brought into clinical use for non-cancer indications. Often, they are available as generics, but this is not a primary consideration.

- The toxicology profile is good, with low toxicity even with chronic dosing. Use for metronomic protocols is seen as an advantage, though no drug is ruled out if it cannot be used in such a schedule.

- There is a plausible mechanism of action. Note that a drug need not be directly cytotoxic, candidate drugs may have putative mechanisms of action that are anti-angiogenic, inhibit particular pathways, or target aspects of the tumor microenvironment.

- Strong evidence: *in vitro, in vivo*, and human data (epidemiological, published case reports, clinical trials).

Human data is scored significantly more highly than *in vivo* or *in vitro* work; results in syngeneic, orthotopic mouse models have the highest weight in preclinical work.

- There is evidence of efficacy at physiological dosing. There are many drugs where there is preclinical work that shows efficacy but at doses, or by route of administration, not achievable in patients, or only achievable at doses with significant toxicity.

When the project started, Pantziarka and his Anticancer Fund's first order of business was to study six drugs for their anticancer potential, including Nitroglycerin, Itraconazole, Mebendazole, Cimetidine, Clarithromycin, and Diclofenac. Dr. Pantziarka called for the fast-tracking of approvals and the use of various repurposed drugs in cancer, and social campaigns to raise public awareness of such drugs.

The First Six Drugs Studied by the ReDo Team were:

Drug	Type	Existing Indication	Availability
Mebendazole	Anthelminthic	Threadworm infections	Generic
Nitroglycerin	Vasodilator	Angina	Generic
Cimetidine	H2-receptor antagonist	Peptic ulcer	Generic
Clarithromycin	Antibiotic	Respiratory tract infection	Generic
Diclofenac	NSAID	Pain relief	Generic

Drug	Type	Existing Indication	Availability
Itraconazole	Antifungal	Broad spectrum antifungal	Generic

Other candidate drugs listed as their research targets included losartan (angiotensin-renin system blockers), chloroquine/hydroxychloroquine, statins, propranolol (beta blockers), omeprazole/PPI, and polysaccharide K/PSK.[41]

The core group of researchers included three Belgians representing the Anticancer Fund, Dr. Pan Pantziarka, Dr. Gauthier Bouche, and Dr. Lydie Meheus. Other authors included Dr. Vidula Sukhatme, Dr. Vikas Sukhatme, and Dr. P. Vikas representing the United States Arm, GlobalCures Inc., affiliated with Beth Israel Deaconess Medical Center and Harvard Medical School in Boston, Massachusetts.

Currently, with the assistance of groups of multiple scientists and grassroots donations, the Anticancer Fund and Repurposed Drugs in Oncology project have completed and published numerous studies and clinical trials ranging from cimetidine to propranolol, from chloroquine to nitroglycerine, and from artemisinin to Baclofen. Dr. Pan's groups partnered up with the US group, GlobalCures, and the SHARE project, which collects and collates vital data among various institutions on cancer research.

But as I write this now in 2020, the ReDO project has cataloged 310 approved drugs that have anticancer effects. They are contained in Appendix E. At the time of this writing, more than 279 late phase clinical trials on ReDO drugs are being conducted.[42]

The U.S. Right to Try Law

Over the last six years, Dr. Pantziarka and company have done an impressive job, but there have been setbacks. The UK's legislation which would have improved access, the Medical Innovation Bill, was defeated at the eleventh hour in parliament.[43]

However, a ray of sunlight was the passage of the Right to Try Bill in the U.S.[44] This was signed into law on May 30, 2018 and helped set the tone for future repurposed drug use. The only problem was that it applied mainly to expensive single agent pharmaceutical sponsored agents.

The principles that apply to repurposed drugs include these criteria:

#1 A terminally ill patient has exhausted all other treatments options ...

#2 The drug has passed FDA Phase I clinical testing...

#3 The patient's health care provider or treating physician must recommend and approve...

#4 The patient must sign a written informed consent...

Repurposed drug combinations legally can be added to the standard care under the off-label use exception without the need to invoke the Right to Try Act. However, drug combinations do not always require the case be terminal as in the first criterion for Right to Try. The second condition is always met with a repurposed drug because, by definition, they have been already passed an FDA Phase I trial. I feel strongly that for patient protection, the third criterion should exist; a physician's approval and prescription. This helps protect the patient from toxicity. Finally, adding the informed consent that meets the fourth criterion is essential for the physician to help prevent liability in the event the outcome is not as expected. This ensures widespread patient access to repurposed drugs.

The Informed Consent Form

There is a standard informed consent form at the end of this book. Feel free to provide this to your doctor. He can print it up, have you sign it, and then he may feel more comfortable prescribing the repurposed drug combination.

Protecting physicians when they prescribe off-label medications will improve access for future patients, and this is essential. Dr. Pantziarka, Dr. Gyawali and colleagues wrote an article in 2018, "Does the oncology community have a rejection bias when it comes to repurposed drugs?" I will let you answer that question after you read his quote below.

Bias Against Repurposed Drugs

Clinical trials have been blocked or cut short early with the heavy-handed application of criteria. At the same time, all kinds of exceptions were made for pharmaceutical-backed expensive drugs.

Dr. Pantziarka comments on the disparity:

> "It is paradoxical that the oncology community, while complaining about higher drug costs, encourages futile trials of expensive drugs and yet does not give the same benefit of the doubt to lower cost repurposed drugs. This is important because even if the expensive drugs...achieve significance in some tumors, they are likely to be cost ineffective and out of the realm of affordability for millions of cancer patients worldwide.

> However, the discovery of better outcomes with repurposed drugs such as metformin, or statins, has the potential to lead to immediate application and the transformation of cancer care access across global boundaries. In conclusion, we strongly urge the oncology community to apply similar standards...in the assessment of the clinical worth of repurposed drugs and newer agents in cancer."[45]

Dr. Pantziarka has identified a regulatory bias against repurposed drugs. The existing forces in the cancer community apparently are discriminating against the repurposed drug trials and approval process.

Why would they do that? Just as in real estate, there are the three most important factors in the cancer drug clinical trial and approval process. Money, money, and money.

The Anticancer Fund is run on grassroots donations and favors effective and inexpensive drugs. Big Pharma, which controls treatment protocols, prefers expensive and profitable drugs that may not be as safe or effective. But such disparities can be resolved with awareness and public education. Unlike the pharmaceutical interests that saw fit to raise the price of mebendazole 100 times after its antitumor actions were discovered, Dr. Pantziarka strives to make inexpensive new cancer treatments an option as soon as possible. Just as AIDS gained awareness through public outcry, solutions began appearing.

The same thing needs to happen with repurposed drugs.

The Inflammation and IR Connection

As I became more familiar with the science surrounding these repurposed drug cancer treatments, I began to see connections to many of the issues I tried to address with my Coffee Cure Diet. As Dr. Pantziarka said in a recent interview:

> "Our view of cancer is that we no longer think of cancer as a disease of the delinquent cell; we increasingly understand that cancers cannot exist without supporting microenvironment. The other thing that we are also discovering is that TP53 is an incredibly diverse transcription factor. It's involved not just as a tumor suppressor, but functions in the immune system, handling metabolic stress, senescence, and aging.
>
> These two things, a new view of cancer that incorporates the microenvironment and a new understanding of the role of the TP53 signaling have not quite made it into our view of LFS.

We know that chronic inflammation is a driver of tumorigenesis. One of the things I'm interested in is the idea of a precancerous niche. This is a tissue environment that is primed for cancer initiation and development. It's a host environment characterized by chronic inflammation, high levels of oxidative stress, the release of proangiogenic factors, immune dysfunction, and so on. Now, these are all things that are associated with the mutated TP53 gene.

Therefore, one of the ideas that I am developing is that cancer initiation is related to the host environment being ready for cancer before there is a cancer present. Cancer initiation (in LFS) may be associated with this chronic inflammation and this highly oxidative and stressful environment that causes additional mutations over and above the TP53, which drives the cancer initiation and progression.

It is very difficult to drug transcription factors, especially something as complicated as TP53 (the tumor suppressor gene). But what we can do is look at pharmacological interventions that address some elements of that precancerous niche. If we can reduce the chronic inflammation, reduce the oxidative stress, and reform the damaged immune system, then we are in a position that fewer cancers may be initiated; therefore, we can reduce the risk of cancer in these patients that have a very high-risk of cancer. There are a number of possible drugs that are attractive in this respect, chief among them, metformin...and also aspirin..."[46]

I immediately recognized this pro-tumor niche. It is similar to the pro-disease niche that exists in insulin-resistant patients. I also recognized his mention of aspirin and metformin, 2/3 of the S.A.M. prevention cocktail. We can all strive to reduce the risk of cancer by lowering inflammation and oxidation and blocking the cancer friendly niche before it develops. Not only can we prevent cancer from forming in LFS, but we can use the same strategy as cancer prevention in all high-risk groups.

In the next section of the book, we will look more deeply at the science to explain how and why these drugs are so effective.

SECTION II:
THE SCIENCE BEHIND REPURPOSED DRUGS

Chapter 5

PLEIOTROPY

The drugs we've discussed so far are able to combat cancer because of their pleiotropic effects. Pleiotropy is the property where a single gene can affect multiple traits. In pharmacology, pleiotropy includes all the drug's actions other than those the drug was designed to treat. For example, I often tell my patients that aspirin is typically used as a nonaddictive over-the-counter pain killer for headaches, joint pain, and muscular pain, but it is also an excellent medication to control fever in adults. In addition, it is often used as an antiplatelet medication, a blood thinner to lower the risk for heart attack. And, as we shall discuss soon, it also has anti-inflammatory and antitumor effects.

Pleiotropy is a principle woven into the fabric of the medications that doctors prescribe. Tylenol can be used to control both pain and fever. And as we shall see, the pleiotropic effects of one particular drug, commonly used to treat diabetes, may make it the most important anticancer drug on the market today.

Insulin Resistance and Bad Genes

In the Coffee Cure Diet, I discussed the differences between those people cursed with the genes for insulin resistance (IR), the so-called thrifty genes that are good at storing fat. Contrast those with skinny insulin sensitive genes who can eat anything and stay lean. Those with IR have thick waists and tend to have higher triglycerides, higher blood sugars, and higher blood pressure levels. They also tend to have a higher ratio of triglyceride to HDL, the ratio I refer to as the longevity index.

It turns out that IR causes 40 % of all cancers.[47] Also, but not always, in general, the higher the triglyceride level, the greater the cancer risk, and the lower the HDL level, the greater the cancer risk. Curiously, it is not overweight obesity that is most related to cancer;

it is the presence of IR. Studies have shown that even those of normal weight who have elevated TG/HDL ratios are at increased risk for heart disease and Alzheimer's and are also at higher risk of developing cancer.[48]

As if that were not bad enough news for me, since I harbor IR genetics, once the inevitable cancer occurs, the treatments do not work as well, and those persons are at higher mortality risk (the risk of dying).[49, 50]

If you are like my wife, Faith, and have a slim waist and HDL of 100 or greater and triglycerides of less than 100, count your blessings. On the other hand, if you are more like me, then do what I do; drink coffee and whey before meals, fast overnight 16 hours, and exercise your muscles daily to get rid of your belly fat.[51] It will be lifesaving to decrease your waist size (measured around the navel) to less than your hip size.[52]

Fasting improves P53's (our main tumor suppressor gene) function.[53] Not eating, otherwise known as intermittent fasting, is a strong cancer suppressive.[54] Exercising your muscles after meals drives glucose into the muscle, effectively stealing it from fat and potential cancer cells. You can reverse insulin resistance with fasting, weight loss, and a low-glycemic diet, even if you have bad genes.

Most people who get cancer share at least one common risk factor. The risk factors of smoking, viruses, and insulin resistance explain the initiation of about 80-90% of all cancers. This leaves about 10% of us with other causes of cancer, including hereditary cancers, the so-called Lynch syndrome, FAP, HNPCC, BRCA mutations, etc.

RISK FACTORS & CANCER

- Cigarette Smoking 40%
- Insulin Resistance 40%
- Viruses 10%
- Hereditary & Other 10%

Familial adenomatous polyposis refers to a hereditary condition that causes colon cancer at a young age. People with FAP develop precancerous colon polyps in their teens. Many chose to have complete colectomies before age 20 rather than risk fatal cancer development. In a study, two medications were able to reduce FAP polyps by 90%.[55] One was the common drug MBZ, the one discovered by Dr. Riggins in treating the mice. The other was a traditional NSAID called Sulindac (a cousin of Aleve). After these two drugs suppressed 90% of the polyps, the 10% remaining were a fraction of their normal size. What were these two wonder drugs one might ask? Were they the subject of $100,000,000 in medical research?

As I stated, they were simple common prescription drugs that have been used for the last 40 years without any difficulty. But they are not in widespread use for FAP patients.

I do not know about you, but if I carried an FAP diagnosis, and no one had told me about these two drugs, I might be upset that I had chosen preventative colectomy at age 20, not realizing there might have been another option.

French Lilac

If MBZ and Sulindac can suppress 90% of colon precancerous adenomata in the worst cases of FAP, what do you suppose those two can do to your risk? This brings me to my next point: metformin, perhaps the best cancer preventative agent of all time. Even scientists on PubMed have referred to its properties as magical.[56, 57]

METFORMIN INHIBITS CANCER

- Leukemia
- Glioblastoma
- Melanoma
- Pancreatic
- Head & Neck
- Nasopharyngeal

* Prostate
* Ovarian
* Endometrial
* Breast
* Salivary
* Non-Small-Cell Lung

Metformin was discovered in France and is derived from the French lilac plant. Its action is not limited to suppressing colon polyps. It has powerful actions against a large variety of cancers: breast cancer, glioblastoma, esophageal cancer, prostate cancer, ovarian cancer, pancreatic cancer, melanoma, endometrial cancer, non-small cell lung cancer, head and neck squamous cell cancer, and nasopharyngeal and salivary tumors.[58] It decreases IGF, induces apoptosis, and targets resistant P53 mutant tumor cells. It lowers insulin levels. It lowers blood sugar levels. It makes regular chemotherapy, such as cisplatin, more effective.[59] It makes tumors more sensitive to being killed by radiation.[60] It helps other drugs create apoptosis in chronic lymphocytic leukemia.[61] It inhibits metastatic spread in prostate cancer.[62] Metformin acts as an activator of AMPK, which suppresses the mammalian target of rapamycin (mTOR), a major starting point for cancer initiation. Metformin also works on halting the division or proliferation of cancer cells through AMPK dependent pathways.

Metformin blocks the cancer cell from using glucose in oxidative phosphorylation (OXPHOS) and also blocks compensatory use of fats through inhibition of lipogenic citrate. The dual blockade of glucose and lipid fuel forces the tumor cell to use reductive energy sources (ketoglutaric acid or alpha ketoglutarate) in the cytoplasm.

HOW METFORMIN HURTS CANCER

- Starves Cancer of Glucose/Fat

- Decreases IGF

- Activates AMPK

- Creates Apoptosis

- Enhances Chemotherapy

* Blocks OXPHOS (glucose)

* Lowers Insulin

* Targets Cancer Stem Cells

* Causes Cancer Cell Death

* Enhances Radiation Therapy

Because metformin effectively blocks OXPHOS in mitochondria, there is a decrease in total citrate levels in the cytoplasm, which ultimately blocks effective tumor metabolism and growth. The longer a person has been on metformin prior to a diagnosis of breast cancer or the progress of breast cancer, the longer the survival (greater than a 35% reduction in mortality with greater than four years of use).[63, 64] A review of 111,000 records revealed an overall 23% cancer survival improvement associated with pre-cancer use of metformin across the board in patients with a large variety of tumors including prostate, lung, colon and breast.[65] This survival advantage occurred in both non-diabetic and diabetic populations. Metformin use reduces the risk of getting cancer by some 31%.[66] The numbers in other studies are even more impressive.

A Taiwanese study reviewed diabetic women and ovarian cancer risk.[67] About one-half million women without cancer were followed for seven years. Of those, 286,106 were never users of metformin, and 193,369 were frequent users. Only 601 out of the 286,106 frequent users developed ovarian cancer. Many more (2,600) of those who never used it out of the 193,369 developed ovarian cancer. With which group would you have wanted to be included? On average, users of metformin were less than one-third as likely, depending on the dose, to develop the tumors. The group taking the most metformin had more than an 80% risk reduction. Of the 601 users who developed cancer in the metformin group, we don't know how many smoked, had IR, or harbored chronic viruses. But one thing is clear— their chance of developing cancer was much less.

TAIWAN STUDY OF OVARIAN CANCER

- Metformin Users   601/286,106 = .21% Cancer Rate

- Non Metformin Users   2,600/193,369 = 1.34% Cancer Rate

- Metformin Use   85% Reduction in Ovarian Cancer Risk

In another Taiwanese study, this time involving men developing prostate cancer, almost 400,000 diabetic patients were studied.[68] The researchers followed 209,269 patients who never used metformin and 186,212 who did over seven years. Only 2,776 metformin users out of 186,212 developed prostate cancer, and a lot more (9,642) of the nonusers developed it. Depending on the dose of metformin, the risk in nonusers was three to four times greater.

TAIWAN STUDY OF PROSTATE CANCER

- Metformin Users   2776/186,269 = 1.5% Cancer Rate

- Non Metformin Users   9,642/209,269 = 4.6% Cancer Rate

- Metformin Use   68% Reduction in Prostate Cancer Risk

Finally, the Taiwanese researchers also studied bladder cancer risks and metformin use.[69] A total of 532,515 patients with diabetes were followed for seven years. Of 532,519 nonusers, 6,213 or 1.17% developed bladder cancer. Of 408,189 metformin users, only 1,847 developed the cancer (0.45%). The ratio was 2.6:1. However, in the longest users and highest dosages of metformin, the ratio was close to 4:1.

TAIWAN STUDY OF BLADDER CANCER

- Metformin Users   1,847/408,189 = .45% Cancer Rate

- Non Metformin Users   6,213/532,519 = 1.17% Cancer Rate

- Metformin Use   62% Reduction in Bladder Cancer Risk

Several studies have examined whether metformin has an anticancer effect in most people, diabetic or not. Because of the multiple mechanisms it employs to suppress tumor initiation, growth, and spread, there is good evidence that metformin is effective in almost everyone. There is now almost uniform agreement in the research community that metformin is highly anticancer. The word, unfortunately, has not gotten out to either patients or most physicians.

I would recommend metformin be considered for anyone who is at high-risk for cancer, whether their risk extends from diabetes, prediabetes, insulin resistance, viruses, smoking, or genetics (with your doctors' evaluation, approval, prescription, and blessing of course). I take 1500 mg per day. Some may notice a benefit at a dose as low as 250 mg per day. The maximum dose is generally 2000 mg per day.

Diabetics taking metformin had lower all-cause mortality than even normal nondiabetics not taking it.[70] Diabetic metformin users also had lower cancer rates than normal nondiabetics who did not take it. This is a phenomenal statistic, as diabetes doubles or quadruples the cancer risk in most people.[71] To think that adding metformin to a diabetic would lower his risk below normal for cancer is all the more impressive.

The results were even more when diabetic metformin user's death rates were compared to diabetic non-metformin users. There was a 32% reduction in death. When diabetic metformin users were compared to diabetic non-metformin users with respect to cancer, there was a 24% reduction in cancer occurrence.

A small study of patients with pancreatic cancer revealed a 34% five-year survival compared to a 14% five-year survival without it.[72] Since it only involved 44 patients, these results were deemed "not statistically significant." In another study of 302 pancreatic cancer patients, the two-year survival for metformin users was 30.1% versus 15.4% in the non-metformin group.[73] The beneficial effect of metformin was seen in pancreatic cancer of all stages. There are currently more than 100 ongoing clinical trials looking at metformin not just in preventing cancer, the reason I take it, but in treating active cancer.

Unlike most standard chemotherapy, metformin suppresses cancer stem cells, the root of cancer.[74] While most toxic metal-based chemotherapies only debulk the tumor (like chopping off the top of a tree), metformin kills the stem cells, the root, which can ultimately prevent the cancer from returning. In addition, metformin inhibits epithelial-mesenchymal transformation (EMT).[75] This is when a cancer cell frees itself from its local tissue tether and becomes a free agent, able to circulate like a bacterium throughout the body. Most toxic chemotherapies fail to kill these metastases.

I take metformin daily because if I happen to have a melanoma or colon cancer cell trying to break away and metastasize, the metformin might just kill it or stop it before it gets started. But by far, the most important effect is that metformin blocks the cancer cells' energy production and fuel, which often results in cancer cell death-apoptosis; it blocks glucose oxidative phosphorylation and fat synthesis.

METFORMIN'S PLEIOTROPIC EFFECTS

- Mimics Fasting
- Has Life Extending Effects
- Reduces Insulin Levels
- Helps Reverse Insulin Resistance
- Lowers Cancer Risk (Preventative)
- Raises T-Cell Immunity
- Improves Wound Healing
* Simulates Caloric Restriction

* Reduces IGF

* Causes Weight Loss

* Reduces Inflammation

* Helps Kill Cancer Stem Cells

* Lowers Cancer Angiogenesis

* Lowers Oxidation

Therefore, you do not want to overload on eating sugar or fat as both of these can "feed" the cancer cell by overcoming the metformin's blockade if you consume enough of the wrong food.

Metformin reduces IGF-1 and insulin, and these decreases can lead to life extension. Metformin lowers insulin levels and insulin resistance in mice. It also extends lifespan and reduces carcinogenesis in rodents.[76] Caloric restriction has increased longevity in rodents by decreasing insulin levels and downregulating mTOR, a pattern that can lead to major increases in longevity.

The opposite of CR or caloric restriction is caloric excess. This is unfortunately associated with excessive insulin secretion, IR, increased rates of cancer, stimulation of mTOR and premature diseases of aging (e.g., cataracts, impaired wound healing), and the development of both diabetes and cancer. Even in patients who do not calorically restrict, metformin will artificially produce a restricted caloric state in the human body.[77] This is why metformin is deemed a calorie restriction mimetic and is now being intensively investigated as an anti-aging compound.

Some say metformin may have already saved more people from cancer than any other drug in history. Some 120 million prescriptions are written annually. Metformin, an antidiabetic biguanide derived from the French lilac, may be even more effective than actual caloric restriction. However, I do not want to take any chances. I do both.

Can Metformin Extend Lifespan?

Metformin decelerates aging in worms or nematodes by increasing lifespan up to 36% in a dose-dependent manner. Metformin increases lifespan in mice by 10-20%.[78] Metformin patients enjoy the benefits of caloric restriction with improved exercise performance, prevention of metabolic syndrome, increased insulin sensitivity, and reduced LDL cholesterol, all without a decrease in caloric intake.

Metformin seems to improve all nine hallmarks of aging which include genomic instability, telomere length, epigenetic alterations, loss of proteostasis, deregulation of nutrient sensing, mitochondrial dysfunction, cellular senescence, stem cell exhaustion, and altered cell-to-cell communication.[79] It also lowers inflammation and oxidation, raises T-cell immunity, reduces cancer angiogenesis, and promotes P-53 tumor suppressive function.

Studies suggest a 31% less chance of getting cancer with long-term metformin use. Instead of 1.8 million new cancers per year, we could be looking at 1.2 million new cases. Studies support a 35% reduction in the death rate. We could drop our US annual cancer death from 600,000 to 395,000 lives. Who exactly has been sitting on this information, and why? I wish I could say that metformin was so dangerous and risky that if everyone took it there could be more problems, but I cannot. Metformin is the most prescribed drug in the world. It has been in use in the United States since 1995 and France since the 1970s. Its worst potential side effect, fatal lactic acidosis, occurs in only three out of 100,000 cases and is no more common in metformin users than in nonusers.[80] It is, therefore, a nonissue.

It originally sold under the brand name Glucophage, but generic versions were released in 2000. Bristol Myers Squibb owned the patent, and profits were close to two billion dollars per year. The company successfully changed the formula a few times and were thus able to extend its patent until 2009.

Today, metformin can be purchased between $1 and $5 per month in the USA. There are no billion-dollar profits to be had, and no one seems to be interested in selling a drug that cannot make them a lot of money. Even if the drug can prevent or, in some cases, cure cancer, metformin is bad for business. If the number of US cancer cases dropped by 1/3, Big Pharma and the chemotherapy industry would stand to lose hundreds of billions.

In addition to suppressing cancer both before and after it forms, metformin is anti-aging. I have taken it for 15 years and plan to continue. Dr. James Watson, co-discoverer of the DNA double-helix structure and Nobel Prize laureate, also takes it for its anticancer effect.[81] Ask your doctor if you should as well.

Chapter 6

THE WARBURG EFFECT

Dr. Otto Warburg found that cancer cells process energy quite differently than normal cells. Cancer cells waste tons of fuel by burning it inefficiently. The easiest comparison would be a gas-guzzling SUV compared with a Prius.

The first might get 14 miles per gallon, while the Prius would get 50 miles per gallon. Cancer cells are like the SUV, though the scale is even more lopsided. The normal cell gets 100 miles per gallon of fuel; the cancer cell averages just 5 ½ miles per gallon.

Cancer Guzzles Glucose

Like a gas hog, cancer wastes glucose freely. Normal cells metabolize glucose in the mitochondria using very efficient aerobic metabolism and oxidative phosphorylation. This process produces approximately 36 ATP (adenosine triphosphate) per glucose unit. Cancer cells, on the other hand, as Warburg discovered, prefer to metabolize glucose in the cytoplasm outside of the mitochondria using inefficient aerobic glycolysis, a type of fermentation that produces only 2 ATP per glucose unit, approximately 94% less.

FEEDING YOUR CANCER

- Warburg Metabolism (Cancer)
- Normal Cell Metabolism
- Cancer guzzles glucose and wastes most of it.

* 5 ½ miles per gallon (2 ATP)
* 100 miles per gallon (36 ATP)
* Cancer Requires Lots of Carbs

This information can be used to help us fight cancer. If we refuse to fill the cancer gasoline tank, the tumor shrinks. It can be as simple as cutting back a lot on both calories and carbohydrates, but as I will explain later, in addition to being a gas hog, the cancer is also smart and can learn to improvise and eat other things besides glucose. The cancer automobile can even learn to run on grease, much like some car engines can be modified to run on vegetable oil. Cancer engines can be converted to run on protein, as we shall soon see.

Experts believe tumors want to reproduce at all costs; they are not worried about being fuel efficient. When fuel is plentiful, as in our current Western diet and lifestyle, cancer cells are seldom deficient. When glucose or carbs are eliminated, as in fasting or low-glycemic diets, the glucose-dependent tumors (the majority) at first shrink, and the tumor will often resort to a variety of compensatory methods for creating energy.

Lactate: Cancer's Bank Account

Warburg metabolism produces large quantities of lactate. Lactate is usually nothing more than a waste product. However, the smart cancer cell can learn to burn this lactate to create more energy if you stop eating.

This lactate is like money in cancer's bank account. Lactate can be drawn out later if the person stops eating. Lactate can be re-used in a reverse Warburg effect where it is taken up by the mitochondria and burned through the more efficient and normal oxidative phosphorylation pathway (OXPHOS). This use of the Warburg lactate can help a tumor resume growth even when dietary fuel is limited.

HOW CANCER OUTSMARTS YOUR DIET

• You Cut Back on Carbs	* Cancer Burns Protein (glutaminolysis)
• You Stop Eating (Fast)	* Cancer Burns Lactate (Reverse Warburg)
• You Stop Eating (Fast)	* Cancer Eats Itself (Autophagy)
• You Go Keto	* Cancer Learns to Eat Fat (ketoglutarate)

In times of low fuel (i.e., fasting), the tumor can also "eat" or recycle old cells for fuels in a process called autophagy. This is also a common strategy for chemotherapy resistance and why repurposed drugs that block CSCs also block autophagy and are so effective in killing cancers.

The antimalarial drug chloroquine or the antihistamine loratadine (Claritin) helps block this.[82] Cancers that have spread or metastasized tend to use an energy pathway that uses amino acids from protein to create energy. This is referred to as glutaminolysis and is common to a variety of tumors: triple-negative breast cancer (TNBC), pancreatic cancer, lung cancer, glioblastoma multiforme, lymphoma, and prostate cancer.[83] Curcumin and resveratrol can help block this. L-asparaginase is also a glutamine blocker.

Butterflies and EMT

Epithelial-mesenchymal transformation (EMT) refers to how a cancer spreads or metastasizes. This is controlled by the cancer stem cell, or the CSC, not to be confused with plain stem cells now commonly used for rejuvenation. Cancer stem cells are present with cancers, while everyone has regular stem cells.

The easy way to understand EMT is the caterpillar to butterfly analogy. Normal cells are like caterpillars. They can only fly in their dreams. But when they are awake, they must crawl slowly to get anywhere. However, after they emerge from their chrysalises, they are transformed into butterflies.

Similarly, normal skin cells, after transforming into melanoma, still cannot travel. Even melanoma tissue is tethered to the skin. However, when the CSC waves the magic wand through special signals (Hedgehog, WnT, and NOTCH), the melanoma's wish is granted, and it becomes a butterfly temporarily. It freely travels throughout the body.

CANCER STEM CELLS

- Control Cancer Spread
- Cause Chemo Resistance
- Killed by Repurposed Drugs
- Not hurt by Chemo/Radiation

* Control EMT
* Can Regrow Tumor
* Slow Growing
* Good at Rewiring

Once settled, the CSC waves the wand a second time, and a reverse EMT known as mesenchymal-epithelial transformation (MET) takes place. The mobile melanoma cell re-roots into the new tissue. In melanoma's case, this may be the brain or liver, and now the cancer cell turns back into the caterpillar (or plain melanoma cell). It is then re-tethered to the new tissue in the new location. As we shall see, blocking this requires repurposed drugs, as there are no current standard chemotherapies that block this entire EMT process. The key to preventing EMT or metastases is by killing the CSC, the roots of the tumor. Unfortunately, standard care with surgery, chemotherapy, and radiation spare these cancer stem cells, which often leaves the person vulnerable to the ravages of EMT or metastasis, continuing the spread of the cancer.

The EMT process can be blocked with drugs and supplements that attack cancer stem cells. Part of the process of EMT involves travel through the body. Normally, there are no good routes to follow if the tumor is not touching a blood vessel. However, the tumor-associated fibroblasts (TAF) receive signals from the tumor to bulldoze a road for the tumor to follow. This involves dislodging or dissolving some of the soft tissue, which allows the tumor macrophages tumor activated macrophages (TAM) to travel. These macrophages help clear obstacles away.

DISTANT TUMOR SPREAD

- New Seeds: EMT
- MET means re-root
- EMT causes travel
- Sprouting in New Tissue

Meanwhile, as the tumor ferments, its pH drops and oxygen levels plunge (hypoxia), triggering the release of a protein called HIF (hypoxia-induced factor), which stimulates angiogenesis. Further stimulating vessel growth is the release of a vascular endothelial growth factor (VEGF), triggering the creation of tons of new blood vessels.

LOCAL TUMOR SPREAD

- Bulldoze New Roads
- Clear Away Debris
- Form New Blood Vessels
- Growth Factor
- * By TAF
- * By TAM
- * By VEGF
- * By HIF

BLOCKING LOCAL SPREAD

- Mebendazole
- Aspirin
- Low Sugar Diet
- * Doxycycline
- * Dipyridamole
- * Low Carb Diet

Avastin, a chemotherapeutic agent that carries some significant toxicity, was developed in 2004 to block this.[84] Repurposed drugs can also block VEGF with less toxicity including mebendazole, doxycycline, aspirin, and dipyridamole.[85]

The S.A.D. Cocktail

Consider blocking TAM and VEGF through the use of repurposed drugs. One of the best drug combinations for fighting this is Jane's cocktail of statin, aspirin, and dipyridamole, which I like to call the S.A.D. cocktail (a variation on S.A.M.).[86] Diet is also a significant factor. In addition to keeping your diet low in glycemia, you will want also to avoid high protein diets to avoid feeding glutamine burning tumors.

First, a word about the ketogenic diet: in my book, *The Coffee Cure Diet*, I discuss my decades-long experience with this. Low carb diets are fine with low saturated fat, but high saturated fats promote the secretion of inflammatory cytokines like tissue necrosis factor alpha (TNFa) and interleukin-6 (IL-6), both of which powerfully promote cancer. High saturated fat diets can also fuel tumors.

I would tend to agree with Jane McLelland's preference for the Mediterranean diet.[87] Avoid all meats except fish and stay away from carbohydrate-rich processed food. The most important change that you can make is to be consistent and exercise your muscles daily. Find something you like, whether it is walking, cycling, lifting weights, and just do it. Even ten minutes each day or after meals will make a big difference.

ANTICANCER DIET & LIFESTYLE

- Low Meat Except Fish
- Low Processed Food
- Muscle Exercise Post Meal
- 16 hour fast
- High Plant Polyphenols
- Low in Sweet Fruit

* Low Concentrated Sugar
* Low Refined Carb
* Low Saturated Fat
* Exercise during Fast
* High in Vegetables
* Low in Sweet Juices

Also, learn how to fast. I swear by 16-hour overnight fasts for at least four to five days a week. When combined with metformin, these fasts can promote apoptosis in tumor cells.[88] Apoptosis is when your cancer cells shrivel up and dissolve; it is cancer cell death.

If you exercise in a calorie depleted or carb depleted state, such as after your overnight fasts, you may improve your P53 tumor suppressor gene function causing apoptosis in precancer and cancer cells.[89] I try to do this at least two days per week.

Some cancers contain MYC mutations. These tumors thrive on glutamine in addition to sugar and fat. If you have an MYC mutation, I would avoid supplementation with added protein. Avoid all meats, even chicken and turkey except for Omega III rich fish. I would even avoid excess dairy protein if you have a MYC tumor. HER2 and EGFR tumors increase glutaminolysis and fat metabolism. KRAS is a mutation heavily involved in pancreatic cancer and is one of the worst of the RAS family of mutations.

Cancer Stem Cells and the War Room

How do cancer stem cells (CSCs) know when to develop resistance to chemotherapy and radiation treatment? What stimulates cancer cells to suddenly break free from a primary tumor and spread to the brain, lungs or liver and then re-root and grow new tumors? There are many complicated growth factors and signaling pathways, but the three most important are the Hedgehog, the WnT, and the NOTCH.[90, 91]

These signals explain resistance to chemotherapy and radiation. Imagine the cancer as a tumor tree. The instant the tree is attacked and clipped above the ground, it cries out for help. These cries are signaled through the three main pathways.

The damaged tree, above ground, sends desperate pleas to the rescuers, below ground, the roots of the cancer, the cancer stem cells.

These stem cells are the guardians of the tumor. Whenever the tree is damaged or threatened in any way, by cutting, chemicals, or radiation, the CSCs will hear about it, and come to the rescue.

Normally sleeping, they are awakened by the screams in the middle of the night. They spring into action. Imagine that they jump out of their bunks and head straight to the war room. They set up shields to prevent further tumor-tree-cell death (apoptosis). The CSCs make the tumor resistant to chemotherapy and radiation. They also send the Special Forces to break away and set up new outposts. These are known as metastases.

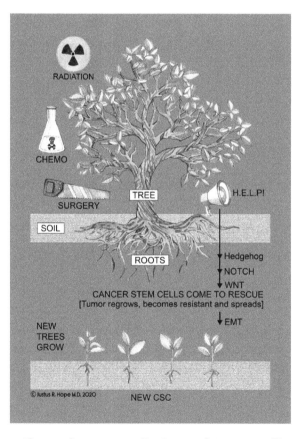

Chemotherapy, Radiation and Surgery all
Stimulate EMT (Metastasis)
Figure 1. The Cancer Tree and the Roots (CSC).

To begin the process, the epithelial-mesenchymal transformation (EMT) must begin. The epithelial cells which have been attached to the tumor lose their adhesions, their polarity, and become detached and set adrift like the Navy Seals. These free-floating cancer cells roam the body.

They travel to distant organs where they then do a reverse EMT and re-root. They stick to the new tissue which may be brain, lung, or liver. They regain their polarity, lose their mobility, and form a new tumor tree. None of this would be possible if we could take out their entire communications network. If we could silence their screams, the CSCs would never come to the rescue, and the tumor tree would die once and for all.

CANCER'S BACK UP PLAN

- Uses CSC to regrow
- Uses CSC to travel
- Uses CSC to fight chemo

* Uses CSC to gain strength
* Uses CSC to rewire
* Uses CSC to resist radiation

Blocking the Hedgehog, WnT, and NOTCH signaling systems is the key to preventing the tumor from returning and becoming resistant to treatment.

CANCER'S LIFELINE

- Hedgehog
- WnT
- NOTCH

* Cancer's Email
* Cancer's Texting
* Cancer's Voice

Because our standard cancer treatments target only the tree, we need repurposed drugs to address the roots and communications network. Surprisingly, many common supplements have major activity against these CSCs and their signaling pathways.

Jamming the CSC Signals

To disrupt these signals, I would start with supplements.

Curcumin, a component in the spice turmeric, is my first recommendation. And not just any curcumin. Most commercially available curcumin has poor absorption and is inactivated by the stomach pH. I would, instead, follow Dr. Kofron's lead and get nanocurcumin. Curcumin inhibits NOTCH signaling.[92] Second, get resveratrol. Resveratrol is found in grapes, berries, and peanuts, and it is anticancer by virtue of blocking NOTCH signaling.[93] Genistein induces apoptosis and inhibits cell growth in pancreatic cancer by downregulating NOTCH.[94]

Sulforaphane from broccoli targets pancreatic stem cells also by suppressing NOTCH.[95] Adding quinoxaline, an antibiotic, also inhibits pancreatic cancers by downregulating NOTCH.[96] Quercetin and Luteolin, both supplements, also hinder NOTCH.[97] The drug niclosamide, an antiparasitic, in particular, suppresses NOTCH-driven cancers, which include gastric, breast, colon, leukemia, glioma, and medulloblastoma.[98]

The mutation MYC is often seen in NOTCH cancers. Experimental studies on various cancers have shown that radiation therapy to the tumor bulk accelerates the repopulation of the cancer via the cancer stem cells.[99]

NOTCH-DRIVEN CANCERS

- Gastric
- Colon
- Glioma

* Breast
* Leukemia
* Medulloblastoma

Following each radiation treatment, the cancer stem cells become stronger and more resistant. This helps explain the failure of radiation therapy. Not only does the ionizing radiation cause the CSCs to grow faster, but they also become super cells, repairing their DNA more quickly and forming 50% less poisonous ROS (reactive oxygenation species).[100]

BLOCKING NOTCH

- Curcumin
- Resveratrol
- Suforaphane
- Quercetin
- Niclosamide

* Turmeric
* Nuts, Grapes, Berries
* Broccoli, Cauliflower
* Luteolin
* Metformin

Like aliens that thrive on nuclear fallout, the CSC feeds on radiation. They behave almost like bacteria that have acquired resistance to an antibiotic with one exception; resistant bacteria don't feed off of antibiotics.

Hedgehog signaling is also present in most cancers. Like e-mail, the Hedgehog has three main pathways: one might be G-mail, another AOL, and still another Yahoo. The three Hedgehogs are Indian, Desert, and Sonic, based on their ligands. They attach to receptors called PTCH. The Hedgehog signaling is heavily involved in pancreatic cancer, as well as EMT and metastasis.[101] Following chemotherapy, the Hedgehog communication pathway e-mails are vital to the recovery of the cancer.

HEDGEHOG-DRIVEN CANCERS

- Lung
- Esophagus
- Prostate
- Liver

* Stomach
* Pancreas
* Breast
* Brain

The signals help prevent cancer cell death and keep the cells dividing and spreading. Hedgehog signals cause stem cell division and transformation into fast-dividing tumor cells.[102] It helps create slower dividing cancer stem cells in the underground war room and more troops in the above- ground tree. Hedgehog is regularly used to communicate to the Seal team to head to remote locations and deploy more troops.

BLOCKING THE HEDGEHOG

- Curcumin
- Sulforaphane
- Metformin

* Cyclopamine
* Quercetin
* Mebendazole

Cyclopamine, a natural compound found in the plant *veratrum californacum*, commonly known as the corn lily, was the first phytochemical found to inhibit the Hedgehog pathway.[103] Sonic Hedgehog is the main form of pancreatic cancer communication and facilitates both tumor invasion and spread.[104] Cyclopamine, in conjunction with the standard chemotherapy Gemcitabine, reduced both the metabolic spread and primary tumor bulk in pancreatic tumor xenografts.[105]

Curcumin downregulates Sonic Hedgehog and can reverse EMT.[106] In other words, it can send the enemy seal team back home. Sulforaphane blocks the renewal of CSCs by suppressing Sonic Hedgehog.[107] Other studies show that quercetin is anti-Hedgehog.[108] Quercetin, when combined with sulforaphane, inhibits Hedgehog in pancreatic CSCs. Both metformin and MBZ strongly interfere with the Hedgehog.[109] Metformin helps block Sonic Hedgehog and gastric cancer and blocks NOTCH in colon cancer.[110]

The so-called NOTCH prefers more personal communication. It is often cell-to-cell. I imagine it is like two people speaking on a cell phone. NOTCH uses transcription proteins SNAIL-1 and SNAIL-2.

They are ligands that attach to receptors known as NOTCH-1, NOTCH-2, NOTCH 3, and NOTCH-4. Cancers with high SNAIL and SLUG activity are more deadly.[111]

Finally, we have reached the WnT signaling tumors. These include many of the viral-propelled cancers related to H. pylori, HepC, EBV, and HPV, like cervical and hepatocellular tumors.[112] Also, MYC driven cancers are often involved in ovarian, colon, and sarcoma. I imagine WnT communicates as text, not so intimate as in NOTCH (voice), but not as distant as Hedgehog (e-mail). WnT signaling (text) is common and is involved from start to finish in the cancer disease process.

WNT-RELATED CANCERS

- Cervical
- Esophageal
- Gastric
- Melanoma
- Non-Small-Cell Lung
- Endometrial
- Multiple Myeloma/Bone

* Liver
* Lymphoma/Sarcoma
* Nasopharyngeal
* Breast
* Colon
* Ovarian
* Viral-Propelled Tumors

Cancer stem cells are signaled as soon as the cancer forms, and WnT signaling keeps them dividing and resistant to apoptosis. WnT triggers EMT at the same time, causing EMT-related cell detachment, motility, and migration with subsequent invasion and metastasis. WnT is often involved in bone metastasis,[113] is often driven by the MYC gene,[114] and WnT tumors tend to down-regulate PPAR gamma. Since PPAR gamma is protective, you want more of it.   One way to suppress WnT is by lowering insulin and inflammation. High inflammation and insulin levels drastically elevate cancer risks.

JAMMING WNT SIGNALS

- Metformin
- Niclosamide
- Statins (Lipitor)

* NSAIDS (Ibuprofen, Celebrex, Sulindac)
* Aspirin
* Ivermectin

Metformin and statins, as well as NSAIDs, help block this effect and protect you.[115] Niclosamide, in addition to jamming NOTCH, can also interfere with WnT signals.[116] Another antiparasitic, Ivermectin, originally only for veterinary use, is approved for human use against river blindness, a tropical disease. It is also increasingly recognized as a WnT antagonist.

***

The bottom line is this: to win your war against cancer, you must not only worry about the chemotherapy radiation battle against the above ground fast-growing tumor. You must also pay attention to blocking the communication networks to the below ground slow-growing cancer stem cells, which control EMT. Metastasis, or the spread of tumor beyond the original location, is responsible for 90% of cancer deaths. To be effective against blocking EMT, one must block the tumor's ability to communicate to the CSCs, which control EMT.

The Double Agent of Cancer: TGF-Beta

Transforming growth factor-beta, otherwise known as TGF-beta, is the growth factor that drives normal cell growth through wound healing. However, like the CSC, it can also promote metastasis through EMT.

I like to image TGF-beta as a double agent in our body's cancer cold war. When we don't have cancer, TGF-beta functions as a tumor suppressor, working for our side and helping to snuff out any cancers before they can get started.

During early stage cancers, TGF-beta signals block tumor growth in epithelial compartments.[117] Epithelial tissue is traditionally derived from the ectoderm, usually skin, hair, and nails.

However, when the cancer is advanced, especially when chronic inflammation is present, TGF-beta turns on us and becomes stimulating to the cancer. Our spy, trusted by us to snuff out cancer, becomes a double agent and now works for the other side, the tumor. TGF helps cancer not only grow but become a more powerful instigator of EMT and tumor spread.

There are three types of EMT. EMT-1 occurs in embryogenesis and is normal when we develop in utero. It helps our cells differentiate and transform from epithelial to various mesenchymal tissues. EMT-2 occurs as a normal transformation in response to tissue injury. For example, when we break our arm, our body creates inflammation in the fracture area to stimulate blood flow and tissue repair.

This inflammation stimulates EMT-2 through TGF, where cells must transform from epithelial-to-mesenchymal to grow new tissue, bone, muscle, and fascia. This helps repair the damage so long as the inflammation is brief and only during the time necessary. In the case of a fracture, the time is between six and eight weeks.

EMT-3, however, is where we see the problem. This causes prolonged inflammation. Scenarios would include chronic infection such as HIV, Hep C, or HPV where there is chronic irritation or damage of cells due to viral replication.

THREE KINDS OF EMT

- EMT-1   *   Normal and Noncancerous

- EMT-2   *   Normal Wound healing

- EMT-3   *   Inflammation, Viruses & Cancer

Long-term inflammation beyond six to eight weeks can promote cancer. We see this with Hepatitis C and H. Pylori with gastric and liver cancers. TGF loses its tumor suppressant effect first and then begins to promote cancer cell motility, invasion, and metastasis.

TGF drives EMT-3. At this point, our double agent can now work alongside other signaling pathways, such as WnT or NOTCH. TGF-beta is notorious for signaling SNAIL-1 and SNAIL-2 to spread our tumor everywhere. Radiation, a known carcinogen, stimulates TGF driven EMT. TGF signaling also plays a major role in cancer stem cell or CSC maintenance. High levels of TGF are associated with poor patient survival and increased CSC survival.

TGF-Beta & CSC

- Both cause Chemotherapy Resistance

- Both cause Radiation Therapy Resistance

- Both Stimulate Metastasis (EMT)

- Remember My Formula: CSC + TGF-beta = EMT

TGF is a bad actor. Chemotherapy also stimulates TGF-beta cancer resistance.[118] Standard metal-based chemotherapies like Cis-platinum increase the level of TGF-beta messenger RNA as well as the secretion of active TGF-beta in the blood. This renders tumor cells resistant to the Cis-platinum drug. Studies from Arteaga and colleagues show that radiation-induced TGF-beta promoted metastasis in cancer cell lines.[119] When TGF-beta was treated with anti-TGF-beta antibodies, the Cis-platinum sensitivity was restored, and resistance was overcome.[120] Repurposed drugs that block TGF-beta include dipyridamole, once again a component of Jane's S.A.D. combination. A common blood pressure agent, Losartan, has potent anti-TGF-beta activity. It enhanced chemotherapy effectiveness in ovarian cancer models.[121]

TIPS TO LOWER TGF-Beta

- Keep viruses away
  * Lactoferrin, Zinc, Vitamin D

- Get Your Vaccines
  * HPV, HVB

- Treat Known Infections
  * Harvoni for HCV, Kaletra for HIV

- Keep Inflammation Low
  * Polyphenols, Green Tea, Coffee

- NSAIDS
  * Aspirin

- Dipyridamole
  * Losartan

Another way to suppress TGF is to keep your levels of inflammation low. Get your infections healed. Treat H. pylori. Treat Hep C. Get vaccinated against HPV. Avoid chronic infections. I like a daily dose of lactoferrin (contained in whey protein) as it suppresses many viruses, bacteria, fungi, and parasites.[122]

Avoid consuming saturated fats and trans-fats as they raise levels of inflammation and C-reactive protein. Drink coffee, as it contains chlorogenic acid and naturally lowers inflammation on a daily basis. Of course, prescription medications like NSAIDs, also lower inflammation and can be taken. Aspirin also lowers inflammation. Inflammation stimulates TGF, which causes cancer.

TGF Loves mTOR

The P13 K mTOR pathway is another major driver of cancer.[123] It is stimulated by nutrient excess, especially a high glycemic diet. These diets elevate insulin levels, which in turn releases IGF, which then stimulates P13 kinase and then mTOR, the mammalian target of rapamycin. P13 K also drives TGF stimulation of EMT. High glycemic diets spike mTOR. mTOR is also activated by TGF beta. The combination of mTOR and TGF together is like jet fuel for driving metastases (EMT-3).

Studies show that blocking mTOR with drugs like RapaLink-1 reduces EMT, after stimulation with TGF.[124] While I don't advise rapamycin as it given to transplant recipients and has lots of adverse effects, metformin lowers mTOR extremely well.

The first step to lower mTOR stimulation is with diet. Diet change works well. Sugar or simple carbohydrate intake like breads or sweets trigger the production of Insulin and IGF. IGF triggers P13K. P13k then triggers Akt which lights up mTOR.

LOWERING mTOR

• Metformin	* Berberine
• Lowering Simple Carbs	* Fasting
• Green Tea	* EGCG
• Plant-based Diet	* Cruciferous Vegetables
• Exercise	* Curcumin

Not everyone produces the same amount of mTOR after eating. My wife is genetically lean, and can eat carbs with minimal mTOR release. If one has insulin resistance like I do, much more is stimulated. That is exactly why 40% of all cancers are linked to the condition of insulin resistance. If you want to continue to eat your carbs, and also keep cancer at bay, then reversing insulin resistance is a great option. Improving one's insulin sensitivity means controlling your diabetes, lowering your A1C, and losing body fat. What is insulin resistance?

In essence, excess weight (in particular belly fat) causes our insulin to work less efficiently. Our pancreas must secrete more insulin to compensate. These insulin-resistant conditions include prediabetes, diabetes, hypertension, elevated triglycerides low HDL, etc. Excess insulin secretion in response to a high carbohydrate meal results in chronic hyperinsulinemia or high insulin levels.

The easiest way to tell if you are insulin-resistant is to look into your triglyceride to HDL ratio. If it is greater than 3.5, you are at risk. If your waist-hip ratio is higher than .8 as a female or .9 as a male, you likely have it. Insulin resistance and how to reverse it is covered in more detail in the *Coffee Cure Diet*. However, to summarize this, diet and lifestyle changes, including building muscle and losing weight, can help reverse this. It is crucial to do everything possible to restore insulin sensitivity if you have insulin resistance.

The best and the easiest first step is to add the prescription drug metformin or the over-the-counter supplement berberine, which will help lower insulin levels by reducing blood sugar levels.[125] I take metformin every day. Other substances that naturally lower mTOR include green tea and its active ingredient, Epigallocatechin gallate (EGCG).[126] Cruciferous vegetables like broccoli and brussels sprouts are good. Lowering animal protein helps, so vegetarians tend to have lower levels of mTOR.[127]

I also do five to ten sets of twenty muscle exercises most days to keep my insulin levels low and to suppress my P13 K mTOR pathway. If you don't wish to get cancer, you need to tame your mTOR. If you already have had cancer, you will want to lower mTOR to keep it from returning.

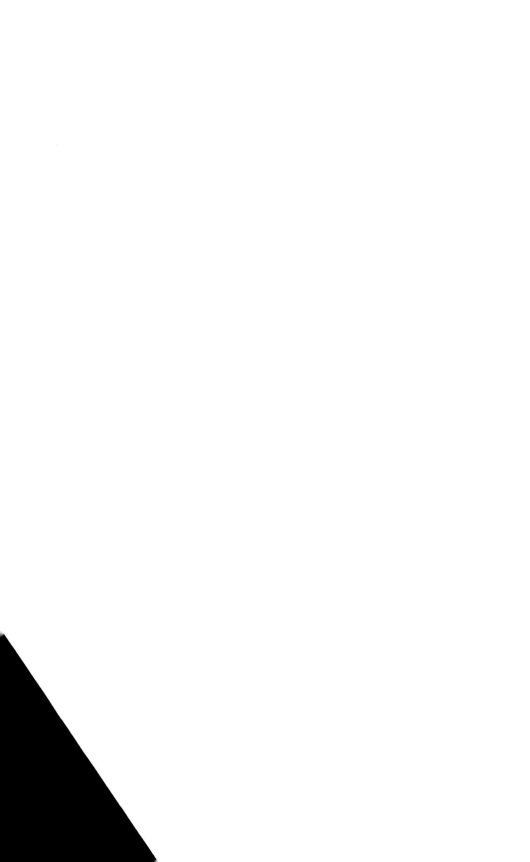

Chapter 7

TUMOR RESISTANCE, EMT and AUTOPHAGY

When you declare war on your cancer and begin treating it, the tumor will fight back. The more it has spread, the more powerfully it responds.

As discussed, attacking the bulk of the tumor often causes resistance by stimulating cancer stem cells through the three major signaling pathways, Hedgehog, WnT, and NOTCH. Whenever surgery, chemotherapy, or radiation is done to the tumor, you should ALWAYS add a repurposed drug cocktail to counteract the stimulation to the CSC population.

However, aside from this CSC, the tumor will also fight back using two other methods: autophagy and EMT. Autophagy is stimulated when nutrients are deprived. When a person with cancer fasts, consumes a low-glycemic diet, or adds Metformin, the tumor is metabolically stressed. Its ability to use glucose is diminished, and it is in danger of starving and dying (apoptosis). This is what we want.

Jane McLelland showed how we can help overcome cancer by depriving it of its nutrients in her book about starving cancer. Metformin drugs the cancer by blocking Warburg metabolism, cancer's preferred and wasteful use of glucose. As explained earlier, cancer simply adjusts, uses other forms of metabolism, or learns to process protein or fat.

If one blocks these compensatory pathways with the combination of metformin, a lipophilic statin (like Lipitor), aspirin, dipyridamole, carbohydrate restriction, and fasting, the tumor will be stressed. It will do what it must.

BLOCKING TUMOR ESCAPE

- Block Autophagy   * Chloroquine or Loratidine

- Block Warburg   * Metformin/Berberine

- Block Reverse   * Metformin/DCA
  Warburg

- Induce   * Pulsed
  Apoptosis/Oxidation   Chloroquine/NSAID/VitC

Often at this point, cancer fights back through the protective process of autophagy. It uses lysosomes to collect dead cellular debris, and fuel is recycled. It is not too far off from plane crash survivors cannibalizing their dead comrades to survive the ordeal. The cancer cells also recycle nutrients like lactate in a reverse Warburg process. The tumor cells essentially burn their trash to gain more energy and conserve fuel.

However, by using repurposed drugs like chloroquine or hydroxychloroquine, you can help block autophagy, which can lead to apoptosis and cancer cell death. But you cannot win the war unless you also block EMT.

Remember my formula CSC + TGF-beta = EMT (metastasis). Never allow your tumor to communicate with its CSC and always strive to block the duo of TGF and mTOR.

The combination of metformin, chloroquine, and overnight fasting with a low-glycemic diet is powerful in blocking the P13 K mTOR pathways. The two drugs, metformin and chloroquine, also help block autophagy.[128] Loratidine also lowers autophagy. But don't forget that you must also kill the bulk of the tumor. This is ideally done with standard treatments, including surgery, chemotherapy, and radiation.

The trifecta of debulking, blocking P13 mTOR, and blocking autophagy is a good strategy in blocking tumor escape. Jane McLelland goes a step further. She uses intravenous Vitamin C as an oxidant to periodically cause cancer cell death, termed apoptosis, along with using NSAIDs. Others oxygenate with pressurized O2, hyperbaric oxygen. Oral vitamin C supplements do not oxidize like the intravenous infusions.

After having weakened it by starving it with drugs and diet changes, oxidizing her cancer is another reason Jane survived. Her use of periodic or pulsed IV Vitamin C may have been the determining factor in her winning her war. Chloroquine (CQ) and hydroxychloroquine (HCQ) are both powerful apoptosis inducers. Later we will discuss pulsing of CQ/HCQ or NSAIDS at crucial times when your tumor is the most vulnerable.

Whenever getting standard therapy, you will also want to target the CSC with repurposed drugs and supplements simultaneously. Since chemotherapy and radiation often done at the beginning of treatment can trigger the CSC, this is the most important time to add the cocktail. This will help prevent resistance from developing. Anti-EMT strategies, like blocking P13 mTOR, blocking TGF, and anti-autophagy strategies, like using drugs like NSAIDS or CQ/HCQ, are smart and strategic.

***

As we have seen, signaling from the fast-growing tumor to the stem cell root is done by three main drivers: The Hedgehog (Hh), WnT, and NOTCH. Together, these three form the communication link between the fast-growing tumor bulk, the metaphorical cancer tree, and the below ground root, the cancer stem cells, CSC.

The CSC, the generals of the cancer army, usually are asleep until awoken by the signals of the tumor bulk being under attack. Whenever the tumor bulk is attacked through surgery, chemotherapy, or radiation, the Hh, WnT, and NOTCH cry for help. The CSC generals spring into action and trigger EMT, metastatic spread, as well as new resistant tumor growth.

Various strategies to cure cancer by targeting cancer stem cells

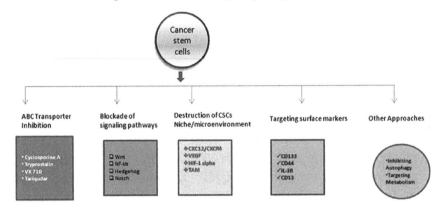

Courtesy of Singh et al, *Front Mol Biosci.* 2017
Figure 2. Targeting Cancer Stem Cells by Blocking WnT,
NOTCH, and Hedgehog

The stem cells and TGF-beta together are the two main drivers of EMT or metastatic spread. CSC can grow and divide by reproducing themselves or making full-blown tumor tissue. CSCs can also almost magically turn anchored epithelial cells into mesenchymal (or free-floating cells) that travel and then again magically transform back to epithelial cells and re-anchor.

These grow into entirely new tumor colonies. The tumor, or bulk, is rapidly dividing, and just in front of itself, it secretes growth factors. The front of the cancer is rich in cancer stem cells and mesenchymal tissue. The area in front of the tumor, the tumor microenvironment, contains more TGF-beta to drive more CSC and EMT growth as well as EGF, the epidermal growth factor. EGF drives many cancers and is notorious in breast cancer and glioma.[129] Targeted therapies include antibodies against EGF receptors, like cetuximab (chemotherapy), which blocks the growth factor action. Naturally, resistance to this tends to develop quickly.

Due to its preference for glycolysis and Warburg metabolism, the tumor develops low oxygen and low pH levels, causing other growth factors to be produced. In addition, there is a lack of blood vessel supply, which can stimulate angiogenesis. New blood vessels form to service the tumor.

Blood vessels can be thought of as the roads that bring in supplies and truck out waste. They help the tumor grow much faster. Low oxygen induces the secretion of hypoxic-induced factor, HIF, which tells the Project Engineer to add more roads. HIF stimulates VEGF, vascular endothelial growth factor, that constructs the maze of new roads, the blood vessels that feed the cancer.

The Tumor Microenvironment

The advancing tumor front is rich in Warburg lactate, and poor in blood supply. It lives in a barren, and oxygen-starved microenvironment. Recall Warburg metabolism is wasteful as it is not done in the efficient cell furnaces, the mitochondria. Instead, it is done by a fermentation process. This uses up the oxygen, and the area around the tumor ends up hypoxic and acidic. Acid and low oxygen stimulate the release of HIF, which stimulates VEGF and new blood vessel growth making tumors bulge with veins and blood.

The development of monoclonal antibodies that attack VEGF has been a major breakthrough in cancer therapy. Avastin, also known as bevacizumab, is a recombinant monoclonal antibody that binds to VEGF and inhibits its activity, thereby inhibiting angiogenesis and potentially halting tumor growth. It works well in many cancers including my friend, Evan's glioblastoma. As with most chemotherapies, it also has some side effects, some severe. In addition, resistance can form, and the addition of repurposed drugs that also block VEGF is valuable. Platelet-derived growth factor also assists.

BLOCKING ANGIOGENSIS

- Block VEGF
  - * Anti-VEGF Antibodies: Avastin
  - * Propranolol, Itraconazole
  - * Curcumin, Resveratrol
- Block EGF
  - * Cetuximab
- Block PDGF
  - * Aspirin, Dipyridamole

Between EGF, HIF, and angiogenesis, the tumor front advances. Repurposed drugs that can block both VEGF and platelet-derived growth factor (PDGF) include aspirin and dipyridamole (i.e., Jane's S.A.D. cocktail).[130] Propranolol also inhibits VEGF.[131] A tumor metastasis often has a hard feel, often ten times stiffer than surrounding tissue. This is due to the special properties of tumor colonies, mainly the specialized fibroblasts that are the building blocks of the connective tumor tissue. Platelet derived growth factor, PDGF, induces fibroblast growth.

TAF & TAM Pave the Way

The TAF, or tumor-associated fibroblasts, secrete various substances, including MMP, metalloproteinases, which help clear the way for paving more tumor highways. Immune cells, TAM, tumor-associated macrophages, contribute to inflammation, which powerfully stimulates tumor growth and VEGF.

All of these growth factors make the local area surrounding the tumor cancer friendly, by being low pH, low oxygen, highly vascular, stiff, and inflamed. Repurposed drugs that counter these conditions include NSAIDs like COX-II inhibitors such as Celebrex or COX general inhibitors like ibuprofen or naproxen. These can reduce inflammation. Treatment with hyperbaric oxygen can increase O_2 levels, which counter the tumor's preferred environment.

BLOCKING THE MMP AND INFLAMMATION

- Block Matrix Metalloproteinases
  - Mebendazole, Doxycycline
  - Aspirin, Propranolol

- Block Inflammation
  - NSAIDS (Celebrex, Ibuprofen)
  - Polyphenols (Coffee, Green Tea)

MBZ and doxycycline can help block MMP.[132] I like the combination of doxycycline and MBZ; however, propranolol and aspirin can also be effective. I always remind my patients not to forget the role that diet and lifestyle play in inflammation. Visceral, or belly fat, triggers macrophages to release inflammatory cytokines interleukin six and tissue necrosis factor alpha in those people with insulin resistance and who are overweight. These can greatly increase the risk of developing cancer.

Plant polyphenols like coffee and chlorogenic acid are strongly anti-inflammatory.[133] I personally drink four cups of coffee per day. Coffee suppresses my appetite in addition to tempering inflammation; controlling both keeps insulin resistance and belly fat in check. How do you know if you have elevated levels of inflammation? Get your CRP, your C-reactive protein, level checked. It is a simple blood test. You will want this key number below 0.5.

HAMPT: Prevent Metastases After Surgery

Dr. Wan and colleagues formulated the HAMPT combination of repurposed drugs. They wrote, "Aspirin, lysine, mifepristone and doxycycline combined can effectively and safely prevent and treat cancer metastases."[134] This cocktail was designed to target CSC and EMT processes. Mifepristone is a progesterone receptor antagonist commonly used as an abortifacient.

It is cytotoxic against various human cancers. It interferes with tumor invasion, migration, and angiogenesis. It also inhibits TGF-beta. One study showed that Mifepristone blocked multiple colorectal cell lines from EMT spread.[135]

Scientists found similarities between the drug's mechanism of blocking embryo-implantation and tumor metastasis. It has the safety record of having been used successfully for as long as 14 years. Aspirin inhibits COX-II and the prostaglandin pathway. It improves survival in colon cancer patients.[136]

HAMPT FOUR COCKTAIL

- Aspirin

- Doxycycline

- Mifepristone

- Lysine

Low doses between 75 and 325 mg per day help its anti-metastatic effects by inhibiting MMP-2 (metalloproteinase-2). It also downregulates EMT and lowers platelet mediated nuclear factor kappa B (NFkB). NkfB enhances inflammation and suppresses immune response to cancer. It is almost always a tumor enhancer, although in rare cases, similar to TGF beta, NkfB can function as a tumor suppressor.

Aspirin, in addition to blocking NKfB, can reduce adhesion and invasion of blood vessels (block VEGF). Long-term aspirin use has been shown to reduce distant metastasis by some 30-40% and reduce the risk of metastatic adenocarcinoma by almost 50%.[137]

Doxycycline is an antibiotic in use for over 40 years. It is considered safe and relatively nontoxic. It is a potent MMP inhibitor and has long been shown to reduce and prevent cancer bone metastasis in various situations.[138]

Lysine is an amino acid that inhibits MMPs and helps destroy tumor friendly acid environments. It buffers the tumor microenvironment. Lysine inhibited metastasis in cell models.[139] Although no clinical trials have been done using the HAMPT combination, Dr. Wan and colleagues feel it is a reasonable metastasis prevention strategy for cancer patients to use following surgical removal of their primary tumors.

Advanced Cocktail: EIS

The EIS repurposed drug cocktail was developed by the U.S. physician Dr. Richard Kast and colleagues. It involves a six-drug combination to block EMT transformation in glioblastoma.[140] The six include pirfenidone, naproxen, rifampin, quetiapine, itraconazole, and metformin.

The first drug is pirfenidone and is a well-tolerated drug approved initially to treat fibrosis. It also blocks TGF-beta signaling, a major driver in epithelial-to-mesenchymal transformation, EMT.[141] TGF-beta, as previously stated, promotes angiogenesis and EMT.

Recall my formula for metastases or tumor spread: CSC + TGF-beta = EMT (spread). The easy way to think about this is that both CSC and TGF-beta must be blocked to prevent metastasis. The common link is the communication network through Hedgehog, WnT, and NOTCH.

Pirfenidone has the added benefit of inhibiting the inflammatory cytokine TNF-alpha.[142] It also blocks PDGF, a stimulator of tumor metastasis in patients suffering from chronic Hepatitis C viral infections.

The cytokines interleukin-6, as well as TGF-beta, are both elevated in cancer. Two years of treatment with pirfenidone (400 mg three times per day) caused both interleukin-6 and TGF-beta levels to drop by approximately 50%.[143]

Quetiapine, a drug initially approved in psychiatry, has antitumor activity through inhibition of nuclear factor kappa b signaling (NKfB) through RANK.[144] RANK is associated with increased

SNAIL activity (involved in NOTCH signaling - a major stimulant of CSC and EMT). GBM secretes RANK, which furthers EMT and glioma cell migration.

RANK is over-expressed in several cancers, including breast, hepatocellular, endometrial, lung, and prostate. RANK causes invasion and migration.[145] Quetiapine helps block the RANK pathway. The EIS regimen attempts to target both RANK and TGF-beta mediated growth.

The third drug, rifampin, is an antibiotic originally indicated to treat tuberculosis as well as resistant Staph. Rifampin is also used to treat H. pylori infections and leprosy (Hanson's disease). Rifampin can exert anti-EMT activity by inhibiting the powerful WnT signaling pathway.[146]

Upregulation of WnT is created in response to either chemotherapy with TMZ, the standard in GBM. WnT delivers signals to cancer stem cells causing EMT transformation and creating resistance to both TMZ and radiation therapy. Theoretically, rifampin should help decrease treatment resistance to both TMZ and radiation.

THE EIS SIX COCKTAIL

- Pirfenidone
- Naproxen
- Rifampin
- Quetiapine
- Itraconazole
- Metformin

The drug Naproxen is a commonly used NSAID with COX inhibiting effects. Interleukin-6 promotes cancer as a co-factor of EMT. GBM cells produce Interleukin-6 (Il-6) as a tumor growth factor. Naproxen decreases levels of Il-6. Miconazole, an old antifungal drug, is a powerful inhibitor of Hh signaling.[147] By downregulating Hh, it has been shown to inhibit metastasis. Hh is upregulated by standard chemotherapy and similarly stimulates EMT.

There is also cross-communication with the SNAIL pathway. Itraconazole helps block both.[148] It has been shown to inhibit Hh signals, which in turn inhibits the growth of breast cancers, melanoma, and endometrial cancer.

The sixth and final EIS drug discussed is appropriately saved for last, and is a component of most cancer cocktails, due to its multiple modes of action. As mentioned earlier, it can both prevent and kill cancer. It has impressive actions against CSC, so it is a natural choice in an anti-metastatic combination. It is metformin.

Metformin: The Rising EMT Star

Metformin, in 2013 was dubbed "a rising star to fight EMT in oncology" by Dr. Barriere and co-workers.[149] As discussed earlier, metformin is associated with both a lower rate of cancer development and a higher rate of survival.

It has many antitumor actions, including raising AMP kinase, which downregulates mTOR along the P13K pathway.

It interferes with the tumor's mitochondrial energy processing (OXPHOS). Metformin also inhibits TGF-beta-induced EMT in non-small cell lung cancer, NSCLC.[150]

METFORMIN'S SUPPRESSION OF EMT

- Reduces mTOR/P13/Akt
  * By Raising AMPK

- Reduces NOTCH Signaling
  * By Reducing SNAIL2

- Reduces TGF-beta
  * By Reducing SNAIL2

- Reduces Interleukin-6
  * Non-Small-Cell-Lung Cancer

- Reduces Chemo/Radiation Resistance
  * By Reducing SNAIL2

- Enhances Chemotherapy Effect
  * To 5-FU and Cisplatinum
  * To Temozolomide (TMZ)

- Restores Chemotherapy Effect

It helps block SNAIL activity and cervical cancer EMT.[151] NOTCH regulates EMT-related genes called SLUG and SNAIL to promote metastatic cancer spread through the EMT process. Metformin can reduce both SNAIL and SLUG. SNAIL and SLUG are collectively known as SNAIL2. Metformin also helps block radiation-induced EMT and chemotherapy-induced EMT through both SNAIL and SLUG pathways.[152]   Standard chemotherapy with Docetaxel, unfortunately, stimulates metastasis-related MMP-9 but metformin partially reverses this.[153]

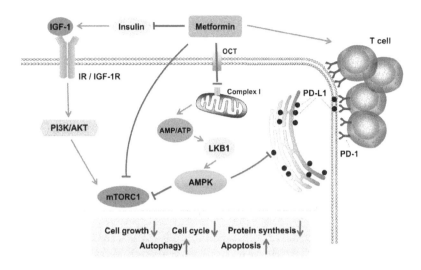

Courtesy of Chen et al. Aging. 2019
Figure 3. Metformin Blocks Key Cancer Pathways.

Metformin reduces EMT changes in lung and adenocarcinoma cells exposed to TGF-beta by decreasing SNAIL-2.[154] TNBC, triple-negative breast cancer has high levels of TGF-beta. Metformin inhibits TGF-beta in TNBC, which reduces cell growth, invasion, and motility.[155] Metformin reverses estradiol-induced EMT in endometrial adenoma via AMPK activation which reduces TGF-beta.[156]

Metformin lowers interleukin-6 in NSCL cancers and lowers TGF-beta in prostate cancers helping inhibit EMT in both.[157]

With NSCLC carcinoma, the addition of metformin to standard chemo 5-FU doxorubicin and Cis-platinum increases treatment sensitivity and apoptosis.[158] Metformin enhanced apoptosis (cancer cell death) along with the agent, Sorafenib (chemotherapy), against glioma cell lines.[159] Metformin worked synergistically in killing glioma cells in vitro (tissue culture).

A tissue culture study revealed the gradual development of GBM cell resistance with nine months of treatment with TMZ. Exposure to metformin for only several days restored sensitivity to TMZ treatment.[160] Metformin also reverses chemotherapy resistance in many cancers.

Evan, my friend with GBM, has already enrolled in the Care Oncology Clinic trial and is receiving their basic four-drug cocktail, comprised of metformin, atorvastatin, doxycycline, and mebendazole, in addition to all standard treatment. The standard treatment includes radiation and chemotherapy with Temozolomide (TMZ). He is also receiving Avastin, the VEGF blocker. Unfortunately, his tumor was too large to remove, so he is considered inoperable.

Because of this, he really needs an advanced cocktail tailored to attack GBM, one that blocks many more pathways, to gain a real chance of beating the odds with his terrible tumor.

This brings me to the CUSP-9 Cocktail.

This cocktail was the brainchild of cancer researcher Dr. Richard Kast, who along with 27 other scientists developed this nine-drug combination in 2013 to extinguish GBM. CUSP-9 is shorthand for "coordinated undermining of survival paths with nine repurposed drugs". Dr. Kast and colleagues have been gathering additional data these last seven years with encouraging results.[325]

After Kast's discovery, the cocktail was applied by many in compassionate use settings. Skaga and Skaga described it as a folk remedy, one that circulated amongst GBM survivors––until it was tested in the laboratory.

The CUSP-9 GBM Cocktail

The CUSP-9 is a nine-drug cocktail for use against glioblastoma. This is an advanced cocktail. Basic cocktails, like the one used by Care Oncology Clinic, the four-drug cocktail used in its METRICS trial, showed great promise with doubling survival times in glioblastoma patients. More advanced cocktails, or second-generation combinations, including the HAMPT and the ESIS the six-drug regimen, were designed to target multiple glioma pathways.

One favorite combination is the CUSP-9 strategy which combines TMZ, the standard chemotherapy for GBM with nine additional repurposed drugs: Aprepitant, auranofin, Captopril, Celecoxib, disulfiram, itraconazole, minocycline, Quetiapine, and sertraline.[161]

The researchers, Dr. Erland Skaga and Dr. Ida Skaga and colleagues, felt that by blocking multiple signaling pathways at the same time, they could block the escape of CSCs seeking to rewire, which would render them sensitive to the cytotoxic effects of TMZ.

Their nine-drug combination was chosen because of its low toxicity parameters. They noted some patients had used this nine drug cocktail on a do-it-yourself basis. The scientists wanted to test this with a formal study. The researchers felt that if CUSP-9 was used in combination with the cytotoxic agent, TMZ, it could be effective. And they were correct.

Essentially, they tested each individual drug's effectiveness against cultured glioblastoma tumor stem cells from five patients suffering from recurrent or relapsed glioblastoma. TMZ, the standard of care, was not effective against any of these cell cultures. They had all developed resistance. However, the combination of CUSP-9 plus TMZ showed substantial benefits.

In 50% of the glioma cells, the CUSP-9 plus TMZ was highly sensitive.

The researchers' goal was to target the CSC population within the tumor by attacking the key signaling pathways, especially WnT, Hh, and mTOR. Two resistant GBM stem cell cultures were tested in silico (i.e., in the laboratory). The CUSP-9 plus TMZ combination was 80-90% effective at reducing WnT signaling. In another GBM cell culture called T1459, the CUSP-9 plus TMZ combination was 100% effective at blocking CS sphere formation. It essentially killed all the cells. Interestingly, each of the drugs alone was ineffective. But the combination was incredibly effective.

The cocktail eliminated the cancer cells.

It was also effective against T1506 GBM cells. In another population, T1502, the combination had limited effectiveness, with 75% of the tumor cells surviving.

The lesson is that depending upon the individual patient and the specific GBM tumor genetics, the cocktail plus TMZ's potential could range from curative to minimally effective. I looked at a photo of the findings against the cell line T1459. Each drug test included a Petri dish showing minimal growth inhibition. There were thriving cancer colony spots present. Each drug by itself had almost no effect.

However, in the Petri dish treated with the combination CUSP-9 plus TMZ, the dish was cancer-free. Not one cell survived. This type of testing should ideally be done in one's cancer cells, whether resistant glioma-blastoma, colon cancer, or pancreatic cancer, etc. Clearly, the combination approach works, and sensitivity testing of your tumor cells takes the guesswork out of it.

I will discuss this more in the final section, on personalized cancer care.

And it makes sense. It blocks key signaling pathways to CSC, allowing the TMZ to debulk the tumor without the CSCs being notified to rewire.

Dr. Richard Gerber, a long-term GBM survivor and repurposed drug advocate, recognized the same logic.

"My approach was based on finding as many agents which could block the sort of pathways which activate glioblastoma, and doing it all at once so that the glioblastoma would have less of a chance to mutate and escape by a pathway because I would always be blocking that pathway."[162]

Indeed, this approach seems the key to the secret of GBM's long-term terminal cancer survivors. This is precisely why Dr. Ben Williams and Dr. Richard Gerber are not freaks of chance, but bastions of a paradigm shift in cancer treatment. When CSC pathways are not blocked, the tumor simply acquires resistance to the chemotherapy and radiation and stimulates EMT and metastatic spread. When repurposed drugs cocktails are added, CSC and EMT pathways are blocked, and the cancer colony root dies, ensuring a long-term survival.

Drs. Skaga and Skaga note the CUSP-9 was chosen based upon the drugs that cross the blood-brain barrier. However, differences in patients' metabolism make blood levels and brain concentrations variable. So, physician supervision remains important to monitor for toxicity.

In general, for a one-size-fits-all approach, the CUSP-9 plus TMZ for GBM is not a bad starting point. However, it is best to identify your tumor's specific genes and biomarkers by sequencing and customizing your cocktail based on sensitivity testing. Again, more on this in the last section, the one on customized cancer care.

If it were up to me, I would be tempted to add MBZ and metformin for good measure. They are nontoxic, and each blocks so many pathways, why wouldn't you? And if it were up to me, I would most certainly add the various supplements nanocurcumin, Quercetin, Resveratrol, Melatonin, turkey tail mushroom, lactoferrin, fish oil, and flaxseed oil.

SECTION III:
PERSONALIZING YOUR CANCER TREATMENT

Chapter 8

CHOOSING THE RIGHT PLAN FOR YOU

There is no question that combination therapy with repurposed drugs holds the key to long-term survival in terminal cancer. But how does one choose the ideal combination of drugs, treatments, and lifestyle changes? It starts by having the right people in your corner.

Selecting Your Medical Team

In medicine, as in life, the wealthy and powerful often have different options than the rest of us. Lance Armstrong, fresh off a one-million-dollar purse after winning the world championships, did not get standard chemotherapy. He researched the proposed standard chemotherapy treatments and side effects and then hired a dream team of physicians at Indiana University. He achieved a cure despite having stage IV testicular cancer, which spread to the lungs and brain. He did not receive the usual protocol. He negotiated.

Although most patients do not have the resources of Lance Armstrong, everyone has internet access. With Google Scholar and PubMed, one can do their own lifesaving research into repurposed drug cocktails for cancer.

You probably have some form of health insurance if you reside in the United States. Your selection of physicians, similar to the selection of a legal team, will play a major role in your cancer survival chances.

You will want an accessible GP or a trusted family physician that is willing to work with you—if the provider you see is a physician assistant or nurse practitioner, even better. I have found that mid-levels are often more compassionate, spend more time, and are usually more willing to listen. And of course, you will want a well-trained oncologist to provide you with the best and most recent cancer treatments.

Optimal chemotherapy, radiation therapy, and surgery to remove the bulk of the tumor are important as long as one attacks the stem cells at the same time. Despite any problems that the modern cancer care system may have with monetary influences, the United States cancer care system remains second to none in the world.

I happen to believe that adding repurposed drugs and supplements makes it even better. More recently-trained oncologists, especially the younger ones, are more receptive to the concept of cancer stem cells and repurposed drug use, although any oncologist that is educated and keeps open to the idea will be good.

Finally, having a nutritionist and/or an integrated health specialist on board will balance your team. A family member with a background in the biological sciences who can take on the task of research and gathering articles for your team is a huge bonus.

If a new repurposed drug like mebendazole is discovered tomorrow, and a benefit to surviving melanoma is found, and you have melanoma, you need to know about it. Chances are your oncologist will not tell you. However, your research assistant or you should find it immediately on PubMed and Google Scholar by simply doing a search, "melanoma + repurposed drugs" or "melanoma + CSC + repurposed drugs." Always pay attention to the most recent articles.

Studies done in the United States and Europe are generally, but not always, more reliable than those done elsewhere. Retrospective studies are less reliable because the groups are often not evenly matched. Studies using large numbers are more statistically reliable than small studies. Prospective studies are more reliable than retrospective in general. Placebo-controlled double-blind trials are the best.

I look for studies that show an improvement in survival, whenever possible. When I see these, it is golden, because not only does this reflect the drug is reasonably safe, but it shows the drug reduces the death rate from all causes. For example, metformin reduces the death rate from all causes. I also like to see agreement with studies from different countries and in different labs.

SCIENTIFIC STUDIES

1.	Retrospective	Chart reviews
		Groups not evenly matched
		Subject to bias in selection
		Investigators can cherry-pick data
2.	Prospective	Criteria set in advance
		Less prone to bias
3.	Placebo/Randomized	Matching control group
		Researchers know who gets drug
4.	Placebo/Randomized/Blind	Matching control group
		Researcher don't know who gets drug
		Eliminates bias

This brings me to the subject of bias. Bias in scientific research can unfortunately occur in many scenarios. It might be innocent. A scientist wants his new drug to show an effect, so he does a retrospective review of charts on drug X and chooses criteria which make it look good. It might be because the study's sponsor or the researcher expects the result to be positive for his company. In either case, the data can be manipulated to show the desired outcome. This is called cherry-picking.

In a prospective review, one where the criteria are set out in advance, this is less likely to occur, UNLESS one changes the criteria at the end of the study. For example, one might begin the study looking at survivorship from cancer, but at the end of the study, change the criteria to improved quality of life. This is known as p-hacking, data fishing, or data butchery.

The randomized placebo-controlled studies are less prone to manipulation; however patients and scientists often know in an open-label study who is getting placebo, and who is getting the drug, so the data can be "helped" along.

The best studies remain the randomized and placebo-controlled type with a double-blind feature. This means neither the researcher nor the patient knows who got placebo until the end of the study when the blind code is removed and the data analyzed.

Whenever the studies don't align with each other, that is when results are diametrically opposed, always suspect bias. If a big company heavily funds a scientist, that could explain a contrary result, especially if the study was retrospective.

Start with S.A.M.

Once you have your team assembled, the first step is to start with a repurposed drug cocktail that carries the highest upside and the lowest risk. As we saw earlier, Dr. Mark Moyad's S.A.M. cocktail, made up of commonly prescribed medications: aspirin, metformin, and a statin may be a good place to start for any patient. For the statin, I prefer atorvastatin, but lovastatin and simvastatin also work well. Typical doses of atorvastatin are 10 to 40 mg per day. Higher doses can elevate liver function tests, but these are usually less than 2x normal (SGOT, SGPT) and considered an acceptable risk.

Even those who don't have a cancer diagnosis should consider this cocktail if they are at increased cancer risk. If one has a history of smoking, insulin resistance, or viral infection, they are at increased risk. Hydrophilic statins do not protect against cancer as well, so I would not recommend rosuvastatin, fluvastatin, or pravastatin. Metformin protects in a dose-dependent manner. The higher the dose, and the longer once takes it, the greater the cancer preventive effect. The lowest dose might be 250 mg per day, while the highest is 2000 mg per day. There is a 31% reduction in cancer risk with metformin use.[66] In the event cancer develops, there is up to a 35% reduction in the chance of death.[63, 64] Either way, it can benefit you.

Attacking the Roots of Your Cancer

Aside from prevention, the best time to begin the addition of repurposed drugs is just after your cancer diagnosis, and the sooner, the better.

Why?

Recall the standard of cancer care targets only the bulk of your tumor, the fast-dividing cells. These are the equivalent of the branches and tree trunk. Most people understand cancer cells multiply rapidly and hoard sugar and other nutrients. Like a parasite, cancer starves the host.

Surgery, chemotherapy, and radiation all attempt to kill or remove most of the tumor. This causes our other fast-dividing cells also to get poisoned: usually the hair, lining of the GI tract, and bone marrow. It is these effects that typically cause loss of hair and nails, nausea/vomiting and diarrhea. Unfortunately, it can suppress the bone marrow leading to deficiencies of red and white blood cells as well as platelets. This can produce anemia and a loss of blood clotting; but worse, it can cause immune suppression, making one vulnerable to infections.

The slow-growing cells are spared. We do not usually see problems with the heart, brain, or muscle tissue, as these are all slowly dividing cells. Unfortunately, the cancer stem cells (CSC) are entirely different than the bulk of the tumor. The CSC colony is slow-growing and resembles normal cells in many respects. This is known as tumor heterogeneity, with fast-dividing cancer cells being one population and the CSCs being another.

Like normal cells, the chemotherapy misses the CSC. Tragically, both chemotherapy and radiation treatment have a stimulating effect on the CSC population, causing them to grow resistant new tumor cells and replace the bulk of what was removed. It is similar to the effect of pruning a tree, stimulating new growth.

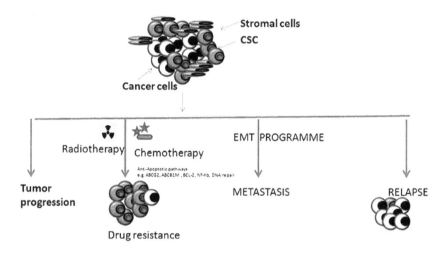

Courtesy of Singh et al. *Front Mol Biosci.* 2017
Figure 4. Radiation and Chemotherapy Create Resistance though CSC Stimulation

Adding repurposed drugs to attack the CSC should be a priority and should be done at the time of chemotherapy and radiation therapy. None of this is done in standard chemotherapy protocols across the country at major medical centers today. Doing nothing to the CSC after stimulating them is irresponsible, in my opinion. We are doing harm with the current standard of care cancer treatment unless we address the cancer stem cells simultaneously.

It would be so simple for doctors to remedy this. Merely add S.A.M. to all cancer patients' medications, taking into account the patients' clinical circumstances.

Common repurposed drugs that can attack cancer stem cells include aspirin, doxycycline, chloroquine, metformin, as well as lipophilic statins like atorvastatin. Additionally, some supplements like berberine, quercetin, melatonin, vitamin D3, nanocurcumin, omega III oils, flaxseed, and extra virgin olive oil have anti-CSC properties.

Dr. Ben Williams added melatonin from the start of his glioblastoma treatment. Dr. Angela Chapman also added chloroquine to her trastuzumab chemotherapy regimen. The was due to the study she found on Google Scholar, "The antimalarial chloroquine overcomes primary resistance to trastuzumab in HER2 positive breast cancer," authored by Dr. Silvia Cufi and colleagues.[163] Adding chloroquine to tumors that were completely resistant to trastuzumab reversed this almost entirely. The addition of chloroquine caused 90% tumor growth suppression when used in combination with trastuzumab.

It was no coincidence that Dr. Chapman beat the odds and survived her tumor. In addition to chloroquine, she noticed the study by Dr. Jixia and colleagues that further added quercetin to block resistance to trastuzumab.[164] She added flaxseed oil to boost the effectiveness of trastuzumab.

By itself, flaxseed oil had no effect on the CSC, but when combined with trastuzumab, it substantially slowed tumor cell division and increased tumor cell death (apoptosis).[165] Dr. Chapman also added melatonin and vitamin D3 which a study revealed could produce complete tumor growth arrest when combined with standard treatment.[166]

Other substances that target CSCs were similarly added: pterostilbene, Omega III oil, flaxseed oil, nanocucurmin, and resveratrol.[166, 168] Do not expect your oncologist to agree with any of this, especially if he works at a major cancer center. Cancer stem cell research is in its infancy, and there are currently no standard treatments to block the effects of this population.

The large and established research centers in the US are currently heavily backed by pharmaceutical interests that fund studies of drugs that attack the fast-growing bulk of the tumor. Physicians have their hearts in the right place but make no mistake, cancer treatment remains big business, and those interests with the most monetary stake do not want repurposed drugs added.

No repurposed drugs to get to the root of your cancer will be added because it takes time to change protocols and thinking, and it will take time for major centers to complete Phase II and Phase III clinical trials on anticancer stem cell treatments. If you want to target your cancer stem cells today, you are best off enlisting the help of your local general practitioner armed with the studies you have printed out from your Google Scholar or PubMed search.

Or simply show him or her this book and the supporting references.

If your GP refuses, follow Ben Williams' advice and find another doctor who will work with you. I do not advise getting the prescription without at least one physician's blessing, due to the potential for drug-to-drug interactions, and the need to factor in your particular medical circumstances. Dr. Ben Williams traveled to Mexico to procure Accutane to treat his glioblastoma. Other patients have taken their relative's prescriptions. Still others have formed social networks and traded their medications.

Obviously, I do not advise these approaches. If you produce a study of chloroquine's benefits against chemotherapy resistance to trastuzumab, a majority of general practitioners will write you the script. It is far easier to secure the supplements as these do not require a physician's order.

But what if you are clueless about supplements?

Get Dr. Mark Moyad's reference guide, *The Supplement Handbook*.[169] It is an excellent starting point for supplement information. Dr. Moyad is arguably the foremost medical authority on supplements in the United States. He is an MD, MPH, and professor at the University of Michigan Medical Center.

Resveratrol, quercetin, flaxseed oil, Omega III oil, nanocurcumin, and melatonin should be a part of most patients' cocktails. Metformin blocks so many stem cell pathways that it is almost always included. It also helps block oxidative phosphorylation IGF, mTOR, and fatty acid synthesis.

Just as the Cancer Care Oncology Clinics selected doxycycline, atorvastatin, and mebendazole to target glioblastoma stem cells, these three agents also have powerful antitumor effects against many types of cancer stem cells and very little toxicity. Ask your general practitioner about adding them. However, if you have an unusually aggressive terminal cancer like pancreatic or glioblastoma, you may want a more aggressive cocktail, one with more medicines that blocks even more pathways.

The C3M3 NSAID2 Pulse Cocktail

While S.A.M. is a reasonable starting point, I am often asked what is a good cocktail to help block as many tumor pathways as possible after a person has developed cancer. An ideal cocktail would do four things:

#1 Impair tumor metabolism or use of fuel. An ideal anti-metabolic cocktail will plug the tumor's automobile engine. A good starting point might be Jane McLelland's S.A.D. cocktail comprised of statin, aspirin, and dipyridamole.

   a. Block Warburg metabolism (cancer's preferred path) aka Aerobic Glycolysis

- Metformin

- Overnight Fasting (TRE) 16 hours

- Low glycemic diet

   b. Block Reverse Warburg Compensation (burning lactate) aka Oxidative Phosphorylation [OXPHOS]

- Metformin

- Doxycycline

- Berberine

- Niclosamide

- N-acetylcysteine [NAC]. This preferentially targets cell with abnormal glycolysis.

   c.   Block Autophagy

- Chloroquine

- Loratadine aka Claritin

#2 Impair tumor blood vessel formation, the building of highways.

   a.   Block VEGF and PDGF

- Statin

- Aspirin

- Dipyridamole

- Mebendazole

- Doxycycline

- Itraconazole

- Propranolol

- Curcumin

- Resveratrol

   b.   Block TAM and MMP

- Mebendazole

- Propranolol

- Dipyridamole
- Doxycycline

c. Block TAF and HIF

- Berberine
- Quercetin
- Luteolin
- Genistein
- Resveratrol

#3 Impair CSC, the root of cancer.

a. Block signaling (i.e., Hedgehog, WnT, and NOTCH) Hedgehog

- Curcumin
- Sulforaphane
- Metformin
- Cyclopamine
- Quercetin
- Mebendazole

WnT

- Metformin
- Niclosamide
- Statins (Lipitor)

- Aspirin
- NSAIDS (Celebrex, Ibuprofen)
- Ivermectin

NOTCH

- Curcumin
- Sulforaphane
- Metformin
- Quercetin
- Niclosamide
- Resveratrol
- Luteolin

b. Block TGF-beta

- NSAIDS
- Dipyridamole
- Aspirin
- Losartan
- Polyphenols (Green Tea, Coffee)

#4 Reduce Metastatic Spread.

a. Block EMT

- Agents that jam NOTCH, WnT, Hedgehog, and TGF-beta

- Agents that reduce Angiogenesis, MMP, VEGF, TAF, and TAM

- Agents that attack CSC

b. Reduce Insulin (Improve Insulin Sensitivity)

- Metformin

- Berberine

- Fasting (TRE)

- Chromium picolinate

- Post-meal muscle exercise

- Low-glycemic diet

c. Lower IGF and mTOR

- Metformin

- Plant-based diet

- Quercetin

- Curcumin

- EGCG

- Fasting (TRE)

- Resveratrol

- Cruciferous vegetables

The C_3M_3 pulse NSAID2 pulse Chloroquine/ Hydroxychloroquine Cocktail is a logical option that combines several cocktails into one. The acronym is an easy way to remember them.

C_1= Cimetidine

C_2= Curcumin

C3 = Chromium Picolinate

M1= Metformin

M2= Mebendazole

M3= Melatonin

N= Niclosamide

S= Statin (lipophilic)

A=Aspirin

I= Itraconazole

D=Dipyridamole and Doxycycline

C3M3 pulse NSAID2 represents a twelve-drug cocktail that is inspired by Jane Williams' S.A.D. with Dr. Mark Moyad's S.A.M. and Ben Williams' Melatonin with Dr. Angela Chapman's Chloroquine/Hydroxychloroquine.

Dr. Richard Gerber, Jane McLelland, and the ReDO project scientists note that Chloroquine blocks autophagy and induces apoptosis. The problem is that it is toxic and can only be used for short periods at crucial times during the treatment, especially during chemotherapy and radiation. HCQ is less toxic and preferred; however, it can still induce retinopathy, so regular eye exams are advised.

Similarly, I do not recommend long-term daily use of any NSAID. They carry some risk of toxicity to the kidney, heart, and GI tract. Therefore, they should be pulsed only during strategic times, for example, when one is going for apoptosis.

Finally, there are some known potential drug interactions and cautions. Cimetidine can interact with metformin to reduce kidney function. Chloroquine and Itraconazole both can lengthen the QT interval. Thus, caution and perhaps a baseline EKG and kidney function testing is advised as well as the usual recommendation of considering this advanced cocktail only with your doctor's supervision, prescription, and monitoring.

The basic terminal cancer treatment repurposed drug cocktail (in addition to and not instead of standard of care) remains the COC four drug regimen comprising metformin, mebendazole, atorvastatin, and doxycycline. This twelve-to-fourteen drug cocktail represents an advanced cocktail that blocks more pathways.

Keep in mind that the basic 12 drugs may be pulsed with the NSAID, usually Celebrex 200 mg/day and HCQ, usually 200 mg twice per day. This pulse can assist in promoting apoptosis, at strategic times. Pulsing the NSAIDs and hydroxychloroquine might be especially useful during chemotherapy and radiation when the CSC and EMT are maximally stimulated.

Chloroquine use is discouraged due to toxicity. In general, HCQ has similar biological action, and is less toxic. With that said, there is some evidence that in GBM, chloroquine may produce better results than HCQ.

The toxicities and drug interactions may vary depending upon the liver, kidney, and immune function of each individual patient. The drug interactions may vary due to other medications a patient may be taking. Subtracting chloroquine and hydroxychloroquine, most healthy patients should tolerate the basic 12 drugs well, as they are generally considered nontoxic and far safer than conventional chemotherapy. Nonetheless, it bears repeating that I do not advise anyone to take these cocktails without close medical supervision.

The baby aspirin might be especially useful just before and after surgery to block inflammation. Cimetidine will be especially helpful during times of immune suppression as it can improve T-cell ratios.

Always monitor your biomarkers during times of remission, and if they rise, consider a 7-day pulse of NSAID and Hydroxychloroquine. You want to know early if the tumor starts to recur to provide an opportunity to adjust your cocktail. Typical biomarkers would include AFP, CEA, HCG, PSA, CA-125, CA 15-3,

CA 19-9, CA 27.29, and other general tumor markers. PET scans are also highly sensitive to the recurrence. In the UK, Jane's physicians measured other markers as well, Tumor Marker 2 Pyruvate Kinase and Matrix Metallo Proteinase-2.

It is worth noting DCA (dichloroacetate). It promotes apoptosis and impairs Warburg and Reverse Warburg tumor fuel burning.[170] Disulfiram, or Antabuse is an option, but obviously carries toxicity and violent reactions if you drink any alcohol, even cough syrup, with it. Feel free to consider the addition of any of the HAMPT or EIS combinations.

If you wish to focus on blocking metastasis, then consider adding the lysine and mifepristone. Also, consider adding quetiapine, pirfenidone, or rifampin.

Finally, do not discount the value of oxidative strategies to essentially "burn" the tumor. This means killing the cancer or provoking apoptosis. Jane and Linus Pauling, Nobel Laureate, swear by high-dose vitamin C. For it to be an effective pro-oxidant, not an anti-oxidant, it may require IV administration.[171] Your goal is not to be scientifically perfect and to wait for the latest double-blind and placebo-controlled study evidence. Your goal is to survive, as Ben Williams bluntly put it. So never be afraid to speak up to your doctors. Don't fear offending their sensibilities. Remember, they work to serve you, not the other way around.

Remember what virtually every long-term survivor has preached, "Attack the tumor from as many angles as possible." This may mean more supplements, more repurposed drugs, or more changes in diet, and always under your physician's careful supervision.

Block Warburg Metabolism

Most of the time, the tumor uses the Warburg effect to burn fuel like an SUV. Warburg processing is wasteful, as we saw in Chapter 6. This requires vast amounts of food, so you want to put yourself and the cancer on a strict diet.

But don't think cutting calories and carbs are going to do the entire job. The liver of an insulin-resistant person is constantly producing blood sugar through a process called gluconeogenesis. Gluconeogenesis in IR happens even if the person consumes a low-glycemic diet, even if they are on the ketogenic diet, and even if they are fasting. As I say in the *Coffee Cure Diet*, a person with insulin resistance can give up all carbs, but their stubborn and IR liver will continue to manufacture blood sugar all night long, even while they sleep.

This gluconeogenesis is just as problematic as eating carbs, so it must be addressed if you want to be successful.

GLUCONEOGENESIS TRAP

- Gluconeogenesis

- Occurs with Insulin Resistance
- Insulin Resistance

- Insulin Resistance

- Reverse Insulin Resistance

* Liver makes sugar even if you don't eat it
* Insulin resistance = Diabetes, Prediabetes
* Also seen in High Blood Pressure
* Also seen with TG/HDL ratios > 3.5
* Metformin, Muscle Exercise, Weight Loss

Metformin can help block this, and is a good reason for any insulin-resistant person to ask their doctor for a prescription. Overnight fasts, low-glycemic diets, and metformin can injure Warburg as can the supplements berberine and chromium picolinate. If a person has Type II diabetes, weight loss can cure the diabetic condition and can suppress cancer metabolism. Lowering blood sugar always helps. Muscle exercise with high reps and low resistance done with light bands after meals can facilitate blood sugar lowering through uptake in the muscle. Up to 70 to 75% of after-meal glucose can be absorbed by the skeletal muscles in this fashion. This lowers IGF, insulin levels, and mTOR.

I like to do two sets of twenty reps after meals. It can be done with elastic bands, small dumbbells, or even using your body weight. Jane preferred walking and doing isometric contractions. Many people do not understand the importance of muscle exercise in lowering insulin resistance. Walking alone may not help your muscle absorb the sugar, especially if you have pasta or potatoes. Whatever you do, avoid the combination of high carb and zero exercise.

If you cut calories, go low carb, and fast 16 hours each night, take metformin, and add muscle exercise, you will force the cancer to abandon Warburg metabolism and burn its lactate (that it has saved just for this purpose). The tumor will escape using Reverse Warburg. More on blocking this soon.

Protein Eating Tumors

A large minority of cancers use non-glucose pathways to create energy. They use other macronutrients such as proteins and ketones for fuel. Those that use protein for fuel include glioblastoma, breast cancer, pancreatic cancer, lung cancer, prostate cancer, and lymphoma. This process is turned glutaminolysis.

If you think the cancer will be starved if you give up protein, be assured, it is smarter than that. The tumor can always find protein sources within your muscle. Just as the tumor can rewire if you deprive it of sugar, it can do the same with protein deprivation. With protein consuming tumors, not only must you go easy on your meat consumption, you may need to add drugs.

Substances that inhibit glutaminolysis include resveratrol and curcumin, as well as BPTES and L-asparaginase.[172] Asparagine-rich food consumption has been correlated with increased metastasis in glutamate using tumors. So, avoid poultry as well as beef.

PROTEIN DRIVEN TUMORS

- Glioblastoma
- Pancreatic cancer
- Prostate cancer

* Breast cancer
* Lung cancer
* Lymphoma

Tumors that are starved of both glucose and protein do not automatically die. Let me apologize in advance to the keto diet followers. These tumors can rewire and learn how to burn fat.[173, 174] They can learn to eat ketones. Anything you can do, the cancer can usually do better.

Fat Eating Tumors

Of course, eating saturated fat, especially more than 37% of your calories, can produce both inflammation and insulin resistance. A ketone metabolizing tumor will be in hog heaven if you are on a ketogenic high fat diet. Fat is loaded with calories. On a high saturated fat diet, cancer will have both the calories and inflammation to fuel its growth and spread.

Fat driven cancers include prostate, breast, TNBC, melanoma, and glioblastoma.

FAT DRIVEN CANCERS

- Prostate
- TNBC

* Melanoma
* GBM

The solution is not to consume more than 10% of dietary saturated fat. Instead, consume more unsaturated fat, but still less than 37% of your daily calories. You will want your fat to be mainly unsaturated in the form of olive oil or fish oil. Mediterranean diet foods work best. You will also want to drug the tumor. Lipophilic statins like atorvastatin or rosuvastatin help block the fat oxidizing pathway. Doxycycline also slows fatty acid oxidation. There is even some evidence that mildronate can do this.

I would always consider the use of doxycycline as a CSC targeting fatty acid oxidation blocking agent to help block the metastatic spread through the EMT pathway.

If you have successfully blocked all three macronutrients: proteins, sugars, and fats from your tumor, and now you think you have it starved, then think again.

Reverse Warburg: Eating Lactate

This is a pathway the tumor can use to survive even if you deprive it of all protein, glucose, fat. The tumor has apparently wasted energy by using the inefficient Warburg process for burning fuel.

But this has produces piles of waste in the form of lactate. Only now do you realize the tumor was actually preparing for this moment, when it will use this lactate, and burn it through conventional oxidative phosphorylation (OXPHOS).

The tumor will rewire itself and burn its own waste, the lactate, the so-called reverse Warburg effect. Fortunately, you have the tool of metformin, which can throw a wrench into this. Metformin blocks complex one and also inhibits hexokinase. It helps block both Warburg AND reverse Warburg compensation. Other drugs, including dichloroacetate (DCA) and 2 deoxy-d-glucose can do this, but it is at the expense of many adverse effects, not the least of which is neuropathy. For most people, Metformin and overnight fasting work very well to block reverse Warburg without getting into trouble.

Jane McLelland found that IV Vitamin C infusions helped block G6PDH. Niclosamide can also block the tumor escape to reverse Warburg metabolism.

The Tree and the Root: Resistance to Treatment

In general, standard cancer care treatment debulks the fast-growing cells only with cytotoxic agents. This involves chemotherapy at the highest doses a person can stand while stopping just short of killing the patient. Sometimes the treatment cuts it too close. While not outright killing the patient, the poisoning of the immune system facilitates the patient dying from bleeding (low platelets) or infection (low neutrophils).

I would strongly suggest talking to your oncology treatment team about dosing your chemotherapy metronomically. This means you take lower doses at more frequent intervals to avoid killing you either fast or slowly.[175]

Secondly, the chemotherapy and radiation treatments are now triggering the Hh, NOTCH, and WnT. The calls for help notify the cancer stem cells that their tumor bulk is under attack. The CSCs will immediately go into fight or flight mode, deploying EMT and metastatic microscopic spread as well as rewiring to become resistant and immortal. Now is not the time to rest, recuperate, and nourish yourself because the CSCs are also doing the same thing, only better. It is also the exact right time to add your repurposed drug cocktail as if your life depended upon it because it does. 90% of cancer deaths are caused by metastatic spread, that is, Stage III and Stage IV advanced cancers. If it were me, I would employ a repurposed drug cocktail affecting every possible pathway in addition to the diet and lifestyle changes and in addition to the standard of care of chemotherapy, surgery, and radiation, albeit metronomically accomplished.

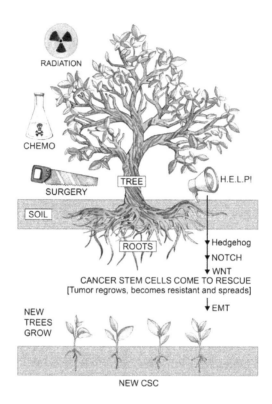

Chemotherapy, Radiation and Surgery all
Stimulate Cancer Stem Cells
Figure 5. The Cancer Tree and the Roots (CSC).

The least toxic, basic cocktail, are the four drugs employed in the METRICS trial by Care Oncology Clinic to treat GBM: doxycycline, mebendazole, atorvastatin, and metformin.[6] This is termed the COC Cocktail.   It contains my two superstars: metformin and mebendazole.

The trio, mebendazole, doxycycline, and metformin together can greatly suppress CSC activity. I might also add supplements. Dr. Kofron and Dr. Chapman already did the research. Start with turkey tail mushroom, which contains polysaccharide K (PSK) and add nanocurcumin. Curcumin is the metformin of the supplement world and blocks multiple cancer pathways. Curcumin's problem is that much of it either does not get absorbed or is chemically altered in the intestinal tract, before it gets to the right tissue. Dr. Kofron felt that nanocurcumin was better than the regular variety.

Allow me to warn you that most common Curcumin preparations will not produce measurable plasma levels. I know of at least one that will. Longvida is a solid lipid curcumin particle and patented formula.[176] It is available online at a reasonable cost. 1000 mg twice daily has produced measurable free plasma levels with good patient toleration. For full disclosure, I have no interest or connection with this company or product.

As always, choose your repurposed medications and supplements with your physician's input and guidance.

Blocking Metastasis

Numerous repurposed drugs can block metastasis. Melatonin worked for Dr. Ben Williams, and melatonin helps block EMT and metastasis. So does aspirin, which I would recommend only if you have no bleeding tendencies and your doctor permits. Throw in Vitamin D3 for good measure as it can help resensitize chemotherapy. Also, remember that chloroquine, when combined with chemotherapy, can resensitize the tumor by blocking autophagy and CSC.

Consider adding it with your doctor's approval and prescription, realizing it is more toxic. Hydroxychloroquine works almost as well and is far less toxic, but it can still cause retinopathy.

My grandmother took Persantine, otherwise known as dipyridamole, for her heart to prevent blood clots. It's considered nontoxic and Jane McLelland swears by it. Itraconazole is an antifungal and is considered nontoxic. It also blocks CSCs. Why not include both?

Autophagy: Cancer's Last Stand

When the tumor has no other recourse because you have used your overnight fasting, vegetarian diet, muscle exercise, statins, metformin, and doxycycline, it does what any smart tumor would when faced with no food. It cannibalizes its dead brethren in a process called autophagy. It ingests various cell parts, including nucleic acid debris using lysosomes in a process called macropinocytosis. The cancer can go on for weeks like this, effectively eating its dead unless you drug it.

AUTOPHAGY DRIVEN TUMORS

- GBM
- Melanoma
- Colon cancer
- Lung cancers
- Prostate

* Pancreatic cancer
* Bladder cancer
* Leukemia
* Ovarian
* Renal

RAS mutation-driven cancers like GBM, pancreatic cancer, melanoma, bladder cancer, colon cancer, leukemia, and lung cancers use this pathway. Chloroquine helps block autophagy and macropinocytosis.[177] So does loratadine.[178] Because loratadine does not cross the blood-brain barrier, chloroquine is a better choice in GBM. There is some evidence that curcumin can reverse autophagy produced by treatment with 5-FU in colon cancer.[179]

Both the tumor and chemotherapy will suppress your immune function. Cimetidine helps reverse this.[180] Cimetidine is ideal for targeting various tumor growth pathways. The more pathways you block (i.e., signaling, growth factors, angiogenesis, metalloproteinases, inflammation, metabolism), the greater the chances of success.

The ReDO Project's Suggested Drugs for Cocktails

Some of the drugs mentioned above have already been studied extensively by the ReDO Project. Their results have shown great promise. Consider some of the following if you have one of the cancers they can fight effectively.

Cimetidine

The first drug studied by the Repurposed Drug in Oncology Project was Cimetidine, the antacid discussed above.[181] It is usually used for treatment of ulcers, reflux esophagitis, or GERD. A typical dose is 400 mg four times a day for one to two months. Some individuals have taken it for ten years with no ill effects.

A Japanese study looked at 64 patients diagnosed with advanced colon cancer and treated with chemotherapy, radiation therapy, and immune therapy. All had surgery with full removal of their tumors. All received chemotherapy with 5-FU for one year. The treatment group which numbered 34 received Cimetidine 800 mg a day for one year in addition to the standard treatment.[182]

At the ten-year follow-up, the survival in the Cimetidine group was 84.6%, whereas that of the control group (non-Cimetidine) was only 49.8%. Cimetidine improved ten-year survival in this study by 70%.

An analysis of five other clinical trials found similar results. The authors concluded, "Cimetidine appears to confer a survival benefit when given as an adjunct to curative surgical resection of colorectal cancers."

Cimetidine can also be used to treat melanoma. One study looked at 1,000 mg per day of Cimetidine in melanoma patients no longer responding to Coumarin treatment. There was rapid regression of the multiple tumors and long-lasting physical improvement. In another study of five cases treated with interferon with failed results, Cimetidine's addition for six to eight weeks led to remarkable improvement. There was complete remission in two cases, partial remission in another case, and stabilization is still another.[181]

Other studies suggested no improvement or mixed results, especially when Cimetidine was used by itself or what is termed monotherapy. That is expected as repurposed drugs work best as part of a multi-drug cocktail in addition to standard chemotherapy. They are not expected to have substantial benefits when used alone.

A double-blinded, placebo-controlled, randomized gold standard study from Denmark followed 181 patients with gastric cancer treated with surgery.[183] The median survival in the Cimetidine group was 450 days compared to the non-Cimetidine group of 316 days.

Cimetidine helps block cell adhesion. It also can help reduce histamine stimulated BEGF. It works through the cycle oxygenase pathway (COX-II). It shows effectiveness against various colon, melanoma, gastric, renal cell, prostate, pancreatic cancers, and GBM, lung, and ovarian cancers.

It also is beneficial if Cimetidine is used before surgery as surgery can facilitate tumor spread through immune pathways. Preoperative and postoperative Cimetidine helped block this.

The Repurposed Drug in Oncology Project suggested many different cocktails that include Cimetidine (CIM), as listed below:[181]

Malignant Melanoma:	Suggested repurposed cocktail:
[Targets: microtubule disruption, inhibition of autophagy, anti-angiogenesis, and immune modulation.]	Cimetidine (CIM) +
	Diclofenac or celecoxib + cyclophosphamide + hydroxychloroquine + mebendazole.

NSCLC:

[Targets: AMPK, mTOR, Hh, signaling, COX-II inhibition, and immunomodulation.]

Suggested cocktail:

CIM + metformin + itraconazole + Diclofenac or celecoxib.

GBM:

[Targets: Inhibition of autophagy, microtubule disruption, Hh signaling inhibition, anti-angiogenesis, immune modulation.]

Suggested cocktail:

CIM +

hydroxychloroquine + itraconazole + mebendazole.

Colorectal Carcinoma:

[Targets: Microtubule disruption, AMPK, mTOR, inhibition, immune modulation, COX-II, antihistamine.]

Suggested cocktail:

CIM + metformin + doxycycline or vinorelbine + mebendazole + aspirin.

Osteosarcoma:
  [Targets: AMPK, mTOR, IGF1, Hh pathway inhibition, tumor vascularization, anti-angiogenesis, immune modulation.]

Suggested cocktail:

CIM +

metformin +
itraconazole +
oral cyclophosphamide.

Breast Cancer (ER plus invasive ductal carcinoma):
  [Targets: Microtubule disruption, AMPK, mTOR, anti-angiogenesis, immune modulation.]

Suggested cocktail:

CIM +
metformin +
cyclophosphamide or
vinorelbine +
aspirin.

Ovarian Cancer:
  [Targets: Microtubule disruption, AMPK, mTOR, Hh, COX-II, immune modulation.]

Suggested cocktail:

CIM +
metformin +
itraconazole +
diclofenac +
mebendazole.

Renal Cell Carcinoma:
  [Targets: Anti-angiogenesis, COX-II, tumor vascularity, Hh inhibition, immune modulation.]

Suggested cocktail:

CIM +
celecoxib +
Losartan +
Itraconazole.

Pancreatic Cancer:
  [Targets: Microtubule
  disruption, Hh pathway,
  anti-angiogenesis, immune
  modulation.]

Suggested cocktail:

CIM +
oral cyclophosphamide +
diclofenac +
mebendazole +
itraconazole.

Gastric Carcinoma:
  [Targets: COX-II,
  anti-angiogenesis, immune
  modulation.]

Suggested cocktail:

CIM +
celecoxib +
itraconazole.

Propranolol

The next drug studied by the ReDO Project was propranolol.[184] Propranolol is a medicine commonly used to treat blood pressure. It also has multiple antitumor effects. It's anti-proliferative, anti-angiogenic, anti-apoptotic, and helps in immune modulation. It has potent anti-metastatic effects in breast cancer as an adjuvant.

Retrospective studies show improved recurrence-free survival in those with TNBC. Improved progression-free survival in eight HER2 negative breast cancer cases is seen. There is some evidence that adding propranolol can reverse resistance to trastuzumab (monoclonal antibody Trastuzumab) in HER2+ breast cancer.

Choy showed in a retrospective study that Stage II breast cancer patients using propranolol had one-half the metastasis rate.[185] In mice experiments, propranolol significantly reduced the number of brain metastasis.

Chloroquine/Hydroxychloroquine

The third drug examined by the ReDO Project was a pair of antimalarials: chloroquine and hydroxychloroquine.[186] These antimalarial drugs affect pathways, including toll-like receptor-9, P53, and CXCR4-CXCL, all major pathways in cancer. They affect tumor blood vessels, cancer-associated fibroblasts (CAF), and the immune system.

Hydroxychloroquine has almost the same biological effects as chloroquine but is far less toxic. It is frequently used in its brand form Plaquenil, abbreviated HCQ. For HCQ, the standard dosage range is between 200 and 400 mg per day.

Toxicity is a consideration, even with HCQ. Toxicity includes retinopathy in doses over 1,000 mg per day. 250-400 mg of HCQ per day for several years is considered within the acceptable risk range. However, it is advisable to have a patient get an ophthalmological exam every three to six months while on the drug as well as blood counts and glucose checks. Keep in mind these toxicities are far less than those of standard chemotherapies. HCQ is often combined with standard chemotherapy, including tyrosine kinase inhibitors, monoclonal antibodies, hormones, and radiation.

A prospective and randomized 1998 study looked at 18 GBM patients. Nine patients received chemotherapy, surgery, radiation plus chloroquine (CQ) at 150 mg a day while nine received chemotherapy, radiation, and surgery without chloroquine. The CQ group's average survival was 33 months, while the non-CQ group's was only 11 months.[187]

The survival almost tripled with the addition of the antimalarial. However, there were slightly more seizures in the chloroquine group. However, these were easily controlled with standard anti-epileptic agents.

A second study by the same research team was even more impressive. They used a randomized, placebo-controlled and double-blind protocol. This involved 15 GBM patients taking 150 mg of CQ each day for 12 months. Because the study used the gold standard protocol, i.e., it was randomized, double-blinded, and placebo-controlled, the results were significant. The median survival time in the CQ group was 24 months, double the survival time in the non-CQ group of only 12 months.[188]

Despite the small number of patients in each study, these data left little doubt about the effectiveness of chloroquine in glioblastoma.

Another case study involved a pediatric patient. This patient had a recurrent BRAFV 600 E mutant brain stem ganglioglioma. The patient lost sensitivity to the chemotherapy vemurafenib. However, once CQ was started, the patient once again became sensitive to 30 more months, an excellent result.[189]

In eight patients with refractory multiple myeloma, 500 mg of CQ was given daily for two-week sessions. This was done in addition to cyclophosphamide and bortezomib. Three in the CQ group experienced partial restoration of bortezomib sensitivity. Another three had a partial response, and one had stable disease while four had progression.[190]

Thirty-five pancreatic cancer patients were given HCQ 1,200 mg per day plus gemcitabine before surgery. There were promising drops in the biomarker C19-9. There was significantly improved disease-free survival only in the eight patients where autophagy was suppressed with the CQ (as defined by at least a 51% increase in the autophagy marker LC3B-II measured in peripheral blood mononuclear cells).[191]

The greatest antitumor effect of both HCQ and CQ is inhibition of autophagy. However, these antimalarials also help interfere with TLR-9 and NFkB signaling, as well as CXCL and CXCR and P53 pathways. Toll-like receptor nine and NFkB both enhance the matrix metalloproteinases MMP2 and MMP7 as well as cyclo-oxygenase.

In pancreatic cancer patients with CSC-derived xenograft, CQ successfully targeted highly aggressive CSCs. This suggested that

CQ could be used in combination with gemcitabine to eradicate tumors.

CQ has been shown to help block glutaminolysis by affecting glutamate dehydrogenase. It was felt there would be a synergistic effect between metformin and CQ. Both CQ and HCQ can activate Caspase-3 and modulate Bc1-2/Bax ratios, including apoptosis in CLL and glioblastoma.

CQ can also target CSC by downregulating the Hh signaling pathway.

CQ can inhibit hypoxia stimulated metastasis by modulating HIF1 alpha, VEGF, and EMT. CQ can also inhibit CAF acting tumors that preferentially use autophagy like STAT3, Akt, and MYC mutants that use autophagy and are more likely to respond to HQ and HCQ.

The one issue is that HCQ has been shown in some cases to promote tumor growth in RAS driven pancreatic cancers developing without P53 (KRAS$^{G12D/+}_{p53-/-}$).[192, 193]

The ReDO author's report states:

"CQ and HCQ have been studied in multiple preclinical cancer models and have demonstrated activity on several cancer supporting pathways and in combination in a broad range of others. Our review has highlighted the multi-faceted action of CQ and HCQ against cancers making these drugs attractive for these complex cases."

The authors drew attention to following for side effects:

"Although the side effects of CQ and HCQ are minor in comparison with conventional chemotherapy, the possibility of retinal toxicity...requires ongoing monitoring."

Nitroglycerine

The next drug the ReDo Project studied was nitroglycerine.[194] Nitroglycerine is a drug commonly used for more than a century to control angina, chest pain due to heart disease. It improved cardiac oxygenation via multiple mechanisms, including vasodilation, decreased platelet aggregation, increased erythrocyte O2 release, and decreased mitochondrial utilization of oxygen.

It can reduce HIF-1 alpha levels, and this may have anti-angiogenic, pro-apoptotic, and anti-efflux effects. It has low toxicity, but must be used with caution if combined with PPDE-5 inhibitors, commonly used for erectile dysfunction such as sildenafil, vardenafil, and tadalafil. It can be used in pill or patch form.

A randomized controlled phase II trial of NTG in combination with Vinorelbine and Cis-platinum looked at 120 patients with Stage III-b, Stage IV inoperable non-small cell lung cancer (NSCLC). The NTG patch group's response was 72% compared to 43% for the placebo group. Median survival was 413 days in the NTG group and only 289 days in the placebo group.[195]

Tumor progression was 327 days for the NTG group, but only 185 days for the placebo. A subsequent study showed a 59% NTG response compared to 24-36% in similar controlled populations.[196] Treatment with NTG resulted in lower plasma VEGF levels. Other trials showed no response to NTG with NSCLC (the Australian NITRO study).

A prospective open-label trial looked at 29 men after surgery and radiation using the NTG patch. The biomarker PSA was followed to determine doubling time (PSADT). Only three out of 29 taking the NTG had the disease by the end of the 24 months. The extrapolated PSADT in the NTG group was 31.8 months compared to a matched non-NTG control group of 12.8 months. The NTG clearly slowed the tumor biomarker PSA's doubling time.[197]

Itraconazole

The next drug studied by the ReDO group was itraconazole (ITZ).[198] This is a common, nontoxic, antifungal agent in use for decades. In standard doses, it can inhibit Hh signaling and may induce autophagic growth arrest. It is usually taken orally in 100-200 mg capsules. It has common mild side effects with nausea, rashes, and pain. Rare significant effects include liver failure, heart failure, and neutropenia.

A retrospective study looked at 23 patients with ALL (acute lymphoblastic leukemia), 11 received ITZ. Disease-free survival tended to be longer in the ITZ group, but the remission rate was similar.[199] In castration-resistant prostate cancer, 29 patients were tested with low dose ITZ at 200 mg per day. This was compared with the high dose arm of ITZ at 600 mg per day. Progression-free survival was 48% at 24 weeks in the high dose ITZ group while only l1.8% in the low dose group.[200]

ITZ had positive effects on circulating tumor cell counts, and Hh signaling was reduced. Toxicity was greater in the high dose arm with the main effects being fatigue, nausea, anorexia, rash, hypertension, hypokalemia, and edema.

In a case report, there was a 65-year-old patient unwilling to undergo castration who had recurrent prostate cancer.[201] ITZ was given at 300 mg per day for 12 weeks. This caused a 50% reduction in PSA levels. The treatment was stopped due to elevated bilirubin (which returned to normal after treatment cessation). The PSA rose again after ITZ treatment was stopped.

In a study involving metastatic non-small cell lung carcinoma, 15 patients were randomized to ITZ plus chemo (Pemetrexed) and eight to chemo alone. Progressive-free survival (PFS) was 67% in the ITZ added group vs. 29% in the chemo alone group.[202] In a study of ovarian clear cell carcinoma, chemo plus ITZ was compared with chemo alone. There was a 44% response rate in PFS at 544 days and median survival of 1,047 days. The authors of the study felt that this was remarkable in a disease that rarely responds to chemotherapy.[203]

The 65% response in TNBC with recurrent disease looked at 13 patients, 12 of whom had metastasis to the lungs, liver, and brain.[204] All were treated with combinations of docetaxel carboplatin and gemcitabine with adjunctive ITZ 400 mg per day on a two-week cycle. The response rate was 65% median PFS was 10.8 months, and median total survival was 20.4 months with data on three patients censored. The authors of this study felt these results were encouraging compared to the typical response rates without ITZ.

Another case looked at a 64-year-old male with inoperable Stage III pancreatic adenocarcinoma.[205] He developed widespread histoplasmosis (bad fungus throughout this body) following his third cycle of gemcitabine. The fungus was treated with ITZ for nine months. His chemotherapy and all other cancer treatments were stopped during that time.

Inexplicably, his pancreatic tumor shrunk and became operable. He had it removed and remained in full remission for four more years. There was no sign of tumor recurrence or metastatic disease. Later he began reporting weight loss and developed a secondary tumor, NSCLC. The treating physicians felt the pancreatic tumor had responded to the antifungal ITZ.

ITZ inhibits endothelial cell proliferation (involved in angiogenesis). Since the Hh is a major stimulator of CSC, ITZ has become a major Hh and CSC inhibitor. The anti-Hh effects occur at very low ITZ doses, and it acts by the secondary smoothened pathway.

"The notion of blocking CSC as well as treating tumor bulk is gaining momentum," wrote the ReDO authors' team led by Dr. Pan Pantziarka. However, it has not yet become common knowledge among either the general public or the medical community.

The Remission Cocktail

If your initial battle with cancer is successful, chances are you will have undergone some form of chemotherapy in addition to the repurposed drug cocktails described above. Chemo takes a huge toll on the body, and you will likely be shell-shocked, battle-scarred, and exhausted. Now is the time to rest, strengthen your immune system, and regroup. Now is the time to enjoy your life and family, but absolutely not the time to drop your guard. You will want to continue most of your supplements, and the majority of your anti-stem cell repurposed drugs.

As we have emphasized, the chemotherapy and radiation will make your tumor scream, and the cancer stem cells will help it rewire, and this is likely if you do nothing. You will want to prevent this.

First, you will also want to pay attention to your diet. Contrary to traditional medical thinking, diet and exercise play a huge role in treatment success or failure. Avoid spikes of blood sugar as these also trigger spikes of cancer-promoting insulin and IGF. Low-glycemic diets work best at this point, and taking metformin will help protect you in the event you slip up on your eating habits.

Keep inflammation levels low by doing muscle exercises every day. In my book, *The Coffee Cure Diet*, I advise the "five and fly," a routine using stretch bands or light dumbbells to get blood into your muscles, which helps stabilize your blood sugar. Walking is great; however, many people recovering from the ravages of chemo prefer not to venture too far outside of the house.

The five and fly can be done in the privacy and comfort or your living room and in front of the television or computer. It is done after you wake up after your overnight fast and before your breakfast for maximum benefit. This will boost your immune system, and it will also increase your natural P53 tumor suppressor function. It will provide you a dose of anti-inflammatory myokines created by your muscles.

While recuperating, please do not make the common mistake of increasing sugar consumption. Fruit smoothies or juices, even containing blueberries, will help cancer stem cells more by spiking your blood sugar, insulin, and IGF levels and mTOR, the mammalian target of rapamycin. Instead, avoid sweets, juices, and fruit smoothies. They usually have high glycemic indexes.

An apple a day will not hurt you, but avoid more than one serving of fruit as stem cells love glucose and high glycemic fruits like watermelon, grapes, pineapples, pears, and nectarines. Instead, learn to love your cruciferous vegetables and green leafy salads. Add extra virgin olive oil liberally. Fish oil and Mediterranean diet foods heavy in nuts and fermented foods are ideal.

I would not overload on saturated fat or meat given the pro-inflammatory effects. I also would not overload on salt as these can trigger your renin-angiotensin system, which has been linked to cancer growth. Although dairy is controversial, and I swear by my Lacto-Mediterranean diet, I would avoid extra protein, including dairy, if you have a tumor that uses glutaminolysis or the breakdown of protein for fuel. If you are a keto diet fan, keep your total fat consumption below 37% of total daily calories in case your cancer adapts to ketones. In my experience, the less saturated fat you consume, the better. Don't be afraid to add a statin to block the tumor's use of fat, especially if you are a keto fan.

Dr. Moyad and I strongly believe in the cancer preventative effects of the S.A.M. cocktail. I think a strong case can be made that S.A.M. should be a part of most cancer patient's long-term remission drug cocktails. They suppress cancer stem cells and EMT, the epithelial-mesenchymal transformation (metastasis).

If you are at risk for GI bleeding, you may not want to include the aspirin, or you may want to take it with an antacid, like cimetidine. Baby aspirin is safer than full dose. As always, never add a prescription medication without your doctor's approval.

The beauty of metformin is that patients without diabetes can take it. It will generally not reduce blood sugar below normal, although it will seriously hamper the tumor's ability to metabolize glucose.

Patients can safely take lipophilic statins like atorvastatin without high levels of cholesterol. It will not harm them even with decades of use but will help block your tumor's ability to synthesize fat, cholesterol in cell membranes, and organelles. It will even help you if you eat too much saturated fat or cholesterol (by accident, of course).

Mebendazole is a repurposed drug with powerful activity against a dozen cancers, including brain, breast, pancreatic, lung, melanoma, and colorectal. Although I would not advise taking it for years, it could be easily part of both your chemotherapy repurposed drug cocktail and your early remission cocktail for three to six months. Chloroquine has a much higher level of toxicity, and its use should be limited to the duration of chemotherapy. Hydroxychloroquine is less toxic. Cimetidine has some overlap with chloroquine and can be continued indefinitely.

The more repurposed drugs we have on our side, the greater the chance we can survive cancer. Simply adding the best four or five repurposed drugs to target CSC and EMT, as well as supplements and lifestyle changes, can provide years of additional survival.

Chapter 9

THE COMING REVOLUTION IN CANCER CARE

Widespread use of repurposed drug cocktails, both for the prevention and treatment of cancer, is coming. Today's patient is better educated, more sophisticated, and more well informed than previous generations.

If the patient finds credible research showing a cocktail of nontoxic drugs will improve his survival, then his doctor should prescribe them. Pure and simple. What is the best advice going forward? In addition to cocktails, drugs, and supplements, the theme will be to lower toxicity. Chemotherapy will be done with the metronomic method, which is a lower dose at more frequent intervals.

Radiation therapy will be done more precisely and sparingly, especially to sensitive tissues like the brain. Tumor treating fields (TTF), the use of electrical fields to disrupt mitotic tumor cell division, effect fast-dividing cells, and spares slow dividing cells. Crucially, it is nontoxic. The FDA has already approved this technology as both a first and second-line treatment for glioblastoma, and so far, it has shown some survival benefits.[206]

Adenoviral vector therapies also show significant promise in the treatment of glioblastoma at this time. In theory, they have the advantage of targeting only cancer cells with low toxicity to healthy tissue.[207]

I was also intrigued by Dr. Duma's gamma knife treatment.[208] This technology has produced substantially increased survival in glioblastoma patients of up to 12% for five years, 7% for seven years, and 4% for ten years. The gamma knife takes advantage of the fact that the glioma grows along white matter pathways. Dr. Duma targets the area where the tumor is expected to grow and provides precise radiation beams to those white tracks. In other words, he does not radiate the tissue where the tumor exits at the current time, but where the tumor is expected to travel in the future.

We must recognize there are thousands of different types of gliomas based on different combinations of genes, gene mutations, and epigenetics. Using the TCGA or Cancer Care Genomics Atlas, some 15,000 tumors have been classified.[209] GBM has been divided into roughly five groups, based upon a study of four genes. However, there are many sub-types, including patients with methylated gliomas, which have better survival, patients with IDH1 mutations, which enjoy improved survival, and still other categories of gliomas, like EGFR mutations, with lower survival.

Incidentally, these can be identified based upon CSC markers like CD133, CD44, SOX2, Nestin (NES), and MYC. It is clear that CSC has a controlling role in GBM survival. Blocking the CSC with repurposed drug combinations is the key to long-term survival in GBM and other terminal cancers.

For my friend with glioblastoma multiforme, I recommended that he also use a combination approach. In addition to repurposed drugs through the Cancer Care Oncology Clinic and beyond the standard chemotherapy, radiation, and surgery, I strongly advised he add TTF and gamma knife with his doctors' knowledge and approval.

One-Size-Fits-All

The traditional oncology community still treats GBM with a one-size-fits-all approach. This approach, of course, involves surgery and chemotherapy, usually with TMZ and radiation. It almost always fails, as there is only a 3% five-year survival rate, which has not changed much in many decades. If you had GBM, would you accept this? I hope not.

I believe Stefan Roever's ingenious strategy of personalized cancer care holds the greatest potential for the future direction of cancer treatment by tailoring nontoxic repurposed drug cocktails to one's precise tumor genetics. Roever, a successful entrepreneur and

German lawyer, owns gene sequencing companies. He co-founded Genia Technologies, a company that makes rapid DNA sequencing systems which he sold to the Swiss giant, Roche, for some 350 million dollars.[210]

At approximately age 50, Stefan Roever was struck with GBM. Did he beat a path to the nearest University Hospital and submit to standard GBM care? If you had hundreds of millions of dollars and the latest genetic science at your fingertips, would you? Of course not.

Instead, he hired a team of physicians who could both select and prescribe for him repurposed drugs. He sequenced his own brain tumor's genetics by using his own company's technology. Then he went a step further. He developed a test of his body's tumor burden, the amount of circulating tumor DNA.

He would draw his blood every week or so, and at the same time, would meet by video conference with his treatment team of physicians. If his tumor blood markers remained undetectable, he would continue his drug cocktail and lifestyle changes. If, on the other hand, the tumor markers rose, reflecting increased tumor burden, he would make a change.

How does one then determine which drug to add or subtract if the tumor markers rise, or which drug to dial up or down? One does a sensitivity test, much like we currently conduct a blood or urine culture to decide on the best antibiotic. We test many drugs against the tumor's DNA to see which one is the most effective. This tells us which drugs the tumor is resistant to, which would not work, and which drugs the tumor cells respond to, the drugs that would benefit most.

Liquid Biopsy

Matt DeSilva, the Notable Labs founder, is developing blood tests that can help patients customize their treatment to determine which are the most active against their particular type of tumor cells.[211]

I spoke to him as his father had died of GBM some five years earlier. "With GBM, it is often difficult to obtain a tissue biopsy. You cannot always get tissue, especially if the tumor is inoperable. Blood testing is not invasive, and you can get largely the same DNA information from blood that you can from the traditional biopsy."

With traditional needle biopsy or surgery, the tumor can be spread. Indeed, liquid biopsy, or testing blood in cancer patients, is the wave of the future on many levels. It is helpful in both the prevention and monitoring of treatment progress.

CTC, which stands for circulating tumor cells, or CT DNA, which stands for circulating tumor DNA fragments, can often be found in lung cancer patients before the person shows any symptoms. It can be used as a screening test. As technology improves, it will become the standard of care, but currently, it is in its infancy.

Only about 20-30% of GBM patients will have circulating tumor cells in their bloodstream, not yet enough for widespread application. There may be only one single tumor circulating tumor cell in ten ccs of blood, a needle in a haystack, or one in a million. So refined analytical methods are needed.

Tumors also shed DNA fragments, which can be highly amplified using polymerase chain reaction (PCR) technology. PCR is often used in forensic cases to take small amounts of a criminals' DNA and amplify them so they can be tested. The same technology can be used to amplify microscopic or minute amounts of circulating tumor DNA.

This technique can improve sensitivity to the 80-90% range, which is where Notable Labs is now operating.

A person can get his tumor DNA genes sequenced without surgery using a standard blood test—a so-called liquid biopsy.

Personalized Cancer Care

One by one, a cocktail of drugs can be selected using sensitivity testing, and this can provide much better guidance than the trial and error approach used years ago by Dr. Ben Williams, Dr. Richard Gerber, and Jane McLelland. This is modernly called personalized cancer care.

Stefan Roever refers to it as "an engineering approach" to solving the problem. If your tumor markers remain low, you stay the course. If they start to rise, you change your cocktail, and you tweak it. Stefan is developing this technology with his new company, NAVIO, Navigating Individual Options in Oncology.

He explains it:

> "The fundamental conviction behind this model is to treat something as complicated as this (GBM), you need to do it through combination therapy... You actually have to hit it from as many different angles as possible. The problem is you don't know what it is that works. You don't know as your treating it if you are making progress or not."

With his company's technology, he gets this feedback:

> "We can see what the tumor burden is. It is a completely different approach to cancer treatment...Let's try something, see if it works; if it doesn't, let's tweak it...An average patient gets one or two shots with standard therapy, if you are lucky, you get a third with a clinical trial, and if you are really lucky, you get put on a second trial. In this model, you get ten or 20 shots where you can constantly tweak your approach...It is impossible to manage if you don't have the feedback (with the tumor burden custom biomarkers)."[212]

Stefan Roever says the custom biomarker testing is currently available only to "people of means." Eventually, the price will come down, and insurance may cover it. What is my advice to the average person? First, contact the Care Oncology Clinic to at least start on a basic cocktail of repurposed drugs. Or, work with your research and your GP in starting with your repurposed drug cocktail.

Finally, take advantage of currently available biomarkers. Now, physicians can draw up different blood tests to monitor the treatment course of different cancers: CA-19-9 for pancreatic cancer, CA15-3 for breast cancer, and CA-125 for ovarian cancer. PET scans are always a good option and are standard in monitoring for tumor recurrence. One can measure CEA carcinoembryonic antigen, LDH or lactic dehydrogenase, or PSA or prostatic surface antigen. I like to measure C-reactive protein (CRP) in all patients; it is a measure of total body inflammation.

If your markers rise, it means the tumor is gaining strength. Check your hemoglobin A1C, which will tell you your body's average blood sugar over the last 30 days—the lower, in general, the better. Lower levels of average blood sugar, in general, mean the tumor has less glycolytic fuel. You will want yours less than 5.7 or 5.8 to keep from stimulating your P13K mTOR pathway.

Dr. Bigelsen's Case

Dr. Bigelsen, a 55-year-old physician in New Jersey and in excellent health developed a stomach ache and jaundice. Tests revealed stage IV pancreatic cancer, the same type that claimed the lives of Michael Landon, Patrick Swayze, and Steve Jobs.

Knowing that the average survival was dismal, Dr. Bigelsen decided to be guided by science, yet use a better approach—personalized cancer care. He felt this would give him the best chances, and he was correct.

First, he partnered with an oncologist, Dr. Allyson Ocean of the Weill-Cornell Clinic, one who was willing to prescribe repurposed drugs in addition to standard of care. He underwent liquid biopsy testing of his cancer's unique genetic markers like Stefan Roever.

This data showed that Dr. Bigelsen's cancer would not have responded to standard treatment, and that a repurposed drug cocktail from the start would be a more effective strategy. Based upon the specific test results, Dr. Ocean designed an individualized cocktail of repurposed drugs including Hydroxychloroquine and paracalcitol, a form of synthetic intravenous vitamin D.

She also targeted the fast growing tumor bulk with the standard chemotherapies of gemcitabine and capecitabine. The oncologist also added the repurposed drug, mitomycin, which is not normally utilized as first-line treatment.

Dr. Bigelsen responded with a 98% reduction in the biomarker CA 19-9 and a disappearance of his metastases previously visible on CT scans. He is alive, well, and practicing medicine four years later.[324]

Quincy's Case

Personalized cancer care means customizing your treatment according to your cancer's specific genetics and avoiding the one-sized-fits-all trap. This highlights the potential of repurposed drugs.

Consider how they saved Quincy's life.

Quincy was the topic of a Ted Talk entitled "Who Lives, Who Dies" given by Dr. Ted Goldstein, a former Apple Computer Company Vice President-turned cancer researcher. After a distinguished career in technology, he returned to school, and become a professor at UCSF. He tells the story of Quincy, a toddler who suffered with a rare form of leukemia, JMML, known as Juvenile Myelomonocytic Leukemia. Quincy's only reasonable chance at a cure was through a bone marrow transplant procedure. This was his only route to living a full life.

However, the disease rapidly progressed making Quincy far too sick to withstand the procedure. Dr. Goldstein, a technophile, was familiar with the TCGA, the cancer genome computer data base, so he decided to test Quincy's tumor genes to find a target mutation to attack, something that might help him. The test revealed an FLT-3 fusion mutation that was common to certain kidney cancers. A drug known as Sorafenib is approved to treat kidney cancers, and it has major effects in blocking VEGF and PDGF. It is effective against

FLT-3 related cancers; therefore Dr. Goldstein and colleagues felt it might be worth a try in Quincy's case.

However, it was not FDA approved to treat JMML. Some researchers had even recommended against its compassionate use in cases of pediatric leukemia. There was no way insurance would cover it; however Dr. Goldstein had a friend and colleague working at UCSF who had an inside track. Dr. Frank McCormick, Chair of Tumor Biology and Cancer Research at UCSF, was also the developer and inventor of Sorafenib. To make a long story short, Quincy got the drug, and it saved his life. His white cell count, dangerously elevated at 80,000, dropped quickly to normal after three doses.

His health rapidly improved, he underwent the bone marrow transplant and was cured. The repurposed and off-label use of Sorafenib, customized through genetic testing, proved to be the key to young Quincy's survival. As we shall later discuss, medical visionaries like Dr. Patrick Soon-Shiong of Los Angeles believe personalized care is the pathway to curing cancer.

The Optune TTF System

Both Matt's father and Stefan Roever decided to include the Novocure Optune System, which employs tumor treating fields to hinder cancer cell mitosis.[213] This is a part of combination therapy for many patients with GBM. It is being tested in many other cancers as they all use mitosis to divide. I believe tumor treating fields will eventually become part of the standard care in combination treatments. Attacking the cancer from all possible angles, including the electrical angle, makes sense.

Whatever you do, if you have terminal cancer, do not settle for average or standard care—the standard care results in dismal results.

Remember to target CSC in addition to the fast-growing tumor bulk. The cancer stem cells will almost always gain strength and resistance from chemotherapy and radiation treatment.

Unfortunately, biopsies and surgeries on the tumor will also often stimulate CSC and EMT metastatic spread.

Barriers to Treatment

My friend and patient, let's call him Luther, asked me for help. His pastor's good friend, another pastor's wife, developed brain cancer. The pastor had asked the congregation to pray for her. Luther asked if I had any advice.

"I believe prayer always helps, but informing her and her physician about the option of repurposed drugs wouldn't hurt either. Get her a copy of Jane McLelland's book. Don't just tell her to order it. You should order it, deliver it to your pastor, and see that she and her husband receive it. Maybe also have your pastor attend the doctor's appointment with her."

When I saw Luther again, he announced he had done it. "Good job!" I said, but deep down, I realized that probably was not going to make a difference in her treatment approach. She would receive standard chemotherapy and radiation and would not get the cocktail. There were just too many barriers. She and her husband were not scientists, and they would simply take the cancer specialist's advice as gospel. Her doctor would likely dismiss Jane's book as just another alternative treatment or form of quackery.

I knew that because of Matt De Silva's experience. Matt had knowledge and resources, but his mom and dad followed the antiquated advice of their regional cancer center team. While his dad received standard radiation and chemo for the glioblastoma, Matt's input was marginalized as nothing more than the desperate musings of a grieving son, wet behind the ears, freshly graduated from Cornell, and not having a stitch of true medical knowledge to contribute.

"Sonny boy," his family seemed to say, "Stick to your stock trading and let your Dad's specialists do the cancer treatment." Within a year, with the usual treatment for GBM, Matt's father became another predictable casualty of glioblastoma.

Well-meaning advice, even if scientifically valid, is typically discounted by family members, unless it's provided by a professional who is also a stronger. We simply don't trust our lives to the advice of family members who have dug up the latest article.

We much prefer trusting our lives to the prominent medical center doctors. But I will tell you from experience; this is not always smart or the best strategy.

At the University Medical Center, the treatment approach is protracted. The medical student evaluates you first to gain practice doing a history and physical examination. This is followed by another one-hour ordeal and exam by the intern, the doctor most newly graduated with the least experience. After sitting through this two-hour experience, the chief resident comes by to review your case, and finally, after presenting it to the attending physician, your treatment begins.

It's not bad care; however, it's also not the best. If you are a biotech company founder, a bank president, or a sports star, you generally don't go to the university medical center. You go straight to the best in the field in private practice and avoid the one-size-fits-all approach. You get the best in modern, customized, and effective care. But the public perception, unfortunately, remains that the best cancer care lies in the university teaching hospital.

When the patient is a scientist himself, like Dr. Ben Williams, or Dr. Richard Gerber, or Dr. Angela Chapman, you don't have the issue of family interference. But if you are an educated friend or relative providing that same information, your lectures will often fall on deaf ears.

What's the solution? Improve awareness of the repurposed drug option. Increase its use. Publicize long-term survivor success stories. Legitimize combination cocktails for mainstream cancer care and prevention.

Getting out books written by credible experts, by practicing physicians, cancer specialists, will be the answer. This book is a start. If Luther could show this book to his friend's family doctor, she might just get a cocktail prescribed. The studies are so clear on the benefits of repurposed drugs.

Dr. Emil Freireich's View

Dr. Emil J. Freireich is an icon in the cancer world. He is currently the Professor of Developmental Therapeutics at the world-famous MD Anderson Cancer Institute. He pioneered the POMP protocol in the early 1960s, which launched the combination chemotherapy era.

Dr. Freireich continues to work in cancer care and supports the concept of using repurposed drugs.

"Is there ever a circumstance where a patient should be denied a treatment which in someone's imagination might help them survive this disease? And the answer is no."[214]

If repurposed drug cocktails are acceptable to Dr. Emil Freireich, who among us should ever deny them to a patient, especially if they are nontoxic?

Dr. Freireich says:

"We could move the ball 100 times faster as we did with AIDS. If you have a response, objective progression-free survival, that's it. The truth is in itself. You have to have reproducibility. You have to have a lack of bias. And once you've got that, that's it. And the AIDS guys did it. Now cancer patients have to do it. We have to force congress to change legislation so that when a doctor and a patient agree that when the benefits exceed the potential risks, that should go."

He goes on:

> "All they have to do is learn to balance benefits against risks. If you have nine drugs that are going to cure glioblastoma and you have a patient who is 100 percent likely to die, let's give him the nine drugs.

> Who is against that? You can't do anything risk-free. You can't walk across the street without taking a chance.

> It's nice to do as well as you can, but you can't be insane. We are insane right now. The regulatory process is insane. They are trying to protect people, but they (the regulators) inadvertently get into a situation where they kill people. But that is not their intent. We are just human, after all."

***

Today, some cancer centers are finally beginning to focus on cancer stem cells realizing they may be the key to curing terminal cancer. Professor Tim Downing of UC Irvine stated,

> "There hasn't been a lot of work looking at how mechanical processes within solid tumors influence properties of cancer stem cells, which likely play a big role in fueling cancer aggressiveness."[215]

This cannot come too soon, in my opinion.

However, we already know now how to both block and kill CSCs using combinations of existing cheap and nontoxic repurposed drugs. Advanced repurposed drug cocktails could and should quickly be added to the standard of treatment in terminal cancer patients. It is not just biotech company founders and scientists that use repurposed drugs for their own cancers.

It is former employees of the National Cancer Institute that are in the know and use them too. Dr. Charlie (Snuffy) Myers, a top US research scientist, formerly with both the National Institutes of Health and the National Cancer Institute, developed a drug named Suramin (an AIDs drug that has anticancer effects). When he developed prostate cancer himself, he was not hesitant to use Suramin off-label to help his own survival.[216]

Dr. Myers also formed a group at the National Cancer Institute looking into repurposed drugs that can be used for others to fight prostate cancer. He looked at phenylacetate, phenylbutyrate, and geldanamycin. He has since retired from running *The Prostate Forum*, a support group and newsletter that is part of the *American Institute for Diseases of the Prostate* based in Charlottesville, Virginia.

The Future of Cancer Care

The biggest obstacle to fight your cancer may not be technology or lack of effective treatment. It may be access.

Dr. Ben Williams, through sheer force of personality, was able to defy convention and procure his drug cocktail. Others, including Dr. Richard Gerber, also a long-term glioblastoma survivor, gained access. He reported that whether it was through relatives, friends, or faking illness, by hook or crook, he got his lifesaving prescription drugs.

Gerber tells the story of how he also did well with an experimental drug that he could not purchase. It was provided through a clinical trial. When the company announced the trial was completed and would no longer manufacture it, he panicked. "I will synthesize it in my own lab," he declared. Gerber, a chemist, knew enough synthetic organic chemistry to make his own custom-designed compounds from basic re-agents. To save his own life, he would produce the medication himself.

Fortunately, the president of the company worried about Richard's safety, implored him to avoid this. The company found a way to provide him with a lifelong supply of the drug before they disbanded.

I realize it is easy for me to advise people to "ask your doctor" for a repurposed drug script after bringing in a study. In theory, it should work, especially if you have known the doctor a long time and have a doctor friend like Dr. David Jennings.

It worked for Dr. Christopher Kofron and Dr. Angela Chapman. As the hundreds and thousands of studies continue to emerge on cancer stem cells and repurposed drugs, it should slowly get easier for people to obtain off-label prescriptions to treat and prevent cancer. However, what do people do who are passive and not willing to argue when their doctor says no?

First, bring them this book. Second, get some help.

Join support groups or activist websites. Start an organization like "Act Up" that helped the AIDS groups gain access to lifesaving drugs. Get the word out. Join Jane McLelland's Facebook page. Get a law passed in the United States similar to the Medication Innovations Bill that failed in the United Kingdom. Simply start a petition on Change.org.

Get compassionate use laws in the United States that cover repurposed drugs and protect prescribers when they are used for terminal cancer. Follow Dr. Richard Gerber's suggestions. He believed we should no longer use cancer care protocols in terminal cases. Instead, they should be treated with personalized prescription cocktails in addition to standard of care.

Standard protocols simply do not work in terminal cancer causes because, by definition, they are not lifesaving. They do not cure inoperable cancers. Why not change the rules and laws to allow customized care in terminal cases?

Of course, the treatment would need to have some evidence basis. But let's not exclude all the wealth of medications we already have in existence that have known anticancer effects. If we know how to block autophagy and EMT and CSC, why not add a cocktail to existing standard care?

Dr. Emil Freireich, and Dr. Ben Williams believe activism may be part of the solution. Also, finding ways to allow pharmaceutical companies to profit from the development of drug repurposing is an important step forward. If we pass laws in such a manner that they provide a monetary incentive, the drug development will follow.

But strength lies not just in money but in numbers.

We have 1.8 million Americans newly diagnosed each year struggling with cancer, and some 18 million new cases worldwide as well. We have 310 existing safe drugs that have anticancer effects. The path forward is obvious. In the future, personalized cancer care will be guided by your own unique tumor's gene sequence. Drugs will be selected based on sensitivity tests to your tumor. Changes to your repurposed cocktail will be based upon your body's specific tumor burden. In the future, we will no longer be using one-size-fits-all protocols. Repurposed drugs will play a major role and become the new nontoxic standard of care.

The practice of medicine and the Hippocratic oath obligates me, as a physician, to serve those who are suffering. It requires me to both inform and advocate for access for everyone, educated or not. Every patient with terminal cancer has a right to be told that the repurposed drug cocktail option is available and can provide a substantial chance for improved survival with a small chance for cure.

Barring Use of Mebendazole

With repurposed medications being cheap and relatively nontoxic, there is no reason to block access, other than the monetary interests of Big Pharma. We should not stand behind regulatory laws to bar a patient from receiving a prescription of metformin or mebendazole. However, the UK did exactly that when Parliament failed to pass the Medical Innovations Act. Organized Oncology wrote in the Lancet that the bill was promoting "precisely the type of emotional response that evidenced-based practice seeks to avoid, and that the bill's provisions threatened to undermine the Hippocratic oath."

Lord Saatchi, the sponsor of the Bill, had lost his wife, the novelist Josephine Hart, in 2011 to ovarian cancer.

Saatchi wrote, "We need to say loudly and clearly that we want to try new treatments for cancer where the old ones are known only to lead to death. We want to escape being doomed to repeat an endless cycle of failure."

The Medical Innovations Bill would have shielded UK physicians from negligence claims, which are the chief reason most will not prescribe repurposed drugs off-label in the UK. It would lead to doctors trying new and promising treatments to change the standard practice of cancer care and ultimately find a cure for the disease that killed his wife.

Saatchi argued, "Cancer patients are routinely prescribed a standard procedure that is degrading, medieval and ineffective and leads only to death." Lord Saatchi felt the Medical Innovations Act would promote responsible innovation.

Many physicians came forward in support of the bill, among them:

- Professor Alastair Buchan, Dean of Medicine, University of Oxford

- Professor Michael Rawlins, President Royal Society of Medicine

- Professor Ahmed Ashour Ahmed, Professor of Gynecological Oncology, University of Oxford

- Professor Stephen Kennedy, Professor of Reproductive Medicine, University of Oxford

- Dr. Henrietta Morton-King, Cumberland Infirmary

- Professor Andy Hall, Associate Dean of Translational Research, Newcastle University

- Professor Mohammed Keshtgar, Professor of Cancer Surgery, Royal Free London Trust

- Professor John Yamold, Professor of Clinical Oncology, The Royal Marsden

- Professor David Walker, Professor of Pediatric Oncology, Nottingham University

- Professor Riccardo Audisio, President, Association for Cancer Surgery

- Dr. John Symons, Director, Cancer of Unknown Primary Foundation

- Professor Dean Fennell, Chair of Thoracic Medical Oncology, Leicester University

These physicians and others authored a letter to the House of Lords stating,

> "This bill legally protects doctors who try out innovative new techniques or drugs on patients when all else has failed. The bill will protect the patient and nurture the innovator. It will encourage safe medical advancement, while at the same time deterring the maverick, thereby recalibrating the culture of defensive medicine. Finally, it will work with evidence-based medicine and provide new data that will inspire and support new research."

In the words of cancer pioneer Dr. Emil Freireich,

> "If you have nine drugs that are going to cure glioblastoma, and you have a patient who is 100% likely to die, let's give him the nine drugs; who is against that?"

Parliament is against that. And so is organized oncology (with their studies backed by Big Pharma).

But not Dr. Emil Freireich, arguably the greatest oncologist who ever lived, the inventor of the combination chemotherapy model.

Fortunately, there is now a worldwide research effort to study repurposed drugs. The genie is out of the bottle. We are in the midst of a drug repurposing revolution. Let's follow the lead of Dr. Ben Williams, Dr. Richard Gerber, Dr. Christopher Kofron, Dr. Angela Chapman, and Jane McLelland. Let's rally behind Dr. Pan Pantziarka and get it done.

Join me and many others in letting everyone you know about repurposed drugs. Spread the word on the S.A.M. preventative regimen. Tell others to read Jane's book, *Starving Cancer*, and Ben's book, *Surviving Terminal Cancer*. Gather a group of friends to watch the movie, *Surviving Terminal Cancer*. Read and study PubMed for your health if you do not have cancer, and for your life if you do. Act Up for your life and the lives of your loved ones today.

The time has come for all patients to have access to both information and repurposed drugs. The doctors are professionals bound by oath to serve us. We do not exist to serve them.

Dominic Hill, director and producer of the film *Surviving Terminal Cancer* said it best:

"Thanks to technology, patients are becoming more equal stakeholders in the decision making process that defines their treatment, and it should be so, lest we forget in premise, doctors are (merely) consultants."[17]

SECTION IV:
REPURPOSING DRUGS
AGAINST CORONAVIRUS

Chapter 10

REPURPOSING DRUGS AGAINST CORONAVIRUS

Repurposed drugs should be used in cancer and other life-threatening diseases, especially when there are no effective alternatives. There is no better example of the need for repurposed drugs than in the current 2020 coronavirus pandemic.

Let me begin with some background on SARS and MERS. SARS is short for severe acute respiratory syndrome, and MERS stands for Middle Eastern respiratory syndrome. Both of these garnered very little United States attention as they did not much affect our country. There were only eight US SARS cases and only two MERS cases.

The Chinese and Saudi Arabian Experiences

In China, the world noticed SARS in a big way. China developed some 8,000 cases, with 774 deaths with a case fatality rate of almost 10%. The theory was that close human contact with animals caused the disease through zoonotic transmission. Zoonotic essentially means the spread of the virus from one species to another. This was similar to the swine flu or H1N1, which originated from birds, yet spread through pigs as an intermediary. The Palm civets, a type of cat, were thought to be intermediaries in SARS-CoV given their close contact with bats, the original reservoir of the virus. Bats harbored a similar strain. Close human contact with the civets facilitated viral evolution and interspecies spread.

SARS, MERS, AND SARS-CoV-2

Virus Name	Intermediary	Origination
SARS-CoV	Palm Civet	Horseshoe Bat
MERS-CoV	Dromedary Camel	Egyptian Tomb Bat
SARS-CoV-2	Pangolin	Horseshoe Bat

Scientists theorized that through a mutational change in the virus, it became infectious to humans, which accounted for the first SARS case in 2002 in China. This was termed SARS Coronavirus or SARS-CoV. The disease spread quickly among humans. It eventually affected 8,439 people. Fortunately, it was contained within a couple of years and ran its course.

However, sometime in 2012, the coronavirus resurfaced in a different form. A camel herder in Saudi Arabia developed respiratory symptoms and fever and was diagnosed with the first case of MERS. He had been grooming the animal's nose before contracting the illness.

It quickly spread, and soon Saudi Arabia had some 688 people infected; 282 eventually died. This carried a much higher fatality rate, at approximately 35% than SARS at 10%. A similar coronavirus virus, MERS, was identified in multiple dromedary camels. It was thought to have passed from the camel to the human. Indeed, the camel viral genetics resembled human MERS. However, unlike with SARS, MERS proved infectious to both camels and humans, and several camels also died. In addition to camel-to-camel transmission, the virus also spread quickly between humans and ultimately affected some 27 countries before running its course.

Coronavirus Basics

Professor Michael Lin, an honors biochemistry graduate of Harvard University and an MD, PhD scientist at Stanford, offers some helpful insights. Dr. Lin runs the Lin Lab at Stanford University and is a world-renowned authority on viruses. He reports the SARS-CoV-2 virus is killed by high temperature, UV light, Windex, Clorox, and hydrogen peroxide. He recommends that face masks can be heated in an oven at 165° F for 30-60 minutes to kill the novel coronavirus.[217]

He observes that the virus can survive on hard plastic or steel up to three days unless it is exposed to heat or bright sunlight when it will be much less. After two to three hours of exposure in bright sunlight, up to 90% of the virus is killed. The virus can survive on masks, cardboard, or porous surfaces less than one day. According to Dr. Lin, the virus has a very thin plasma membrane and is destroyed easily by soap and water or detergents. He notes that Windex contains a detergent that makes it effective.

The novel coronavirus is the third fatal human coronavirus. There have been a total of seven known human coronaviruses, four of which are mild and produce slight diseases such as the common cold, and three are known to be fatal: MERS, SARS, and SARS-CoV-2. The most common mild one has been known since the 1960s as CoVOC43, which causes the common cold.

Coronaviruses all have spikes that give the virus the appearance of a crown or corona. The virus in animals can have very different effects than in humans. For example, the common cold CoV-OC43 coronavirus in humans can be fatal in mice, causing severe hepatitis. By contrast, the potentially fatal respiratory disease the novel coronavirus produces in humans is known as COVID-19. Because of the virus's similarity to SARS-CoV, it is also known as SARS-CoV-2.

It is much more easily spread than either SARS or MERS, making it far more life-threatening. There is a lower case fatality rate originally estimated at only 3%. More recently scientists on PubMed have revised the rate upwards to between 4.21 and 6.16% in Spain and France.[218] This high case fatality rate coupled with the exponential spread has made this one of the world's most deadly pandemics. The disease is following a trajectory eerily similar to the Spanish flu world pandemic that started in 1918 and claimed between 25 and 50 million lives.

In 1918 the world's total population was around 2 billion people. Five hundred million, or 25% became infected. As I like to tell my patients who believe that the coronavirus fears are exaggerated, it is truer than ever that those who fail to learn from history risk repeating it. We all need to take caution from the 1918 Spanish flu and realize that because the novel coronavirus is also a zoonotic-type of virus, it is capable of Spanish flu level calamity.

Hence, there is a need for interim solutions until we can develop a vaccine, which is at least 12 months away. There has never been a more urgent need for repurposing existing drugs to save human lives on a global scale.

But before we delve into antiviral drug strategies, let's look at basic infection prevention.

The World Health Organization advises that everyone adopt stringent infection prevention strategies such as handwashing, sanitizing, maintaining a six-foot distance between people, and avoiding mass gatherings. Also, the common supplement lactoferrin can help prevent viral entry into your cells. A study reported on PubMed shows that lactoferrin binds with heparin sulfate proteoglycans and interferes with the viral binding in SARS.[219] Since SARS-CoV-2 is quite similar, lactoferrin should also help prevent the infection. The higher the dose, the more viral entry is blocked. However, more is not always better. Three grams per day is a typical dose, but higher doses (7.2 grams/day) can produce skin rash, anorexia, fatigue, chills, and constipation.

There is also evidence that supplemental Zinc can help. Since too much Zinc can be harmful, my preferred dose is 30mg per day. Zinc is long known to modulate antiviral and antibacterial immunity. It can also regulate the immune and inflammatory response through inhibition of NKfB and modulation of T-cell function. Lab experiments have shown that Zn2+ has antiviral activity through its suppression of SARS-CoV RNA polymerase.[220] Its action can be improved by adding an ionophore. HCQ and CQ are both powerful Zinc ionophores. Dr. Skalny and Dr. Rink discuss this in more detail in their journal review published in April of 2020.[221]

Dr. Seheult, a critical care specialist, and former ICU director, has lectured extensively on the subject of zinc, hydroxychloroquine, and COVID-19 through his MedCram lecture series. He has also discussed the possible use of other supplements such as vitamin C, vitamin D, quercetin, and N acetylcysteine (NAC) for prevention. He has found evidence for antiviral activity by a number a supplements, and he mentioned that he takes these himself during this pandemic. His videos can be either viewed on YouTube or on his MedCram website.[222] He is board-certified in Internal Medicine, Pulmonary Diseases, Internal Medicine, Pulmonary Medicine, Critical Care, and Sleep Medicine. He provides courses for physicians to aide in studying for their board exams, and is exceptionally knowledgeable, scientific, and easy to understand.

SEHEULT COVID SUPPLEMENT COCKTAIL

- Quercetin Vitamin C
- Vitamin D3

* Vitamin C
* Zinc

Dr. Paul Marik and others in the field of Pulmonary and Critical Care Medicine at the Eastern Virginia Medical School have reported on the potential synergy of Quercetin and Vitamin C for the prevention and treatment of SARS-CoV-2 related disease.[340] The authors state, "Due to their lack of severe side effects and low costs, we strongly suggest the combined administration of these two compounds for both prophylaxis and the early treatment of respiratory tract infections, especially including COVID-19 patients."

I would strongly agree.

What are the symptoms of COVID-19? Many people have few or no symptoms, especially younger ones. The common signs are fever, dry cough, shortness of breath, aches, fatigue, and loss of taste and smell. At the end of seven days of symptoms, a person may become short of breath with signs of pneumonia. This is when some are so severe, they wind up in the hospital or the intensive care unit. This is where many people, especially those older than 50, or with other health problems, die. There is a fatality rate of approximately 15% in those individuals 80 and over, 9% in individuals in their 70s, 4% with individuals in their 60s, and less than 0.4% for those aged 50 or less. The disease is considered mild in those under age 30 with less than a 0.2% case fatality rate.[223]

In my opinion, no one over age 50 should ever wait a week to get treatment. The sooner you get treatment, the better, and that would be with the first sign of any fever or shortness of breath. What is the best treatment, in my opinion?

The Search for SARS Drugs

A computer searched a database of 348 FDA-approved drugs.[224] A half dozen agents were identified as being good candidates against MERS, a related fatal coronavirus. One of these was chloroquine and its cousin, hydroxychloroquine.

These two antimalarials are roughly equivalent in action, but hydroxychloroquine is less toxic. Chloroquine has broad and powerful antiviral action against a broad range of conditions. Preliminary results show that it is active against multiple flaviviruses, influenza viruses, and even Ebola.[229]

It has been shown in the lab to be effective against MERS, SARS, and even HIV-1.[225, 226, 227, 228]

In 2005, CDC scientists Dr. Vincent, Dr. Nichols, Dr. Erickson and colleagues wrote, "Chloroquine, a relatively safe, effective and cheap drug used for treating many human diseases including malaria, amoebiasis and human immunodeficiency virus is effective in inhibiting the infection and spread of SARS-CoV in cell culture. The fact that the drug has significant inhibitory antiviral effect when the susceptible cells were treated either prior to or after infection suggests a possible prophylactic and therapeutic use." [229]

Chloroquine accumulates in lysosomes, where it sequesters protons and increases the pH. It modulates the immune response and suppresses autophagy. It is hostile to both cancers and viruses.

Its major pathway is in blocking COVID-19 viral entry; in other words, preventing the infection.

The computer also identified a pair of protease inhibitors called lopinavir and ritonavir, sold and marketed as Kaletra. Kaletra is FDA-approved for the treatment of HIV-1 infection. It is such a powerful AIDS antiviral, that it is routinely given to healthcare workers after an accidental needle stick injury to prevent subsequent infection. Whereas chloroquine blocks viral entry, Kaletra tends to block viral division and replication. Lopinavir is the most active of the two, while ritonavir functions mainly to reduce lopinavir metabolism, which effectively boosts lopinavir levels.

Some feel ribavirin should be added to the combination for maximal effectiveness. Dr. Chu and colleagues studied 41 SARS patients treated with a combination of lopinavir, ritonavir, and ribavirin.[230] The treatment group had only a 2.4% mortality rate compared to 29% in the control group. In other words, deaths were reduced by 90% with the addition of Kaletra and ribavirin.

Dr. Chan studied 75 patients treated with lopinavir, ritonavir, and ribavirin.[231] The treatment group had a 2.3% mortality rate compared to the control group at 16%.

Dr. Park studied post-exposure prophylaxis against MERS.[232] This involved trying to prevent individuals exposed to the virus from getting sick. This retrospective study treated 22 patients with high-risk exposure to a single MERS patient with the combination lopinavir, ritonavir, and ribavirin. The ritonavir dose was 400 mg/100 mg twice a day for 11-13 days. The ribavirin dose was 2,000 mg loading dose followed by 1,200 mg three times a day for four days, followed by 600 mg three times a day for six to eight days. These were then compared to an untreated control group. Surprisingly, no one of the 22 developed MERS.

A famous SARS researcher and head of Peking Hospital's Pulmonary and Critical Care Medicine Department, Dr. Wang Guangfa, developed COVID-19 infection.[233] He was treated with lopinavir, ritonavir combination, and credited this with saving his life.

Other drugs that have shown strong activity against COVID-19 include chlorpromazine, an antipsychotic and loperamide, an antidiarrheal, also known as Imodium. The matrix metalloproteinases are active in the COVID-19 respiratory infection and ramp up inflammation. Blocking them with doxycycline and glucosamine sulfate, therefore, might be an additional strategy.[234]

The problem with Loperamide, known as Imodium, is that it does not concentrate much in tissues outside the GI tract. 99% accumulates in the intestines, with less than 1% getting into the lung tissue. The problem with chlorpromazine, an antipsychotic, is that effective blood levels were difficult to achieve at standard human doses. One would have to take ten times the maximal dose used clinically, which could lead to toxicity. That might be enough to kill the virus, but it also might harm the patient. Also, no studies on coronavirus outside the lab have ever been done using loperamide or chlorpromazine.

Dr. Michael Lin notes that Japan has also researched a few other repurposed drugs, Camostat and favipirivir, both widely used abroad, but virtually unknown in the US. Camostat (CM) is a repurposed drug in Japan that treats symptoms of pancreatitis.[217] It has been approved in Japan since 1985. It has been approved to treat esophagitis since 1994. Camostat inhibits TMPRSS2, which is required by SARS-CoV-2 to enter cells.[235] It is a serine protease inhibitor, and it also has activity against influenza, including H1N1. It has already been approved and stockpiled in Japan for use in pandemics.

REPURPOSED DRUG CANDIDATES FOR SARS/MERS

- Lopinavir/Ritonavir
- Camostat
- Loperamide
- Chloroquine

* Ribavirin
* Favipiravir
* Chlorpromazine
* Hydroxychloroquine

William Henry Gates III, better known as the founder of Microsoft, Bill Gates, warned the world about the need to prepare for future viral pandemics in a prescient presentation he made in 2015 on the TED Talks platform.[236] Japan was one of the few countries that took heed, resulting in Japan's camostat stockpile. Camostat, while potentially an option overseas, is not available or FDA-approved for use in the United States.

Favipiravir has been approved in Japan to treat novel influenza and has activity against SARS. Novel influenza is considered severe flu, much more than the average or common variety. It is a selective inhibitor of viral RNA polymerase. On 03/18/20, China announced its results of favipiravir against COVID-19 in a trial. The virus cleared faster in the favipiravir group, and there was a measurable improvement in the chest CT scans. The improvement rate was almost 50% faster in the favipiravir-treated group.[237] Like camostat, favipiravir is not FDA-approved or available in the United States. However, for the Chinese, it is approved and stockpiled to be rapidly available for influenza or pandemic outbreaks.

This brings us back to chloroquine (CQ) and hydroxychloroquine (HCQ). These drugs are FDA-approved and available in the US. Even standard human doses produce plasma levels many times greater than necessary to kill SARS-CoV.[238] Moreover, the drug concentrated well in most tissues like the heart and lungs where the ACE-2 receptors are located.

Recall the 2005 findings by Dr. Vincent and the CDC researchers, "When chloroquine was added after the initiation of infection, there was a dramatic dose-dependent decrease in the number of virus antigen-positive cells. As little as 0.1–1 µM chloroquine reduced the infection by 50% and up to 90–94% inhibition was observed with 33–100 µM concentrations. At concentrations of chloroquine in excess of 1 µM, only a small number of individual cells were initially infected, and the spread of the infection to adjacent cells was all but eliminated."[225]

The half-life of HCQ is so long at 40 days that even a once-weekly dose could theoretically accumulate and have both a preventative and treatment action. For many reasons, even before human trials began, HCQ looked like a natural and perfect fit to fight COVID-19.

Chapter 11

HUMAN TRIALS AGAINST COVID-19

As in any repurposed drug discussion, it is always the scientists versus the regulators; it boils down to the doctors versus Big Pharma. Here the scientists are led by Dr. Didier Raoult, the Dr. Pan Pantziarka of the anti-coronavirus movement, who brings the spotlight to the effectiveness of HCQ and CQ against SARS-CoV-2. Raoult, a larger than life medical luminary physician and professor, is the top expert in the world in communicable disease. He looks the part.

With silver shoulder-length hair, the 68-year-old mustache sporting Frenchman never worried about offending the old guard. Professor Raoult completed residencies in both internal medicine and infectious disease and earned both MD and PhD degrees. His laboratory boasts a team of more than 200 researchers who publish between 250 and 350 papers per year and have produced more than 50 patents. He publishes more in one year than most do in a lifetime. His team has isolated 380 new bacterial species and 63 viruses and sequenced 290 bacterial genomes.

In November of 2010, he was awarded the Grand Prix de L'Inserm. This is the equivalent of a Nobel Prize. He shared $450,000 in prize money with the biologist Christopher Bowler. According to many, he is the foremost microbiologist in the world and the principal reference for both Q fever and Whipple's disease.

He has been referred to as the most productive and cited microbiologist in Europe. He directs the IHU Mediterranean Infection Institute in Marseille, France, a world-renowned research and teaching center dedicated to the management and study of infectious disease. Dr. Didier Raoult, both controversial and outspoken, is one of the world's most influential and productive scientists. As of this writing, he is listed as either the author or co-author of 2,909 Pubmed citations.

He is also the antithesis of Dr. Anthony Fauci or any regulatory body. So, when Dr. Raoult published his landmark HCQ study, the first detailed human trial to show the benefit of hydroxychloroquine and chloroquine and those afflicted with COVID-19, he ignited a firestorm. Chloroquine and hydroxychloroquine were long known to block both cell entry and replication in SARS and MERS. They should also work well against SARS-CoV-2.

However, these early studies were confined to lab testing only, testing the activity of these drugs in the test tube. Didier was among the first, along with the Chinese, to show that HCQ worked in live human subjects with coronavirus infections. But the Chinese declined to produce their data.

Didier, on the other hand, was quick to unveil stunning results. In his pilot study, he treated 20 infected patients with hydroxychloroquine and compared them with 16 infected controls that were not treated.[239] By the third day, 50% of the treated group were negative for the virus. By the sixth day, 70% of the hydroxychloroquine group were viral negative.

Six of the 20 patients were treated with Zithromax in addition to hydroxychloroquine. Most impressively, these six patients tested 100% negative for the virus on day six. Only 12.5% of the non-treated group, however, was virus free. These results suggested a 100% cure rate for the group receiving the hydroxychloroquine and Zithromax by day six compared with a 90% infection rate for the group untreated.

For reference, the Chinese had already shown that untreated COVID-19 patients could remain infectious for some 19-20 days; in some cases, up to 34 days.[240] Dr. Raoult felt that the information contained in his study was so significant, that he was ethically bound to release the results immediately, prior to the usual peer-review process. Dr. Raoult recommended that COVID-19 patients be treated with hydroxychloroquine and azithromycin to both cure their infection and to curb the spread. He freely admitted that although better and more scientific therapy, such as a specific vaccine, might later be developed, the current treatment was imminently necessary to treat the COVID-19 threat in real-time.

By eradicating the virus at day 6, Raoult had shortened the time for contagiousness by 66% from 19 days to only six. The implications were staggering. If his results held up, that meant quarantines and isolation times could end 70% sooner. It meant quicker recovery times in infected patients. It also implied lower rates of death. It meant health care workers could take the drug preventatively and not pass the virus to patients. Dr. Raoult had given the world a gift, a crucial tool to stem the pandemic, a discovery worthy of a Nobel prize.

Raoult and his colleagues wrote, "We therefore recommend that COVID-19 patients be treated with hydroxychloroquine and azithromycin to cure their infection and to limit the transmission of the virus to other people in order to curb the spread of COVID-19 in the world. Further works are also warranted to determine if these compounds could be useful as chemoprophylaxis to prevent the transmission of the virus, especially for healthcare workers." [239]

Raoult's study found what the CDC researchers working on test tubes in 2005 had strongly suspected. Chloroquine and hydroxychloroquine might work against the coronavirus in vivo just as well as in vitro, in life just as well as in the lab; it might just be the answer to SARS-CoV-2 and the pandemic: a repurposed drug that might attack not only cancer but also the novel coronavirus.

Dr. Fauci's Reaction

Here we had the result of an open-label non-randomized clinical trial involving 36 patients studied with a drug the CDC knew killed the SARS virus. How would the US task force respond? On March 20, 2020, I watched as they commented on the news. The head of the NIAH had one word.

"Anecdotal."

Without so much as a blink, I stared at the television in disbelief. I replayed the recording to make sure I had heard correctly. Yes, Dr.

Fauci had used the word anecdotal to describe the results of a clinical trial, perhaps the most critical pilot study in the pandemic. As a medical professional, I was struck that something was amiss. Dismissing Raoult's data as anecdotal was neither fair nor accurate. As I would soon discover, many of my colleagues felt the same. I would refer the reader to Appendix F for a collection of their comments.

Like Fauci, the CDC was also not impressed. They had lost their former enthusiasm. They preferred to wait, even as millions more became infected. But why wait with a medication already certified safe in FDA Phase I trials, a medication used for decades to treat lupus and malaria, and a medication that could save tens of thousands of lives?

[To be fair, the dose of HCQ used for the treatment of lupus is 200 mg twice per day, and it is in this context that it's use was considered safe in the FDA trials.]

Meanwhile, Rome burned. As of March 21, 2020, the cases in Italy had increased from 1,700 to 53,000 in less than three weeks. The deaths in Italy had risen from 41 to 4,825. Hospitals in Italy were being overwhelmed with patients dying in the hallways and doctors having to choose who would get ventilators and who would not. Patients were dying due to a lack of hospital resources.

The New York City cases ballooned similarly. However, the CDC had declined to recommend hydroxychloroquine and azithromycin combination. "We need more studies."

I was once again reminded of Dr. Emil Freireich's words regarding repurposed drug use in terminal cancer,

"You cannot do anything risk-free. You cannot walk across the street without taking a chance. The regulatory process is insane right now. They are trying to protect people, but they (the regulators) unfortunately get into a situation where they kill people. But this is not their intent. We are just human, after all."[17]

Ivy League Doctor

What do wealthy, highly educated medical experts say and do in a coronavirus pandemic? If one had millions of dollars, was trained as a heart surgeon, and works at a top Ivy League Medical Center like Harvard or Columbia, what would he do?

Dr. Mehmet Oz is that person. He immediately recognized the potential of hydroxychloroquine. Dr. Oz interviewed Dr. Didier Raoult, the lead physician of the French study. Dr. Raoult felt that it would be unethical to withhold the hydroxychloroquine treatment based upon what he knew. Dr. Oz then interviewed the Vice President, who clarified that hydroxychloroquine, otherwise known as Plaquenil, could currently be legally prescribed on an off-label basis.

Dr. Oz highlighted that US physicians were currently allowed to prescribe Plaquenil for their high-risk coronavirus patients. It did not take a rocket scientist to know exactly what Dr. Oz would recommend for himself, his family, or his patients.

Unfortunately, politics intervened. Because President Trump had personally endorsed CQ and HCQ as promising treatments, anti-Trump news sources went overboard to demonize the drugs. It was no longer just the regulators and Big Pharma who opposed them. It was also left-wing journalists, newspapers, and Trump opponents.

Newspapers uncharacteristically took the low road to attack both Dr. Oz and Dr. Raoult. Ad Hominem attacks usually reserved for criminally-accused politicians were levied against any scientist who had positive words for the antimalarials.[339]

Overnight, CQ and HCQ went from safe and effective drugs used for decades to nothing more than poisons. Headlines began appearing daily about an Arizona man who had died from chloroquine poisoning. However, in reality, it was not prescription chloroquine; in truth, the man had drunk a toxic aquarium cleaner. Other headlines appeared that two Nigerians had been hospitalized due to chloroquine toxicity. Dr. Oz's comments were drowned out by media reports that Plaquenil and chloroquine could stop the heart. These drugs were cast as so risky that tens of thousands of virus deaths might be preferable to risking a single life with HCQ. One had to wonder why all these lupus and rheumatoid arthritis patients were not advised to stop the toxic drugs immediately. Why weren't we seeing law firms advertising class action suits against the drug?

Curiously, at the same, the need for these supposedly toxic medications was also argued.

Media reports circulated about how lupus and rheumatoid arthritis patients were suffering due to a run on Plaquenil, never mind that these cheap pills can be mass-produced in days by the millions.

The politics of HCQ was suddenly painfully obvious.

Was a propaganda campaign at work against HCQ and its use against COVID-19? And why? Who was behind it, and what was the goal? Soon it becomes transparent to any specialist even remotely familiar with CQ and HCQ. I would refer the reader to more detail on this in Appendix F.

Hydroxychloroquine, the kinder gentler brother of chloroquine, the original antimalarial, has found many pleiotropic uses in India, a country where malaria is rampant. There it has been available without a prescription, over-the-counter, for decades, similar to our Aleve or aspirin.

Cinchona Bark

CQ, derived from the bark of the Cinchona tree, has been grown on Indian plantations for generations. HCQ long been known as a safe and effective drug against both lupus and rheumatoid arthritis, but Indian scientists also discovered it was a cheap and effective treatment for type II diabetes. Studies, done as early as 2014, began to show that HCQ could both drop blood sugar and inflammation.

It could also produce healthy weight loss in diabetics. In 2014 the Indian Ministry of Health approved hydroxychloroquine for the treatment of type II diabetes. The US chose an expensive alternative, canagliflozin. At a recent US conference of the American Association of Clinical Endocrinologists, the two drugs were compared.[241] Studies showed an equivalent benefit between HCQ and canagliflozin, as measured by a drop in hemoglobin A1C, a measure of diabetic control.

Dr. Amit Gupta of the GD Institute in Kolkata, India, reported at the meeting. In a head-to-head clinical trial comparing canagliflozin 300 mg once a day to HCQ 400 mg per day, both groups saw their fasting blood sugars drop an average of some 30 points. However, the BMI or weight of the HCQ group dropped from 27.2 to 25.69, while the canagliflozin group's weight remained the same.

The CRP, a marker of inflammation, dropped from 2.8 to 1.9 in the HCQ group, while not lowering in the canagliflozin group. Drops in inflammation and weight are desirable in patients with diabetes. Dr. Gupta also noted, in addition to HCQ being a better metabolic drug than canagliflozin, it was also much cheaper. A month's supply of canagliflozin runs around $600, while a month of HCQ costs only $10.

Dr. Lance Sloan, a US diabetes expert based in Texas, said that most doctors in the US knew nothing about HCQ's benefit in diabetes. He reported that HCQ is not even on the radar to be studied for this purpose. Dr. Gupta concluded, "HCQ is an effective and safe medication in diabetes so it can be used as a cheap add-on drug in cases of resistant diabetes."

I did some math. India has a population of over one billion people. They now have about 10% or 100 million diabetics, many of whom take HCQ or Plaquenil. About 30% of those ages 65 and older are diabetics.

What does this mean? First, it means that many Indian diabetics, especially those older than age 65, probably will not contract malaria, as HCQ has powerful antimalarial effects. Second, many of these Indians will enjoy up to a 15-20 pound weight loss as a beneficial side effect of HCQ. Third, many will notice their arthritic joints do not hurt so much because of the anti-inflammatory benefits. Finally, and most importantly, many will mysteriously be resistant to the ravages of COVID-19.

In reality, we notice that India is one of those "charmed countries" similar to Africa, where coronavirus just cannot seem to gain a foothold. The answer becomes obvious. When India's coronavirus load was almost 50 to 100 fold less than Europe or the US, could the reason be due to the many millions of diabetics in India on HCQ? Or due to widespread antimalarial use? Could this produce a "population resistance" with the virus getting so hamstrung that HCQ patients can easily overtake this pathogen? Let us take this one step further.

The Indian Health Ministry has mandated the use of HCQ.[242] They initially placed a ban on all exports of HCQ, preferring to keep it all for themselves in their own country. They ordered high-risk healthcare workers who come in contact with coronavirus patients to be placed on a regimen of one HCQ tablet per week as prevention. High-risk contacts are also required to take it. All household contacts of infected persons must take it.

Could it be that Indian physicians were more enlightened not only about diabetes but also about COVID-19? Watching India would prove instructive as the pandemic unfolded.

Chapter 12

WHITE COATS VS BLUE COATS

Dr. Colyer describes the fight between the blue coats and the white coats, those in the ivory tower who insist on randomized controlled trials vs. those in the trenches who treat the sick and dying. It is nice to pontificate about the need for absolute certainty before giving your blessing about the validity of a specific course of treatment, but in the middle of a pandemic, Dr. Colyer feels that you need to go with the army you have not the one you wished you had.

And Dr. Colyer is not your average GP. He was also the 47th governor of Kansas. Trained as a surgeon, he has volunteered with the International Medical Corps and provided care in Kosovo and Sierra Leone. He has volunteered his surgical services in Afghanistan and Iraq, and Rwanda during the country's genocide. Dr. Colyer is a leader, a doctor's doctor. He is currently working along with Dr. Daniel Hinthorn, Infectious Disease Director at the University of Kansas Medical Center, in treating patients and health care workers with hydroxychloroquine.

Dr. Didier Raoult describes the issue as a battle between the methodologists and the doctors. The methodologists insist on perfect science, while the doctors use common sense and good clinical judgment to do what is best for their patients. Dr. Raoult describes the methodologists as using cold numbers or "purely mathematical reflection," while a doctor uses ethics and moral principles guided by the Hippocratic Oath. Dr. Raoult applies "Tom's method."[243]

He explained that Tom is his son. The principle of the method is the substance of the Hippocratic Oath, "treat everyone as if they were your own son." Dr. Raoult explained that if he were infected with the coronavirus knowing what he knew, he would take the drug hydroxychloroquine to save his own life; therefore, he would also prescribe it to save his son, Tom, or his patients as well.

As a fellow blue coat and physician, I can relate more easily to Dr. Raoult than to a methodologist or regulator. If my favorite uncle lived in a Texas nursing home, I would want a Dr. Robin Armstrong, a blue coat, to treat him, not a Dr. Anthony Fauci, the quintessential white coat. That is precisely what Dr. Robin Armstrong did. During the COVID-19 outbreak, he treated his 39 infected nursing home residents with a five-day course of hydroxychloroquine.

The 56 residents of the resort at Texas City contracted the novel coronavirus. Thirty-nine gave their informed consent to get the emergency hydroxychloroquine treatment. After the treatment, all patients have done well, according to Dr. Armstrong. "I thought the risk of seeing 15% of the nursing home die was just not acceptable," he said.[244]

Dr. Armstrong admitted that two patients receiving HCQ had to go to the hospital for unrelated conditions, one a woman who had a fall, and the other a man who got dehydrated for not eating and drinking. All survived the COVID-19. Statistically, given their older ages, the results would not have been nearly as positive as the group treated with HCQ. If we look around the country, at the time of this writing, fully one-fifth of the deaths are seen in nursing home patients.

What about the lack of a control group, you might ask? With the mortality being anywhere from 15-40% in the senior population, most blue coats would say that not offering the HCQ would be unethical and dangerous. I have listed several representative comments by fellow physicians in Appendix F.[245, 246]

Most blue coat physicians report that if they or their family members got infected, they would opt for HCQ. Why is the average non-physician more worried about the dangers of HCQ than the average blue coat physician? The simple answer is the media. The complicated answer is the media driven by powerful political and economic interests.

The biggest reason is that doctors have a feel for how likely the risks are. Non-medical people fear complications like vision loss and cardiac arrest after reading a media article and assume it is likely to occur. We blue coats realize, given our experience, that visual loss is extremely rare in HCQ patients. It is something that occurs in less than 2% after ten years of taking the drug twice a day, based on the studies.[247]

We also know that heart complications or cardiac arrests are even rarer, less than about three in one million. Based on this, your chance of winning the lottery would be greater than dying of cardiac complications of HCQ.[248] However, your chance of dying of COVID-19 if you get hospitalized and placed on a ventilator is 50/50.[249] Even if you survive, you may have permanently scarred lungs. Thanks, but no thanks. I would rather chance HCQ for five days than the virus, or its after effects for a lifetime.

The biggest problem with regulators or their white coat relatives, especially in the United States, is that their decisions are often not dictated by science. All too often, the policies are influenced by politics or economics.

Consider this: colchicine has been prescribed by the blue coats for centuries to treat gout. It was not based on randomized controlled trials or the FDA's blessing. Physicians did not need randomized controlled trials to show its effectiveness against gout. It cost pennies per pill and was widely available and effective from 1961 at least until 2009 when the FDA decided to regulate it. This came about because of the passage of the unapproved drugs initiative. On 07/30/09, after new trials were completed, the FDA finally approved colchicine officially and gave its stamp of approval.

It is not surprising that the FDA-sponsored randomized controlled studies proved what everyone else had already known for the last 50 years that it was effective against gout, both preventatively and treatment wise. The price raised from nine cents a pill to $4.85 a pill. The drugmaker Takeda-URL earned 1.2 billion dollars in revenue. Meanwhile, gout sufferers across the country could no longer afford the drug. They were forced to take other less effective and more toxic remedies for their gout. Eventually, the American College of Rheumatology had to step in and sue the FDA.[250]

In 2015, the FDA was sued in federal court to introduce a generic version of colchicine so that the average patient could once again afford it.

SECTION V:
THE SCIENCE OF CORONAVIRUS

—

Chapter 13

ZOONOTIC TRANSFER

Like cancer, viruses love to replicate and spread. Like a tumor, they continuously evolve, change, and adapt to any countermeasures the host may make. For eons, the coronavirus was locked in a competition with the bat's immune system, which is far stronger than a humans. Bat systems are quick to deploy alpha-interferon, the signal that deploys the antiviral army.

Dr. Cara Brooks of the University of California at Berkley, an expert, stated, "When you have a higher immune response, you get these cells that are protected from infection, so the virus can ramp up its replication rate without causing damage to its host. When it spills over into something like a human, and we do not have the same sorts of antiviral mechanisms, we could experience a lot of pathologies." [252]

The Leap to Humans

A vanishingly-small percentage of viruses make the leap to a human host, usually through a protein mutation. This occurred with AIDS coming from chimpanzees, and Ebola, SARS, and MERS, as well as the novel coronavirus all coming from bats. Intense physical activity from flight supercharged the bat metabolism leading to higher levels of tissue damage. Greater levels of free radicals created a more hostile host environment, and ultimately led the coronavirus to mutate into a super virus.

In humans, these viruses have little competition compared to the fierce struggle they had with bats. RNA viruses like coronavirus are more unstable, and errors form more frequently, leading to rapid mutation and evolution. This may explain why the spike protein binding efficiency to the ACE-2 receptor in the novel coronavirus is 10-20 times stronger than in SARS, a massive improvement in infectivity over 18 years.

Why is it that viruses prefer a higher host response or infection? Because massive inflammation, copious secretions like profuse coughing, sweating, and diarrhea facilitate spread. Zoonotic viruses are those that transferred from one species to another and in our case, from animals to humans. Because these viruses are used the harsh bat immune system, they often find child's play in a human host. This is precisely why the great pandemics of 1918 and 2020 were both caused by zoonotic spread. The Spanish flu was a zoonotic virus called H1N1 and transferred from a bird to humans.

Today's novel coronavirus ultimately started with a horseshoe bat. The 2012 MERS virus began with an Egyptian tomb bat, which later transferred to a dromedary camel and then found a haven in humans. The 2002 SARS virus originated in horseshoe bats, spread to civets as an intermediary, and ultimately infected humans.

Although the intermediary for today's novel coronavirus is suspected to be a pangolin, it also originated in a bat, the Chinese Rufous Horseshoe, now scientifically accepted as the natural reservoir.

All of these zoonotic coronaviruses, as well as the H1N1 culprit, produced a particular type of pneumonia, one that features a cytokine storm. Autopsy tissue samples confirm the 1918 pandemic deaths were similar to today's pandemic casualties; both came from the cytokine storm.

Ordinary annual influenza does not cause this. It is a phenomenon common to zoonotic viruses.

The cytokine storm is an overwhelming host immune response that is often effective in killing the virus. The problem is that the flood of cytokines also often kills the host. Even if the host survives, the cytokine storm often leaves the lungs scarred and dysfunctional.

Like all viruses, the novel coronavirus is comprised of a nucleic acid genetic core covered with a protective protein capsid. It has a spike protein that locks to our human ACE-2 receptors.

ACE-2 Reflects Symptoms

Many human tissues contain ACE-2 binding sites to enable viral attachment and entry. These include heart, lung, tongue, kidney, intestine, and brain. Binding to these tissues explains many of the signs and symptoms. Tongue binding explains the loss of taste and smell. Kidney binding explains why many suffer renal failure. Intestinal binding is why 20% suffer diarrhea.

Heart binding is why many suffer heart attacks (No, it's not the chloroquine). Finally, the most lethal binding occurs deep in the lungs with the type II pneumocytes, the lung tissue involved in oxygenation. The more binding sites or ACE-2 receptors one has, the worse the initial infection.

Once this fusion between viral and host cell occurs, the next step is the transfer of the viral contents into the interior of the human cell. Imagine it like a tiny balloon bumping into a large balloon, the virus colliding with the human cell. The small balloon dents the larger, the viral fusion, and ultimately blebs inside it until this small balloon is completely free floating inside the larger. Both membranes remain intact. This process of creating a new protective enclosure is called endocytosis. As we shall see soon, both of these steps, receptor attachment and endosome formation, are blocked by chloroquine.

The endosome opens, and protease enzymes remove the protein coat of the virus. These enzymes depend on an acid environment to work. Because chloroquine prevents this acid environment, it can block protease action.

The viral RNA is translated and transcripted to create a new copy. More viral envelopes are formed to protect the delicate, newly created RNA. The formation of these pouches can be stopped by chloroquine. Finally, after the new viruses are completely formed, the delicate envelopes merge back to the host cell membrane, and the contents are released in exocytosis. Naturally, any endocytosis or exocytosis can be blocked by chloroquine as it opposes the formation of vesicles, lysosomes, and endosomes.

In simpler terms, chloroquine stops pouches from forming. And without these pouches, the virus cannot multiply.

During the coronavirus's attachment phase to spike protein to the ACE-2 receptor, a glycosylation or sugar molecule attachment must occur. Chloroquine tends to interfere with ACE-2s glycosylation, which can effectively prevent attachment. In other words, chloroquine can prevent the coronavirus from ever infecting the cell. Once the cell has become infected, chloroquine concentrates in the vesicles.

Normally, these bags contain a nurturing level of acid, conducive to the viral replication process. Chloroquine turns this acid to alkaline, which proves both hostile and lethal to the virus. The high pH prevents the protease enzymes from working. This is similar to protease inhibition in the AIDS virus, where the protease inhibitors block the final step in HIV infectivity.

In summary, chloroquine helps prevent coronavirus infection and also replication after infection.

Since chloroquine and hydroxychloroquine have been safely used for many decades, why would we not use them to benefit in this great pandemic period like better prepared countries have already done?

The Perfect Weapon

Recall that Dr. Pan Pantziarka likes to look at several factors first before repurposing a drug. He first wants to be assured that it is safe to use in humans. Since chloroquine and hydroxychloroquine both have passed phase I FDA safety trials, there is a check here. Second, he wants to see if it has worked in vitro (or in the lab). Dr. Keyaerts conducted the first in vitro study on SARS and chloroquine in 2004. He found that the typical human antimalarial dose overwhelmed the virus yielding a concentration many times greater than needed to kill it.[253] Another check.

As already described, additional in vitro studies by Dr. Vincent of the CDC confirmed the effects of chloroquine against the SARS coronavirus. Other studies showed chloroquine to be effective against a related fatal coronavirus, MERS.[254] Finally, repurposed drug experts wanted to see human trials to verify that what worked in the lab translated into actual human results against the disease.

Dr. Didier Raoult conducted the first famous pilot study comparing 20 treated infected novel coronavirus patients with 16 controls.[255] The hydroxychloroquine treated group had 70% viral eradication by day six, while the untreated group had only 12.5% eradication. The Chinese human trial looked at 100 infected hospitalized patients, all treated with hydroxychloroquine, and found the quicker resolution of fever, milder disease course, and shorter hospital stays than in the untreated group.[256] Once again, check. So, what is the hold-up?

***

More (Flawed) Human Trials

What followed next was most unexpected and noticed by most of my colleagues. There was a slew of HCQ/CQ publications in big-name medical journals, like the New England Journal of Medicine, The Lancet, and JAMA. Top journals known for their quality suddenly published implausible studies. These were uncharacteristically flawed and used questionable data, or poor methodology. Most of these, quite surprisingly, was associated with no benefit when treating hospitalized COVID-19 cases with HCQ. Once again, as I previously discussed in a prior section, when a retrospective study reveals results diametrically opposed to what the science suggests, one must first question the study design or bias.

For the layperson, it seemed that HCQ was not going to be effective in helping with the pandemic. Worse, the network news portrayed HCQ as deadly.

Many non-medical people began to fear HCQ and wanted nothing to do with a drug the media had cast as so risky, that COVID-19 death would be a preferred alternative. Even many lupus and rheumatoid arthritis patients, who had been previously stable for years on HCQ, suddenly stopped taking their medicine. The dramatic media alarmism seemed to be driven by Trump opponents who wanted to see it buried. But that did not explain the medical journal reports, which one would think were above politics. But were they?

As always, the truth was hiding in the details.

Almost without exception, the data in these curious retrospective reviews were cherry-picked to show a poor result with HCQ. A few researchers even suggested a harmful effect of HCQ, but almost without exception, these studies employed HCQ or CQ in excessive or dangerous doses, certainly not the doses usually used for lupus or arthritis.

For example, the Borba study used chloroquine, the riskier of the antimalarials. In the prior cancer section of the book, I detailed these risks and advised choosing the less toxic HCQ as an alternative.

BORBA, SOUTH AMERICA [335]

DESIGN: Prospective, Double Masked, Randomized

RESULTS: Study halted to due adverse effects in High Dose Chloroquine group

FLAWS: Potentially toxic doses of Chloroquine administered to ICU COVID-19 cases

- Study not completed

- Small sample size of 81 patients limited to ICU cases

- Study design produced "self-fulfilling prophecy"

However, the Borba team chose CQ, but they also employed it at almost ten times the usual dose. How could a drug that is usually life-saving when applied to malaria and cancer suddenly become a villain overnight?

The World Health Organization published data in 2017, indicating CQ is safe with no serious cardiac effects in malaria-related patients at standard doses despite millions of doses being used over many decades.

Could the toxicity of the drug really have worsened overnight in contrast to the decades of data showing it to be safe, or were we looking instead at a political agenda now being furthered by the leading medical journals?

I was not sure, until I starting seeing studies being retracted.

A nominal CQ dose is 200 mg once or twice per day, yet the Borba study administered 1200 mg per day in the sickest ICU cases of COVID-19. Not surprisingly, there was a 39% mortality rate. This was either from the Cytokine storm or the COVID-related cardiac damage with a toxic dose of CQ thrown in. The Borba study was so small with only 81 enrolled, that no helpful conclusions could be drawn. It could not be completed because of the high death rate, a death rate that had nothing to do with proper use of HCQ, a drug the study character-assassinated effectively but indirectly.

A similar study, RECOVERY, used potential toxic doses of HCQ, and when deaths were seen, this study was also halted and used as ammunition to discredit HCQ.

LANDRAY, RECOVERY [326]

DESIGN: Prospective Randomized

RESULTS: Study halted after preliminary results of HCQ patients were compared to control and rates of mortality from COVID-19 were similar. No decrease in death associated with HCQ

FLAWS: Unusually high doses of HCQ, 2400 mg first day, 9600 mg ten day course

- Other drugs in the study did not get interim review. HCQ singled out.

- Usually studies are halted due to adverse outcomes, not neutral ones.

- Study design produced "self-fulfilling prophesy"

- Study not completed

Safe doses of HCQ are considered 400 mg twice a day for loading, then 400 mg per day for lupus or 400 mg once per week for COVID-19 prophylaxis. RECOVERY administered 2400 mg of HCQ on the FIRST DAY, an unheard-of dose, which some experts claim is life-threatening.[326]

HCQ is considered safe by the WHO.

Another study by Mehra and colleagues appeared in a prestigious journal, The Lancet. The Mehra study was so flawed that it was retracted after a group of more than 200 academic physicians exposed its biases.[327]

MEHRA, LANCET [327]

CONFLICT: One author founded Surgisphere, the company that compiled the data

DESIGN: Large Retrospective Data Review

FINDINGS: HCQ with or without macrolide associated with increased in-hospital mortality and death. <u>Study Retracted.</u>

FLAWS: Inconsistencies in the data prompted a request for data audit by the scientific community.

- Major conflict of interest with CEO of Surgisphere as coauthor

- When data could not be verified, the authors could no longer vouch for the veracity of the data sources, and the paper was retracted.

The Mehra study was the most extreme of the flawed anti-HCQ reviews. It purported to show that HCQ was associated with higher death rates in institutions around the world. Media, government, regulators, and anti-Trump pundits seized the moment and immediately published front-page dire reports associating HCQ with death. World Health bodies immediately halted any use of HCQ in COVID-19 in the hospital, outside the hospital, or in any setting outside a clinical trial. Meanwhile, the institutional review boards were reluctant to approve any new clinical trials in a drug that might kill patients.

The only problem was that the data were impossible.

A group of scientists blew the whistle on the data. They noted that the Australian deaths reported in the study cited could not have occurred as they didn't fit the known number of cases reported by the government. There were too many cases for just five hospitals and more in-hospital deaths than those in the entire country during the study period. The authors explained that it was due to a simple mix-up in transposing data from Asia to Australia.

But soon, other glaring problems appeared. There were implausible ratios of chloroquine to hydroxychloroquine in some continents. The authors claimed that in Australia, 49 received chloroquine and 50 received hydroxychloroquine. However, chloroquine was not readily available in Australia, and the administration required special approval from the government. The data were internally inconsistent, and the normal baseline variables were absent. It appeared the data had been cooked.

Busted!

Like a court witness suddenly impeached on cross-examination, the entire study collapsed. An independent audit of the data was demanded.

This review was denied due to confidentiality. Instead, the study was retracted.

Like a public figure who has been unfairly accused and then convicted through front-page headlines, only to later be exonerated with barely a whisper on the back page, HCQ was acquitted.

But the damage had been done. And no one would ever consider HCQ again for COVID-19. That is no one with a closed mind.

However, new results appeared showing clear benefits with HCQ. The retrospective review from New York by Dr. Carlucci showed that the combination of HCQ and Zinc was associated with reduced in-hospital COVID-19 mortality, decreased need for mechanical ventilation, decreased admission to ICU, and increased frequency of being discharged home.[328] The reduction in the death was significant at almost 50%.

CARLUCCI, NYU GROSSMAN [328]

DESIGN: Retrospective Review

RESULTS: 50% reduction in mortality of COVID-19 with HCQ and Zinc

FLAWS: Retrospective design

- Results not peer-reviewed

A second study then found similar results, with more than a 50% reduction in hospital death with early use of HCQ. This study was done at the Henry Ford Hospital Group, and was one of the best designed and higher-powered studies. In contrast to the flawed Geleris Study, where HCQ could be used in varying doses and at any point late in the hospitalization, the Henry Ford study employed HCQ at strict dosing early and consistently. 82 % received their initial dose within the first day of admission, and 91% within the first two days.

ARSHAD, HENRY FORD [334]

DESIGN: Retrospective Review

RESULTS: Reduced mortality in early treated HCQ group of hospitalized COVID-19 patients

FLAWS: Retrospective non-randomized review albeit with better numbers and more consistent application of HCQ dosage with frequency, dose, and time (a strength, not a flaw).

Whereas there were only 1371 patients in the Geleris group, Henry Ford studied 2,541 cases. In Geleris, even a patient given a single dose of HCQ on his last day of life could be counted as an HCQ failure, while Henry Ford required the full five-day early course. Naturally, Henry Ford patients treated with HCQ fared better. They had a 13.5% mortality rate compared to the untreated group at 26.4%.[334]

GELERIS, NEJM [331]

DESIGN: Retrospective Review

FINDINGS: HCQ associated with no effect on death or intubation in hospitalized COVID-19 patients.

FLAWS: HCQ group was sicker.
• Small sample size of 1376 patients.
• HCQ could be given late in disease and just before death.

They saw no major cardiac arrhythmias, which made perfect sense as the doses were low. FORD dosed 400 mg HCQ twice the first day followed by 400 mg per day for the next four days, unlike the RECOVERY trial, which dosed 2400 mg the first day, followed by 800 mg per day for nine more days.

The FORD patients received 2,400 mg in total, while the RECOVERY patients got hit with a whopping 9,600 mg. Did you know that even water, given in high enough doses can cause death by water intoxication? I would bet, if a scientist was motivated, he could design a study that could make water look dangerous.

The infamous Magagnoli VA study looked at only 384 male veterans, and the dose of HCQ was not disclosed. This was another study, similar to Geleris, where a patient could be given a single dose of HCQ on their deathbed, yet still counted as an HCQ failure. Based on the study design, a patient could have been unconscious, on the ventilator, and the HCQ could have been administered through a nasogastric tube. With the death rate approaching 90% in these patients, such use of HCQ is neither fair nor good science.

MAGAGNOLI VA [332]

DESIGN: Retrospective Review

FINDINGS: HCQ alone or in combination with Azithromycin not associated with death or need for mechanical ventilation in hospitalized COVID-19 patients.

FLAWS: HCQ treatment group was sicker.

- Small sample size; only 384 patients

- Sample not representative; all males.

- Results not peer-reviewed.

- Study conducted by Opthalmology Department: Infectious Disease not involved.

- No consistent HCQ dosing. Doses not included in data.

- HCQ could be given late in disease, and just before death.

One had to wonder if the rushed trials were designed to set up HCQ for failure. That is an opinion shared by the majority of my colleagues. Once again, I refer the reader to their comments in APPENDIX F.

An additional study reported in the Indian Journal of Medicine suggests that healthcare workers who use HCQ prophylactically every week have a lower risk of contracting COVID-19 infection.[329] Doses were 400 mg twice the first week, followed by 400 mg once weekly. This was a prospective controlled study.

CHATTERJEE, IJMR [329]

DESIGN: Case Controlled Review

RESULTS: 80% reduction in COVID-19 infection in HCW with weekly HCQ use

FLAWS: Small sample size

- Non-blinded design

This was unlike the Boulware study, which found no benefit with HCQ in prevention, yet conveniently failed to confirm most COVID-19 cases with testing.[330] The Indian Prevention Study confirmed all their cases with PCR, and HCQ worked well.

BOULWARE, NEJM [330]

CONFLICTS: Funding by NIAD

DESIGN: Prospective   Randomized   Placebo-Controlled Double Blind

RESULTS: After suspected SARS-Co-V-2 exposure, the incidence of suspected COVID-19 did not differ significantly between the HCQ and non-HCQ groups.

FLAWS: Only 3% of suspected COVID-19 cases were confirmed by PCR testing

- No HCQ started for up to four days post-exposure

- Subjective reports were the basis for diagnosing COVID-19

- Many subjects were aware they were taking HCQ

- Groups were younger, and none were hospitalized

- Small sample size of 821 and lack of disease certainty

Indian health care workers who took more than four HCQ doses experienced a 40% reduced risk of infection. Those who took more than six doses experienced an 80% reduction in the infection rate.

Of the 172 cases who used HCQ at normal doses, no significant drug reactions were reported. The three most common side effects were nausea, headache, and diarrhea at around 5% each. There were no harmful arrhythmias. Less than 2% reported skin rashes.

The Indian researchers noted a slight INCREASE in the rate of infections after the first two and three doses in the healthcare workers thought to be due to a "false sense of security" where those who took the drug felt they might be more protected and became sloppier with their PPE use.

It would behoove anyone who chooses HCQ prevention with their doctor's full supervision and support, to continue strict PPE and infection control and not rely solely on the drug.

Finally, Dr. Vladimir Zelenko, who had observed remarkable success anecdotally with the triple therapy of Zinc, Azithromycin, and Hydroxychloroquine, published results of a clinical trial in on July 3rd, 2020, exactly one month after the Mehra retraction.

In this retrospective case study involving 712 confirmed COVID-19 outpatients, 141 were treated with triple therapy within about four days of symptoms.[336] They were measured against a control group of 377 untreated and infected patients. Four of the 141 required hospitalization (2.8%). This was significantly less than the 58 of 377 untreated (15.4%) patients. One patient (0.7%) died in the treatment group versus 13 patients (3.5%) in the untreated group. The conclusion was that treatment of COVID-19 outpatients as soon as possible after symptom onset with triple therapy was associated with significantly less hospitalization and five times less all-cause death.

In sum, the lab studies of HCQ's expected benefit against COVID-19 have been confirmed by the better-designed, non-biased trials, namely the Henry Ford study in the U.S., the Chatterjee case series in India, and the Scholz, Derwand, and Zelenko series in New York.

Again, what science suggests should occur in studies usually does, UNLESS the data are cooked, or there is a consistent review bias, which unfortunately has been the case with HCQ and COVID-19. Many of my colleagues suggest in APPENDIX F that had Trump not mentioned HCQ, we would not have seen such a violent backlash against it.

Would most doctors use it or prescribe it for their high-risk patients or themselves? The answer is a resounding yes. Doctor Oz, Dr. Amen, Dr. Colyer, are prominent and highly visible examples of this, but the rheumatologists, cardiologists, ophthalmologists, and family physicians quoted in APPENDIX F remain the hundreds of others that I base this conclusion on.

You, the reader, must ask yourself that if a cardiologist isn't worried about cardiac issues with HCQ, and an Ophthalmologist isn't worried about eye issues, then why would a non-medical person be so convinced the drug was too dangerous to consider? You, the reader, must also ask yourself why most practicing physicians like myself, and most in APPENDIX F don't agree with the media interpretation and party line that "HCQ has no place in the treatment of COVID-19."

Why is it that rheumatologists, those who specialize in treating patients with lupus, notice that COVID-19 is rare in these patients? Why is it that patients who take HCQ daily for their lupus are so protected that even if they contract COVID-19, they rarely die? Read Dr. Olga Goodman's comments in APPENDIX F in this regard. She is a triple board-certified rheumatologist and an expert voice.

Why Appendix F?

There are more than 100 physician comments in this section. Why should you read it when most people skip the Appendix?

Consider this comment:

Dr. Michael Rosenblatt,

"Fair point. However, if you look at the comments made by physicians and nurses regarding this issue, you will find it is consistently against this Lancet "study". Since I have been posting on Medscape, I have found posters to be dispassionate, logical thinkers, even if I disagree with some of them sometimes.

This opens the possibility that the Lancet "review" was very poorly constructed and politically motivated. And Mainstream press ran with it.

Medscape opinions are not accessible to people without degreed medical training. Perhaps it should be opened up to allow more people to read it."

Through this book, you can now see these comments, usually unavailable for viewing by the public. I am convinced that if everyone in our nation had access to practicing physicians' thoughts and opinions, and not just the "talking heads" on television or the internet, they would have a different view of this crisis.

Please take the time to read the physician's comments in APPENDIX F.

I would ask everyone to use their critical thinking in this regard because I am not trying to win any debate or influence any election. I merely want to help patients and doctors use repurposed drugs to save lives, whether a person is threatened by cancer or the coronavirus.

We may be facing a second wave of the pandemic cases this fall, witnessing the infection of not just millions more, but billions more worldwide. The issue of HCQ is not trivial or political. It is medical and scientific.

Everyone should ask their doctor if they are at high risk, and whether they should be prescribed HCQ early or preventatively.

What remains disturbing is the rash of non-peer-reviewed studies and halted trials that used HCQ at excessively high, or inconsistent doses, often in near-death patients. These studies were not fair or up to usual scientific standards, and were done so poorly that some merited retraction.

What remains annoying is the damage done by these flawed studies to the reputation of a drug that basic science told us should work and that China and France showed us did work. As one colleague stated about the distortions, "It would be laughable if the results were not so devastating."

As with antibiotics, early treatment is more effective than late. As one physician put it, saying HCQ is associated with poor outcomes simply because it was only given to the sickest cases late in the disease is like giving an aspirin to someone about to jump off a bridge, and claiming that aspirin use is associated with death.

Indeed, no reputable medical journal would publish such a study linking aspirin with fatalities, but strangely and inexplicably that occurred more than once with HCQ and late-stage COVID-19. These strange publications did not pass "the smell test."

HCQ & HUMAN STUDIES ON SARS-CoV-2

Time Given	Name of Study	Effectiveness
As an Outpatient		
Very Early:	Pre-Exposure (Chatterjee[329])	80% Reduced Infections
Early:	First Symptoms (Scholz[336])	80% Reduced Deaths 84% Reduced Hospitalization
As an Inpatient		
Early: 1st Hospital Day:	Henry Ford[334]	50% Reduced Deaths
Late: ICU or Ventilator.	Geleris[331]	0% Reduction in Deaths

Studies not included: Gautret Series[255, 320], Yao[338], Carlucci[328], Magagnoli[332], Borba[335], Rosenberg[333], and Mehra[327] due to lack of peer review, small size, poor design, cherry-picking, lack of data transparency, retraction, or use of toxic, excessive or unclear dosing. Gautret, Yao, and Carlucci all found benefit, while Magagnoli, Borba, Rosenberg, and Mehra all found detriment or no benefit.

I would encourage interested readers to see the APPENDIX F physician comments, which describe in vivid and unvarnished terms the medical community's interpretation and reaction to these studies. The above review represents a fair and overall summary of my colleagues' response to the studies to date, and their views on HCQ after reviewing more than one hundred of their comments. Clearly, HCQ has a beneficial effect on either preventing or treating the infection, and the studies strongly suggest that the earlier it is used at normal or low doses in high-risk cases, the better.

This is perhaps the best time to point out that all drugs have potential adverse effects, some serious and some mild. One potential toxic effect of HCQ is vision loss; however, this is known to occur rarely at less than 2% of patients with long-term use, that is five to ten years of daily use or longer; certainly not in a five-day course. The other potential serious effect is Torsades de Pointes or life-threatening cardiac arrhythmia. However, this is almost unheard of in HCQ as it occurs more with chloroquine. I do not recommend anyone use chloroquine if HCQ can be used instead. Even with chloroquine, as I will discuss later, its occurrence is so rare that this cardiac arrhythmia is more likely to happen with a Z-pak. If Z-paks don't worry you, then neither should a properly prescribed dose of HCQ.

Finally, if one has an inherited condition called G6P deficiency, one should take HCQ with extra caution as there is a greater chance for a condition termed hemolytic anemia. However, recent studies state there is no data to support G6PD testing before prescribing HCQ or withholding it among African American patients with G6PD deficiency.[337] Once again, your doctor will review this with you before deciding whether to prescribe it.

Most of my colleagues believe that Zinc is a necessary addition to HCQ. HCQ functions as an ionophore, which means that it helps Zinc enter the cell to prevent viral replication. Zinc supplementation, without an ionophore, is not expected to be useful as the Zinc ion is a charged particle, and cannot easily enter the cell. Once again, I do not advise anyone take HCQ or any other drug to prevent or treat COVID-19 without the close counsel, supervision, and agreement by their personal physician.

***

Much like oncologists, virologists are vehemently opposed to the use of repurposed drugs to treat viruses.[257] Virologists much prefer vaccines, a more precise way to target them. Like oncologists, virologists do not want a dirty drug, one with multiple or pleiotropic effects. Oncologists prefer the targeted expensive laser approach, such as monoclonal antibodies. Virologists prefer the targeted approach with vaccines. The problem is that a vaccine, like an FDA phase II or phase III clinical trial, can take years to develop.

EFFECTS OF HCQ AGAINST SARS/MERS

• Interferes with Viral Fusion	Under-glycosylation of ACE-2 receptor
• Interferes with Viral Entry	Inhibiting Endocytosis
• Inhibits Viral Replication	Alkalinizing Lysosomes
• Inhibits Proteases	Alkalinizing Lysosomes
• Inhibits Viral Exocytosis	Alkalinizing Lysosomes
• Modulates Cytokine Storm	Reducing TNF-alpha and Cytokines

President Trump stated, "I think Tony (Anthony Fauci) would disagree with me... (but) we have a pandemic, we have people dying now." Trump added that he had already spoken with the FDA and been frustrated by the agency's pace. "They indicated they would start working on it right away. It could take a year. I said, what do you mean a year? We have to have it tonight."

The FDA relented and issued approval for HCQ to treat COVID-19 in selected cases.

Dr. Keyaerts, the Belgian scientist who first studied chloroquine's inhibition of the coronavirus in 2004, proposed that chloroquine could also benefit those infected by modulating the immune system. Since the hosts' over-reactive immune response, not the virus per se, kills most of the casualties, this made great sense.

Indeed, the science suggests immune modulation by chloroquine may work. In addition to preventing and treating the coronavirus infection, CQ and HCQ can normalize the immune response to increase survival. That is one reason that Belgium's protocol was instituted which mandated hospitals to treat COVID-19 infected patients with hydroxychloroquine barring any contraindication.[258]

Numerous anecdotal reports have surfaced about hospitalized patients on death's doorstep, finally receiving the drug and then experiencing a relatively rapid recovery. Some scientists dismiss these off as unscientific and anecdotal reports; however, the best researchers believe that scientists have an ethical obligation to look into why terminal cancer survivors beat the odds with reasoned investigation. Scientists should not simply sweep inconvenient data under the rug. Similarly, when patients amid a cytokine storm suddenly improve when HCQ is added, perhaps scientists should look closer.

Chapter 14

THE CYTOKINE STORM

The cytokine storm was responsible for most of the 1918 Spanish flu deaths and is also responsible for most of our current casualties in the 2020 coronavirus pandemic. Recall the cytokine storm is why the zoonotic viruses are so lethal and why they can lead to pandemics. The cytokine storm can be likened to gunfire. Your body fires bullets at the virus, with some hitting their targets, and some missing and ripping through normal tissue.

While a normal viral response might be a few bullets with very little collateral damage, the cytokine storm is more like massive machine-gunning in a war zone. In very little time, lungs and heart can be damaged and scarred beyond repair by our own immune system. This is what makes the cytokine storm so deadly and why it must be avoided.

What exactly is the cytokine storm, and what can we do to stop it? The answer has to do with exactly why those with diabetes, heart disease, cancer, and those older than 50 die at a much greater frequency. Why are children and young adults under age 20 relatively safe and protected from this? No one is sure of the reason.

Dr. Didier Raoult, one of the greatest minds in the viral community, offered an opinion. He proposed that it might be through the process of ADE (antibody-dependent enhancement) due to prior exposure to other coronaviruses.[259] ADE modulates immune responses and can cause sustained inflammation in a cytokine storm. Dr. Raoult noted that the first four strains of coronavirus were non-lethal and began appearing in the 1960s. They are genetically similar to the three lethal strains.

Many Americans test positive for antibodies to these first four strains. However, the coronavirus spiked protein epitopes seem to be remarkably similar through the coronavirus strains and can produce ADE in theory. Since older people are generally more likely to have been exposed to the 1960s or 1970s early coronaviruses, it makes sense why older people are at higher risk for the cytokine storm. While this may not be the full explanation, the reality is that those who survive the cytokine storm often develop pulmonary fibrosis or scarring of their lungs.

One study revealed that survivors of SARS, one year later, had a 33% incidence of residual pulmonary function deficits.[260] Pulmonary fibrosis can be reduced with the addition of chloroquine. Along with the cytokine storm, overactivity of TGF-beta can precipitate the development of pulmonary fibrosis. Recall that TGF-beta is our bad actor in cancer. However, TGF beta can also harm us in a pandemic; it can facilitate pulmonary fibrosis in zoonotic influenza. As it blocks TGF in cancer, chloroquine can also help protect us from the viral wrath of TGF-beta in this pandemic.[261]

Blocking Interleukins and TNF-Alpha

It can soften the immune response by a variety of mechanisms. Both hydroxychloroquine and chloroquine help reduce harmful signaling. It helps block p38 MAPK. Activation of MAPK is frequently required by viruses to replicate.[262] Chloroquine inhibits a variety of inflammatory cytokines such as interleukin 1, interleukin 6, and TNF-factor alpha—all integral parts of the cytokine storm.

Chloroquine helps reduce thrombosis or blood clotting, which is thought to be a major complication of the cytokine storm. Studies show that the antimalarials increase survival in lupus patients by decreasing the rate of thromboses by up to 80%.[263]

In the Dengue virus model, chloroquine inhibits alpha, beta, and gamma interferons. It helps inhibit interleukin six and interleukin 12, all inflammatory cytokines.[264] The action of chloroquine helps normalize the immune response. Chloroquine is well-known in immune models to reduce inflammation. It acts against a range of viral diseases, as well as rheumatoid arthritis, systemic lupus, and sarcoidosis.

Macrophages and monocytes can produce harmful cytokines. Chloroquine can help neutralize lethal damage caused by the cytokine storm as well as prevent and treat novel coronavirus pneumonia.

However, nothing can reverse the scarring to the heart and lungs once the cytokine storm has inflicted its damage. Therefore, HCQ must be started early in the disease, preferably before the storm takes hold. What is the main reason for some getting the cytokine storm, while others avoid it? My hunch is that it is related to how much ACE-2 one expresses, and this is related to the angiotensin-renin system.

Too Much ACE-2

A most significant risk factor, in my opinion, is the novel coronavirus portal of entry, the ACE-2 receptor. ACE-2 is also known as angiotensin-converting enzyme 2, not to be confused with the more commonly known ACE or angiotensin-converting enzyme 1. ACE-2 was not even discovered until after 2000. ACE-1 is commonly known to block the over-reactive renin-angiotensin system, which is a common pathway in the development of hypertension or high blood pressure.

ACE1 inhibitors like enalapril, captopril, and lisinopril or other "prils" are blood pressure lowering drugs that block the conversion of angiotensin I to angiotensin II. Angiotensin II is a potent vasoconstrictor and instigator of high blood pressure. Renin is converted to angiotensin I with angiotensinogen. Angiotensin I is then converted to angiotensin II with ACE-1. Therefore, an ACE inhibitor works great in reducing blood pressure with a minimum of side effects except for chronic cough, its most common side effect.

ARBs, angiotensin receptor blockers, work just as well or better by blocking the renin-angiotensin system, but they do not block angiotensin I conversion to angiotensin II. Instead, they block the action of angiotensin II combining to the receptor. In so doing, this lowers blood pressure without producing a cough.

Either ARBs or ACE-1 inhibitors are prescribed to almost 20% of the US population. With the discovery of ACE-2 was the discovery of a parallel and distinct renin-angiotensin system pathway. ACE-2 is an enzyme that converts angiotensin II to A1-7. This is a hepatoprotein that binds to the MAS receptor and has opposing effects to angiotensin II. A1-7 lowers blood pressure, reduces inflammation, and works as a vasodilator. This makes ARBs a bit healthier than ACE-1 inhibitors because ARBs stimulate ACE-2 conversion of angiotensin II to A1-7.

The potential problem we see is that both ACE-1 inhibitors and ARBs upregulate ACE-2 in animal models by as much as three to fivefold.[265] ACE-2 is considered healthy as it tends to favor healing in inflamed lungs.[266] With extra ACE-2 portals, the novel coronavirus has a much easier time entering and infecting cells. The more ACE-2 one has, the quicker and worse the initial COVID-19 infection.

A prominent Australian cardiologist worries. Dr. Murray Esler, director of the Baker Heart and Diabetic Institute of Melbourne, Australia, is a cardiologist and cardiovascular neuroscientist. "The crucial point is that angiotensin receptor blocker drugs increase ACE-2expression remarkably, which is a significant demerit, emphasized by the fact that one favored path of vaccine development is immunological antagonism of the ACE-2 binding site for the SARS-CoV-2 virus spike protein. We have presented the hypothesis that prescribing of angiotensin receptor- blocking drugs during the COVID-19 pandemic might possibly be harmful, and suggests that other antihypertensive drugs are preferred."[267]

Most medical societies including the European Society of Cardiology have warned patients not to discontinue or change their blood pressure medications as the evidence is unclear at this time.[268]

Human studies do not show upregulation of ACE-2 in all cases with ARBs or ACE-1 use.

Some research suggests that continuing the use of ARB and ACE for hospitalized COVID-19 patients might actually improve outcomes because elevated levels of ACE-2 can facilitate the healing of ARDS (adult respiratory distress syndrome).[266] It is a complicated issue as having too much ACE-2 early in the COVID-19 disease facilitates viral infection and entry. However, late in the disease, more ACE-2 can actually help heal the inflamed lungs. The SARS-CoV-2 infection downregulates ACE-2 by damaging cells, thereby causing their destruction and disposal.

High Blood Pressure and ACE-2

Therefore, we see a double whammy with a high blood pressure patient on ACE or ARB. He has too much ACE-2 early on in the disease, which speeds the COVID-19 infection. Late in the disease, when he needs ACE-2 to heal, it has been destroyed already by the virus. Beyond the question of changing medications to calcium channel or beta blockers, there is an alarming fact.

A human study by Dr. Tomos Walters found the patients with atrial fibrillation had higher levels of ACE-2.[269] Indeed, ACE-2 is upregulated in cardiac remodeling as occurs in patients with LVH (left ventricular hypertrophy) or long-standing hypertension. Additionally, a study by Dr. Ramchard revealed that the higher the ACE-2 activity, the greater the chance of major cardiac adverse event or hospitalization.[270]

Likely, older patients with long-standing high blood pressure (over decades) have greater cardiac remodeling, LVH, and atrial fibrillation and, therefore, higher levels of ACE-2 regardless of the medications they take. What are the implications?

First, look at the data. Hypertension was considered the major risk factor for coronavirus death by a prominent Chinese researcher. The director of the Intensive Care Unit of the Peking Union Medical Center Hospital, is Dr. Du Bin. He stated, "From what I was told by the other doctors and the data I can see for myself, hypertension is a key dangerous factor among all the underlying diseases."[271]

Dr. Bin is one of the most respected critical care experts in China. He said, "Though there is no research published on that yet, we believe hypertension could be an important factor in causing patients to deteriorate, leading to a bad prognosis. We keep an eye on older people and those with high blood pressure. They are the key focus."

If we look at the deaths in Lombardy, Italy, perhaps we can gain another clue. Lombardy is a prosperous region in Northern Italy and harbors an older geriatric population. Italian authorities looked at medical records to see why the death rate was so high. At the time of this writing, it was in excess of 10%. This was more than double China's.

One source from Bloomberg reported that the average age of Italian death was 79.5, with over 75% with high blood pressure.[272] Indeed, the greater age and incidence of hypertension compared with China might explain the greater death rate in Italy. Side-by-side comparison of Italy and China is suggestive that hypertension combined with old age are the key factors, just as Dr. Du Bin suggested.

For example, between ages 70 and 79, the Italian death rate was 12.8%, while in China, the rate for the same age group was 8%. For example, in Italy, the death rate for the age 60-69 age group was 3.5%, while it was 3.6% in China. Between ages 50-59 the Italian death rate was 1.0%, whereas in China it was 1.3%. In the oldest group age 80-89, the Italian death rate was 20.2%, whereas in China it was only 14.8%.[273]

The incidence of hypertension in those older than age 65 in China is approximately 55%. However, in the US and Italy, it is more like 70%. However, in the US, hypertension is better controlled, and there is greater awareness in the US than in Italy.

Old age, high incidence of hypertension, and poor blood pressure control all seem to be major factors in explaining Italy's high death rate. Metabolic syndrome or insulin resistance is heavily related to the risk of diabetes, hypertension, and even cancer and was the subject of my other book, *The Coffee Cure Diet*.[274]

At the beginning of this book, I noted that 40% of all cancers are spawned by insulin resistance. Now it appears that insulin resistance has a major impact on the lethality of the COVID-19 infection by increasing risks for hypertension and activation of the renin-angiotensin system. There is no question in my mind that anyone age 50 or greater is in a high-risk group. Male deaths outnumber females in Italy by more than 2:1. Being male and over age 50 makes a person high-risk. Being female and under age 50 creates a lower risk situation.

If hypertension is added to any of these groups, the risks increase. It is tempting to recommend that any one male greater than age 50 and with hypertension or insulin resistance be treated preventively with hydroxychloroquine.

Basic prevention calls for the dosage used in India at 400 mg per week, the dose they use in healthcare workers or high-risk individuals.[275] The data on humans are not in for the optimal dose in coronavirus prevention. The preventative dose may need to be adjusted higher in those with all risk factors (i.e., greater than age 50, male, hypertension).

Rather than reduce the number of ACE-2 receptors by changing blood pressure medications, which might not make much difference in those at high-risk, prophylactic treatment with antivirals might be the most useful strategy.

SECTION VI:
THE POLITICS OF THE CORONAVIRUS

Chapter 15

THE DEMONIZATION OF HYDROXYCHLOROQUINE

The real obstacle to resolving the coronavirus pandemic has not been science. In Michigan on March 27, 2020, the governor issued an order that doctors and pharmacists who prescribe and dispense HCQ for COVID-19 might face a loss of license.[276] The governor of Nevada issued a similar directive that prohibited the dispensing of HCQ for coronavirus.[277] Other states followed suit. In California, despite a prescription, many pharmacies refuse to dispense the drug citing company policy.

Dr. Zelenko, a New York physician, treated 669 COVID-19 patients with a cocktail comprised of HCQ, zinc, and azithromycin. He achieved a 99.9% success rate with only four patients requiring hospitalization and two requiring ventilation or intensive care.[278] There was only one death. Dr. Zelenko reported that with this cocktail, he saw symptoms of shortness of breath resolve within four to six hours.

Our greatest enemy in this pandemic has not been the science or a lack of studies. It remains overzealous regulation. HCQ has been proven in vitro to both prevent and treat novel coronavirus infection. It softens the cytokine storm. Our country's strategy has been sanitizing, quarantining, and social distancing. It has been to create more make-shift ICUs and to build more ventilators.

An Ounce of Prevention

What if we followed the protocol set by India's ministry of health? Health care providers would be required to take HCQ once per week as prophylaxis.[279] All infected patients and their household contacts would be treated with a one week course of HCQ. It certainly has worked for India. They have among the lowest per infection and death rates as a country in the world. And no one in India is dying from HCQ despite what you may hear and read in the US media.

Our country could re-open. We would be able to function well until a vaccine is developed.

As for the scientific basis for arbitrary regulation and rules concerning coronavirus, studies in China show that coronavirus patients shed a virus for an average of 19-20 days with some remaining infectious for up to 34 days. So much for the US policy of fourteen-day quarantines.

One day, the government reports that masks are unnecessary for non-medical personnel. Later, we find that they really are necessary, but that the recommendations were made only to ration the supply.

Furthermore, on the one hand, we hear that it is far too dangerous to consider chloroquine as the drug can cause sudden cardiac arrest, blindness, or kidney failure. At the same time, it is freely dispensed to millions around the world every day and has passed Phase I FDA safety trials. Which is it? Either the drug is safe, or it is not.

But, please do not mislead everyone.

The bottom line is that in our brave new world of the 21st century, we must question everything the government and regulators tell us. We must do our own due diligence. I might add, conduct your own scientific research on PubMed because the standard news channels will not lead you to the truth. Rally for laws that allow doctors and patients together to decide what should be prescribed free of pharmacy and government interference.

That interference is usually not coming from a valid scientific basis, but instead from a financial, political, or regulatory standpoint. Stand up for your right as a patient to receive your Zelenko treatment. Speak up for your right to receive the most effective repurposed drugs for your disease, whether it be terminal cancer, coronavirus, or even diabetes. Perhaps, start with insisting upon access to HCQ now for both prevention and treatment of coronavirus infection.

The Simplest and Cheapest to Treat

In the words of Dr. Didier Raoult, "A movement to reposition drugs has been initiated in recent years. In this strategy, it is important to be able to use drugs that have been proven to be harmless and whose pharmacokinetics and optimal dosages are well-known. In the current episode of novel coronavirus, COVID-19, we find a spectacular example of possible repositioning of drugs particularly chloroquine. If the current data confirmed the biologic results, the novel coronavirus associated disease will have become one of the simplest and cheapest to treat and prevent infectious respiratory disease." [280]

Anecdotes become Antidotes

Regulation is like government. We need a reasonable amount of each to protect society. The problem comes with overly-harsh restrictions that deprive society of access to potentially life-saving repurposed drugs. Regulators traditionally favor the development of expensive and dangerous chemotherapies over cheap non-branded repurposed drugs that may work better.

Remdesivir, although not currently widely available and still in testing, does not have decades of safety data like HCQ. At $50 per month, HCQ is cheap and there are no large profits to be had. The old guard typically will use fear to herd the lay public in their direction. "Do not use aspirin for cancer treatment, it might cause bleeding," as Jane McLelland with stage IV cancer was warned. "Do not use Celebrex as it could cause kidney failure," as Matt De Silva's father with terminal glioblastoma was warned. "Do not use HCQ as it can cause blindness and fatal cardiac arrhythmias," was the drumbeat pounded by the media over these past few months.

Never mind that the drugs aspirin, Celebrex, and hydroxychloroquine have been used for decades safely and passed FDA phase I human safety trials.

When world-renowned researcher Dr. Didier Raoult announced the results of his coronavirus hydroxychloroquine trial, they were quickly dismissed as "anecdotal." When Dr. Ben Williams took a repurposed drug cocktail and survived his glioblastoma, this was described as a "coincidence." When Jane McLelland survived her terminal cancer using off-label drug cocktails, her survival was also considered an interesting fluke. When Dr. Angela Chapman survived her terminal cancer by strategically adding repurposed supplements and drugs, you guessed it, another anecdote.

Repurposed drug use in cancer is no longer considered anecdotal evidence. The hundreds of studies pioneered by Dr. Pan Pantziarka and the ReDO project researchers have gone global. The evidence in favor of using repurposed drugs for cancer is monumental, including the use of chloroquine. The Care Oncology Clinic is collecting data on scores of GBM patients who are living longer because of it. Now with the coronavirus pandemic, we hear, once again, the familiar refrains of danger and anecdotes.

Dr. Jeff Colyer wrote an Op-Ed in the Wall Street Journal calling for the widespread use of hydroxychloroquine.[281] "We have a drug with an excellent safety profile, but limited clinical outcome and no better alternatives until long after this disaster peaks." He writes that it would be a mistake not to use it quickly.

Dr. Anthony Cardillo, director of the MEND Urgent Care Clinics based in Los Angeles, has had similar experiences with many of his patients.[282] "Every patient I have prescribed it to have been very, very ill, and within eight to 12 hours, they were basically symptom-free." More anecdotes.

Dr. Rob Richardson faced a catastrophe when nine patients at the Allworth Veterans' Hospital developed COVID-19.[283] With almost 150 elderly residents, Dr. Richardson did what any responsible physician would do. He used hydroxychloroquine to stem the outbreak. Eight of the nine survived, including 104-year-old William Lapschies, who also had survived the Spanish flu pandemic in 1918. When the Oregon Medical Board attempted to outlaw the use of hydroxychloroquine, Dr. Richardson protested citing his success in the Lebanon, Oregon, nursing home. The Oregon board made an exception to allow HCQ for nursing home patients.[284]

Staten Island Borough President James Oddo petitioned Governor Cuomo to allow the use of HCQ in New York nursing homes due to the extreme risk in close-quartered elderly.[285] Cuomo agreed. In Florida, Dr. Marlow Hernandez, CEO Cano Health in Miami, uses it across 45 facilities and encompassing some 60,000 patients.[286] "We are using it selectively for those who do not have contraindications, for those who have high-risk symptoms." She addressed the usual regulatory objections as follows:

> Question: "What about concerns about the drug, doctor? The CDC has removed it from its guidance. It does have serious side effects with the function of the heart. How can you be sure even if it is helping patients in the short run that it perhaps is causing them more long-term problems with their health?"
>
> Answer: "Sure, and that is why it should never be self-administered. It should not be used as a "preventative drug" different from if you were exposed, and you were a very high-risk patient, and then, maybe have a role for prophylaxis, then, and only then, but never in the case of self-administering without consulting a doctor."

Mixing Politics with Medicine

Dr. Hernandez focused on the real issue, "I know there is a lot of opinion out there and unfortunately, the introduction of politics into the mix. This is a medical issue, not a political one. Like for example, when I hear some say that there are no studies to support its use. This is just simply not correct."

Dr. Dave Lacknauth, Director of Pharmacy Services at Broward Health added, "We are a healthcare team. We have assembled a group of infectious disease physicians, intensivists, pulmonologists, and our chief medical leadership meets three times per week. This medication is medication where we, after looking at a lot of data, are using it. Its role in therapy is really kind of where we have been on the back and forth.

Right now, we are trying to get this initiated earlier on with our patient treatment once we get a confirmed positive case. Because we think that the effects of decreasing viral load will have a bigger impact if we can get this medication on board earlier. But of course, only in clinically appropriate patients. In the hospital, we have methods to monitor heart rhythm through EKG. We have cardiologists, who are also on our teams who have reviewed this and given our physicians guidance on the appropriate use of the medication based on those rhythm rate readings."

Over time and with higher numbers of studies and mounting evidence with hundreds of "anecdotes," the evidence will become obvious. This is what has already happened with repurposed drug use in cancer. It is rapidly occurring with the use of hydroxychloroquine in the current pandemic. Read the comments by the medical community in APPENIDX F to gauge the degree to which this has already occurred.

Dr. Daniel Amen is a noted California psychiatrist and founder of the Amen Clinics. He regularly appears on television and is somewhat of a celebrity. He has authored eight New York Times best-selling books.

When his parents Louis and Dolores contracted COVID-19, they received a prescription of HCQ from their son, and they both recovered within five days. His father, age 90, suffered from heart disease, and his mother at age 88 suffered from recurrent pneumonia. Dr. Amen stated that because he had graduated from medical school and had read the studies showing promising results, he decided to act. He was not content with sitting back and hoping for the best.

In retrospect, his mother, Dolores, is convinced the HCQ saved her and her husband's lives. "Thank God. It's a miracle," she said.

Her daughter Mary reported, "Hydroxychloroquine stopped the COVID in its tracks."

"I'd do it again." Daniel Amen said of prescribing HCQ for his parents.[287]

PubMed Citations

I can hear many readers asking themselves who to believe. The answer for me was easy. Beyond any science that I know, I had the most powerful truth detector at my disposal, the National Library of Medicine. It has proven immune to political agenda, fake news, conspiracy theories, social media, and all kinds of lunacy. PubMed will always lead one to the truth if one searches long enough.

For my readers, please do not base your opinion on the newspaper, internet, FOX, CNN, or even Lester Holt. I can assure you, currently the mass media is missing the mark on this subject.

Base it, instead, on PubMed. Consider this, Dr. Didier Raoult has authored or co-authored 2,909 PubMed scientific papers, and at least 30 on chloroquine, and another 49 on hydroxychloroquine.

If you examine any scientist who speaks out against Dr. Raoult's overwhelming body of research on viruses and chloroquine, simply go to PubMed and search his or her credentials. Type in their last name followed by first initial and search, and the number of their articles will come up. Hands down, Dr. Raoult is the world's foremost scientific expert on hydroxychloroquine, chloroquine, and viruses. If anyone else claims to know more, simply search their PubMed publications. Actions speak louder than words.

No one else even comes close. His treatment team was the first to use hydroxychloroquine for the treatment of intracellular micro-organism infections. His team has 30 years of such experience. He is considered the world expert on the use of chloroquine for treating Q fever. His teams have also pioneered hydroxychloroquine for the treatment of Whipple's disease, where it has become a referenced standard drug.

Dr. Raoult has personally treated 4,000 cases of Q fever with hydroxychloroquine.

I understand some of my colleagues may disagree and state that the number of publications does not translate to content accuracy or lack thereof. I fully appreciate that simply because someone has become a world authority on a drug or disease grouping, that everything he publishes may not be accurate or scientifically correct.

With that being said, I believe it is logical that such an authority's studies and opinions should be given more weight than financially-biased authors and publications lacking the same level of experience and knowledge.

In 2007, some 13 years ago, Dr. Raoult co-authored the landmark paper, "Recycling of chloroquine, and its hydroxy analog to face bacterial, fungal, and viral infections in the 21st Century."[288] When it comes to viruses and chloroquine, no other scientist equals Dr. Raoult. When evaluating criticism of Dr. Didier Raoult'studies, always consider the source of that criticism.

First, is the author even a physician? Second, how many studies have they published on PubMed? Third, how many patients have they treated with HCQ? Fourth, are they funded by any institutions or companies that might bias them? Fifth, are they a competitor of Dr. Raoult? Finally, do they know enough to attack Dr. Raoult's research with a straight face?

Chapter 16

GETTING TO THE TRUTH

This journey through repurposed drugs has taken us from cancer to coronavirus. When it became confusing with cancer treatment in terms of knowing who and what to believe, I turned to the smartest, most accomplished minds on earth. I discovered Stefan Roever, the billionaire biotech mogul who contracted GBM and treated himself. He used his company to sequence his cancer gene genetics. He hired a team of personal physicians who prescribed a cocktail of repurposed drugs. He shunned the oncology community's mediocre standard of care.

Now during the age of the 2020 coronavirus pandemic, I encountered the coronavirus equivalent of Stefan Roever. Meet Dr. Patrick Soon-Shiong, perhaps the brightest mind on the subject and the voice of optimism. Dr. Soon-Shiong, a transplant surgeon, pioneered pancreatic tissue transplants and, like Roever, went on to found multiple biotech companies. He has published 100 scientific papers and holds 230 patents. He invented the cancer drug Abraxane which is effective against lung, breast, and pancreatic cancers.

Words from the Vaccine Doctor

He sold his first large company for 4.6 billion dollars in 2008 and later sold Abraxis BioScience (maker of the drug Abraxane) for 3 billion dollars in 2010. His current company, Nantworks, a cancer research firm, is rapidly developing a vaccine against COVID-19 using natural killer T-cells.[289] His vision helped launch the National Immunotherapy Coalition to encourage pharmaceutical companies to collaborate to test drug cocktail combinations in the fight against cancer. Dr. Soon-Shiong uses supercomputers to search genome sequencing databases, much like Stefan Roever, to find solutions to cancer and viruses.

Dr. Soon-Shiong has advocated strongly for the use of repurposed drugs in this coronavirus pandemic. Until a vaccine is found, we must use medications that either prevent viral attachment, viral entry, or viral replication. Dr. Soon-Shiong feels HCQ may play a role in this.[290] In the cytokine storm, where the fatality rate is highest at about 50%, Dr. Soon-Shiong feels optimistic that mesenchymal stem cell transplants may offer hope and save many lives. Recall that mesenchymal cells are intimately involved in cancer metastasis. However, they can also be used to heal damaged lung tissue with TGF-beta, our double agent, which is tissue healing most of the time and cancer-promoting only when things go wrong.

In a controlled study of H7N9 influenza patients with ARDS, 54% of the control group died while only 17% of the MSC (mesenchymal stem cell) group died.[291] In an early non-controlled Chinese study of COVID-19 pneumonia, seven patients were treated with MSC. They tolerated the treatments without adverse effects and all improved within two days.[292] The MSC rapidly lowered the harmful C-reactive protein and helped neutralize the overactive CD 4+ cytokine secreting immune cells within three to six days.

The worst inflammatory cytokine, the TNF-alpha, was also significantly decreased by the action of the MSC. This may be the best place to add that HCQ also has immune-modulating effects that help dampen the cytokine storm. HCQ helps lupus patients by dampening their TNF-alpha levels. It does so by inhibiting toll-like receptor signaling. HCQ also helps reduce similar harmful activation in HIV patients.

HCQ DAMPENS THE CYTOKINE STORM

- Reduces TNF-alpha
- Inhibits Blood Clotting
- Reduces T cell Activation

Inhibits Toll-like Receptors 7 and 9

Inhibits Interleukin 6

Inhibits Interleukin 1

The antimalarial drug, HCG, is endowed with immune-modulating effects. However, the HCQ must be utilized at the earliest stages of the COVID-19 infection, preferably before the cytokine storm takes hold. Once the cytokine storm has begun to damage lungs, antiviral therapy has much less chance of working, and our only hope may be blocking the cytokine response through monoclonal antibodies, the use of MSC, or even donor plasma. Dr. Soon-Shiong's company is rapidly developing stem cell therapies for COVID-19, but he also reports, "Our goal is not to wait for patients to get to this stage. Our goal is to prevent patients before they get here."

He goes on, "When the cell is overtaken by the virus, the body reacts, which allows the virus to create fibrosis and damage." He further notes that it is not the virus that does all the damage. It is the body's immune response that creates a significant amount of the scarring. I truly believe that with the early use of HCQ at the milder stages of coronavirus disease, as soon as symptoms emerge, the cytokine storm can be avoided in almost all patients.

Dr. Soon-Shiong states, "Indeed, there are drugs that needed to be in clinical trials and now have recently been approved in the emergency setting: chloroquine and hydroxychloroquine."[290] Dr. Soon-Shiong feels that these may play a major role in helping in the early stages of the disease.

Metformin and HCQ Parallels

The parallels between metformin and HCQ are many. Both medications are pleiotropic with major health benefits, not just against their chosen disease. For metformin, this means diabetes. For hydroxychloroquine, it means malaria and lupus. Metformin and hydroxychloroquine both have major activity against multiple cancers.

Metformin is active against head, neck, brain, endometrial, pancreatic, colon, liver, and prostate cancers. Hydroxychloroquine has major activity against brain, breast, liver, colon, melanoma, lung, and prostate cancers. Additionally, metformin helps people live longer by reducing all-cause mortality, the chance of death from all causes.[293] Similarly, HCQ in lupus patients has been shown to help lengthen life and reduce the chance of death from all causes.[294]

METFORMIN AND HCQ

	Metformin	HCQ
All-cause mortality	Reduces	Reduces in Lupus Patients
Blood Sugar	Reduces	Reduces
Insulin Resistance	Improves	Improves
Weight	Reduces	Reduces
Inflammation	Reduces	Reduces
Risk of Heart Disease	Reduces	Reduces
Cholesterol	Reduces	Reduces
Activity Against Cancer	Strong (mTOR, Glycolysis)	Strong Autophagy blocker)

Metformin slows atherosclerosis.[295] HCQ reduces the risk of heart attack in lupus patients by 30%.[296] Metformin reduces general inflammation and specifically the C-reactive protein levels.[297] HCQ reduces general inflammation and specifically the cytokine tissue necrosis factor alpha.[298]

HCQ reduces the chance of thrombosis or fatal blood clots, a major contributing cause of death in the cytokine storm.[299] Metformin helps normalize blood sugar and reduce insulin resistance, which is a major cause of disease. HCQ, likewise, reduces blood sugar, insulin resistance, and is in widespread use in India as an antidiabetic agent.[300]

No one seems to understand the mystery of India. Why is it that exactly six months into this pandemic they have so few cases and deaths of COVID-19 in a country of 1.2 billion people?[301]

Let's look closer at the cases and deaths per million by country. As of 07/07/20, the United States suffered some 9,000 cases per million while India had only 587.

By comparison, most of Europe hovers around 3,000 cases per million. Sweden is about 7,000, while Nigeria is only 153 per million. I will let you ask yourself if anti-malarial use just might account for the difference.

I can hear the critics already. "But they don't have as much testing in India." Okay, granted. But you cannot hide ARDS deaths. They are not occurring in India with a fatality rate of only 16 per million. The US fatality rate is 30 times higher at 407 per million. The United Kingdom's fatality rate is about 684 people per million. Nigeria's is barely 3 per million. While these rates continue to rise both in India and in other countries, India's death rate per million remains far below most European and Western countries.

No one in India is dying of HCQ, and the Indian Ministry of Health continues to use it widely and effectively for prophylaxis. Their data speaks for itself.

Mighty Metformin

Let's return to metformin and HCQ for a moment. For decades the regulators worried about fatal lactic acidosis, a common feature of the biguanide class of medication. In 1978 Dr. Luft wrote, "Of the patients that developed lactic acidosis 50.3% died. From our observation, we conclude the treatment of diabetes mellitus with biguanides should be reserved for specially selected patients."[302] The fear over lactic acid and acidosis in metformin continued. In 2003, Dr. Chan wrote, "Lactic acidosis is a serious reaction to metformin and, and hemodialysis should be done urgently to prevent serious complications."[303]

Finally the issue was put to rest in 2003. Dr. Salpeter reviewed some 35,000 patient-years of data on metformin. The rate of metformin-associated lactic acidosis was only 8.1 cases per 100,000 patient-years, while the rate of non-metformin lactic acidosis was higher at

9.9 cases per 100,000 patient-years. This data revealed clearly that metformin was not associated with lactic acidosis, unlike phenformin.[304]

A similar situation of mistaken identity has occurred with HCQ. We have heard repeatedly in the media that it is associated with potentially fatal QT interval prolongation making everyone fear it. However, this fear may be costing many tens of thousands of lives as HCQ probably is our best solution. In reality, it is another antimalarial, halofantrine, that is most associated with cardiotoxicity when used at high doses.[305]

HCQ, by contrast, has been studied for decades. The data on hundreds of thousands of patients have been scrutinized. The fact of the matter is that HCQ reduces the risk of heart attack by 30% in lupus patients. There is a decreased risk of coronary artery disease in rheumatoid arthritis patients taking it.[306] Finally, a study of lupus patients revealed no increase in cardiac death compared to non-takers of HCQ.[307]

By comparison, other drugs increase the QT interval and the risk of sudden death. However, these are not in the media. Imodium, commonly used to treat diarrhea, is an over-the-counter medication. In overdoses, it can cause prolongation of the QT interval and life-threatening cardiac arrhythmias.[308, 309]

The Real QT Raising Drugs

What other medications can raise the QT interval? The common antibiotic, levofloxacin, does.[310] Azithromycin, a common antibiotic, increases the risk of fatal cardiac arrhythmia. There is a 48% increase with azithromycin used alone, and there is a 150% increase in the risk of arrhythmia using the antibiotic, levofloxacin, a relative of Cipro.[311]

In another study, there was an increased risk of cardiac death by 2.8 times with azithromycin. The author, Dr. Chou, stated, "Health professionals should consider the small but increased risk of significant increased risk of ventricular arrhythmia of cardiac death when prescribing azithromycin and moxifloxacin. Additional research is needed to determine whether the increased risk of mortality is caused by the drug or related to the severity of the infection."[312]

The bottom line is you are at greater risk for cardiac arrhythmia from common antibiotics taken every day by millions of people than by HCQ taken at normal dosage. HCQ is relatively safe, but it can help many patients live longer through decreased inflammation, improved blood sugar, and reduced coronary artery disease. India and Africa have shown us that HCQ might just be the key to blocking the coronavirus.

And if you still doubt a double standard, ask yourself why we do not see widespread media coverage about the known cardiac risks of azithromycin, which by far exceed those of HCQ? We do not hear on the nightly news or anywhere else in the headlines that the commonly-prescribed Z-pak can stop your heart. The CDC and the WHO have not mounted any media campaigns against these antibiotics.

Why exactly is that when 60 million Z-pak prescriptions are written annually? And no one ever warns you about antibiotic-related QT prolongation, Torsades de Pointes, or arrhythmia. If you are not a health care professional, I will wager that you have never heard about those conditions before the pandemic, but I'll bet you took a Z-pak. And what's more, I'll bet you didn't die from it.

Governor's Decree Against HCQ Use

In this final section, we shall examine the regulatory obstacles to repurposed drug use and possible solutions. In almost all cases, repurposed drugs are used in addition to the existing standard of care. By definition, a repurposed drug is one that has been deemed safe for human use and past rigorous FDA safety trials. Also, there is usually a wealth of additional data from years of clinical use and study. Therefore, the assumption that the drug is safe is justified.

The only criteria lacking is that the drug may or may not be effective for its new proposed use. In Evan's case, we do not have data on thousands of glioblastoma patients to yet prove the efficacy of a four-drug Care Oncology Clinic combination against GBM. However, with basic science and in vitro studies suggesting a benefit, the risk/benefit ratio is favorable. "It may help, or it may not help, but it won't kill you" is a fair statement when prescribing the prospects of any repurposed drug.

I promise you, that if you are grappling with terminal cancer, and come to an agreement with your personal physician (one whom you have developed trust through years of treatment), you will want a repurposed drug that he suggests might help. In that case, you do not want interference from the governor, politicians, or pharmacists. You simply want to live.

In America, we are all guaranteed that right to live under our US Constitution and Declaration of Independence. We are guaranteed the rights to "Life, Liberty, and the pursuit of Happiness."

"If you and your doctor agree on a prescription medication, that should go," as Dr. Freireich reminds us. No governor's "decree" should stop you, but in 46 states, that is exactly what happened with repurposed drug use of HCQ. Governors (not medical authorities) unilaterally made prescribing HCQ for COVID-19 illegal. If you were a front-line healthcare worker required to face COVID-19 infections daily, and you and your doctor decided on a prescription for HCQ to be used preventively as they do in many countries, the US pharmacist likely would not cooperate. They would not honor that prescription, and you would be forced to risk your life without it.

Consider this, at a presidential briefing in April 2020, it was announced that an IV antiviral drug, Remdesivir, had shown modest results in hospitalized COVID-19 patients. The very next day, the FDA issued an EUA (emergency use authorization) for Remdesivir to be used in seriously ill hospitalized patients.

This emergency drug authorization was unusual for a drug with no prior FDA approval. The drug had not been FDA-approved as safe, unlike HCQ. HCQ had been used since 1955 to treat malaria and later lupus. When promising results came from studies in China, South Korea, and France on HCQ, fully two months was required before the FDA granted it (the EUA) for use in hospitalized patients.

After the EUA was granted, you might have expected increased availability of HCQ.

Quite to the contrary, governors Cuomo, Sisolak, and Whitmer led the charge to impose prohibitory orders against its outpatient use. Forty-three other states followed suit. Dr. Oz stated that one could get a prescription for HCQ in New York, but "you would have to be hospitalized" to get it filled.

Double Standard

Remdesivir was declared the treatment of choice, the standard of care, both highly unusual for a drug that had not passed FDA trials, and not survived the usual peer-reviewed publication process. It was most surprising for an unapproved drug that had reported some patients seeing potentially severe adverse effects including organ dysfunction, septic shock, acute coronary syndrome, and low blood pressure.[313]

Up to 23% showed evidence of liver damage based on laboratory tests.[314] Gilead's press release commented on Remdesivir's side effects of acute respiratory failure in some 6% in the five-day treatment group, and 10.7% in the ten-day treatment group.[315] Dr. Steven Nissen, a cardiologist at the Cleveland Clinic, stated, "The disclosure of clinical trial results in a political setting before peer-review or publication is questionable."[316]

Dr. Michele Barry of Stanford warned about the government's praise of Remdesivir.

"It is unusual to call a drug the standard of care before the publication of peer-reviewed data and before the studies have shown a benefit in mortality."[317]

Professor Didier Raoult commented, "Deaths as the primary outcome was moved to a secondary outcome, and days to recover became the primary outcome measure. Changing the primary outcome before trial results are completed is highly unusual and suggests p-hacking, a manipulation of the data to get a statistically significant p-value."

By contrast, the multiple studies throughout China, South Korea, France, and the US consistently have shown that HCQ in the treatment of COVID-19 prevents infection, reduces the severity of illness, viral load, number of hospitalizations, the need for the ventilator, and time to recovery. The data on HCQ is far from anecdotal.

Dr. Elizabeth Lee Vliet wrote, "HCQ has been off-patent for decades, is available from a dozen US generic manufacturers, and is also produced in China, Israel, India, and other countries. HCQ costs the average patient less than $10. Remdesivir costs upward of $1000 per dose, plus the added cost of having to be hospitalized to receive it." Dr. Vliet felt that HCQ was unfairly passed over by regulators in favor of Big Pharma's choice.[318]

She highlights a table to support her contention. In those countries where HCQ is used early and prophylactically, they have less than a small fraction of the death rate compared to the US. The US has a 50-100 fold greater death rate than India, Costa Rica, and Australia (the countries that employ early and prophylactic use of HCQ).

Fortunately, the FDA has softened its stance. On May 19, 2020, FDA Commissioner Dr. Stephen Hahn stated, "The decision to take any drug is ultimately a decision between a patient and their doctor. Hydroxychloroquine and chloroquine are already FDA-approved for treating malaria, lupus, and rheumatoid arthritis."[319]

As of this writing, I am encouraged that we are closer to a vaccine, which I feel will turn the tide on COVID-19. In the meantime, I need to report that the weight of science, aside from bias, confirms that HCQ is not effective in the most advanced COVID-19 disease, in the throes of the cytokine storm. However, it continues to be used preventatively every week in health care workers in India with major success, and it likely has some added benefit when combined with Zinc and used early.

As in all repurposed drugs, prospective studies MUST be done to confirm promise in the lab and to make the leap to actual benefit when used in clinical practice. Dexamethasone has shown some substantial benefit in survival when used later in the hospital in advanced COVID-19 disease. Remdesivir, although not technically a repurposed drug, has also shown some benefit later in the condition. Why not be smart and ask your doctor if you might be a candidate for HCQ + Zinc prevention if you are at high risk and don't wish to contract COVID-19?

Why not consider Dr. Seheult's COVID Supplement Cocktail of Quercetin, Vitamin C, Vitamin D, and Zinc if you want to do more than wear masks and isolate in fear? Dr. Paul Marik and Dr. Roger Seheult both are critical care specialists, and they take care of the sickest ICU cases of COVID-19. Above all, they do not want to get infected. They both believe the benefits outweighs the risks in taking Vitamin C and Quercetin. Do you think they might know something most don't?[340] It is far better to prevent cancer or COVID-19 than contract it and try to cure it.

THE COVID SUPPLEMENT COCKTAIL

Quercetin 400mg	Vitamin C 90mg
Zinc 30mg	Vitamin D3 2000 IU

I cannot help but imagine if everyone took the COVID Supplement Cocktail. Would we still be seeing the current degree of pandemic carnage? I think not. If everyone with terminal cancer received repurposed cocktails in addition to their chemotherapy, we would see many more long-term survivors. If S.A.M. were widely adopted as a cancer prevention cocktail, imagine the drop we would notice in both disease and death rates.

Who's against that? You already know the answer.

Rally For Repurposed Drugs

My friend, Evan, did everything right in life. He worked hard, studied, and became a healthcare professional. He helped patients for 40 years and raised his family. He coached soccer and little league. He deserves the right to try all the repurposed drugs he and his doctor decide upon to save his life from glioblastoma.

No governor's decree should prevent that. That is exactly what is occurring now in COVID-19. A lupus patient can fill a prescription for 180 tablets of HCQ with no questions asked. If you are an ICU nurse and want to stay alive for your family's sake, your doctor's prescription for 14 HCQ tablets will be refused in Arizona, Michigan, and New York and up to 43 other states.

Dr. George Fareed is a hospitalist who practices medicine in the Imperial Valley of California where COVID-19 is rampant. He has successfully prescribed HCQ to over 1,000 patients with no deaths and rapid recoveries. Fareed believes that physicians have a moral obligation to inform and offer this option to patients. He believes it should be available in all states if a physician and patient should choose it.

Dr. Pantziarka identified a "regulatory bias" against the approval of repurposed drugs, which is a polite way of saying, the government discriminates against cheap, non-patentable medications whether they save lives or not.[45] This repurposed drug bias affects us all.

I guarantee you that one day the issue will touch you or a loved one.

Whether it is to save your life from terminal cancer or in a pandemic, the time to advocate for everyone's right to receive repurposed drugs, free from governmental interference, is now. Let us pass a law in the US, UK, and other civilized nations that ensures a person's access to repurposed drugs prescribed off-label. Call it The Right to Repurposed Drugs Act. Make it illegal to prevent a valid doctor's prescription for an FDA-approved drug from being denied for any off-label purpose provided the patient and doctor agree. Allow repurposed drugs to save lives.

AFTERWORD

Today marks six months into Evan's glioblastoma diagnoses and treatment. The good news is that there is realistic new hope for both Evan and every patient with terminal cancer.

Personalized cancer care is already here. What was originally only available to the very wealthy, like Stefan Roever, is now covered under Medicare and available for Evan, you and me.

As I write this, I am arranging a full genetic sequence of Evan's tumor to guide the addition of future repurposed drugs. Dr. Soon-Shiong started a company called NanOmics, which allows people to get their tumor DNA and RNA sequenced. Mutations can then be targeted with existing drugs like Sorafenib that was used for Quincy. Dr. Soon-Shiong has had great success with his patients in this fashion. Other companies like Gardant Health now offer liquid biopsy testing by mail. In most cases, these liquid biopsies are also covered by insurance and Medicare. You can sequence your circulating tumor cell genetics without ever having to undergo a surgical biopsy and risk spreading cancer.

You can determine if you have MYC, BRAF, or HER2 and KRAS mutations and then treat them accordingly.

This is especially crucial as the tumor may mutate during treatment, and serial testing may be needed to update the treatment plan against the evolving tumor cells. Dr. Soon-Shiong tells the story of a woman with end-stage cervical cancer who came to him and had her tumor genetics sequenced. She was on her fourth round of chemo and the resistant tumor was spreading with no hope in sight. The test came back showing that a virus had created a HER2 mutation. The monoclonal antibody, trastuzumab, is FDA approved to treat breast cancer, not cervical cancer. However, it made great sense to Dr. Soon-Shiong to repurpose it in this case to fight cervical cancer, which was driven by the HER2 mutation. Insurance would not cover it. Standard oncology would not support the off-label use.

Dr. Soon-Shiong persisted, and the patient agreed. The treatment was administered, and the patient responded. She was blessed with remission and enjoyed a cruise and another year of quality life with friends and family.

Dr. Soon-Shiong tells the story of another patient, David Roy, an executive that he met by chance on an airplane. When David Roy developed end-stage pancreatic cancer and had no other options, he contacted Dr. Soon-Shiong. Roy was in his last days, and no drugs and chemo were working. Dr. Soon-Shiong first sequenced David's tumor genetics, targeted his mutations with repurposed drugs, including Abraxane, and gave Roy immediate remission and a new lease on life.

The lesson is that repurposed drugs targeted and based upon genetic tests work extremely well. Repurposed drugs also work even without genetic testing by suppressing cancer stem cells.

Dr. Stephen J. Bigelsen used Hydroxychloroquine (HCQ) off-label to treat his Stage 4 Pancreatic Cancer. He is a Cornell graduate and a board-certified physician specializing in Allergy and Immunology. He has beaten the odds and survived his cancer for four years, but he also continues to teach at Rutgers University Medical School and maintain a private practice in New Jersey.[321]

Today, let me say loudly and clearly that all terminal cancer patients and their doctors must be informed about these options. This is vital information, not just for Evan, but for us all.

On a final note, I would also state that regulation, unfortunately, holds us back. When regulators deny HER2 tumor patients their trastuzumab, it is tragic and counterproductive. When Quincy was denied his Sorafenib (the drug that ultimately saved his life); that was short-sighted, dogmatic, and cruel.

If we are to beat cancer, we must think differently – in Apple computer parlance – and follow visionaries like Patrick Soon-Shiong and Stefan Roever.

Every patient facing a terminal cancer diagnosis MUST know about cancer stem cells, repurposed drugs, and the option of cocktail treatment. Gone are the days when it was acceptable to mislead the public into believing that such treatments were unscientific or dangerous. Gone are the days when patients blindly followed outdated and medieval advice. And gone are the days when cancer patients must simply "get their affairs in order" and submit to the standard of care.

Today we can all fight back as the wealthy, powerful, and educated do. It should not only be Senators and Biotech millionaires that live; let it be all of us.

We must use repurposed drugs to save lives when a doctor and a patient together decide, based upon careful analysis, that the treatment is warranted. Dr. Harvey Risch is an understated voice through all of this. He graduated with a Bachelor-of-Science degree from the California Institute of Technology in 1972. He went on to earn both his MD and PhD degrees before making health care policy at Yale. He edits several peer-reviewed scientific journals.

The following is what he had to say in support of using repurposed drugs like HCQ for COVID-19.

"It is our obligation not to stand by, just carefully watching, as the old and infirm and inner-city of us is killed by this disease and our economy is destroyed by it and we have nothing to offer except high mortality hospital treatment. We have a solution, imperfect, to attempt to deal with this disease. We have to let physicians employing good clinical judgment use it, and informed patients choose it."[323]

-Harvey A. Risch, MD, PhD
Distinguished Professor of Epidemiology
Yale School of Public Health and Yale School of Medicine
Associate Editor, *Journal of the National Cancer Institute*
Editorial Board, *International Journal of Cancer*

EPILOGUE

Since this book was completed, Dr. Harvey Risch has spoken out further. His comments provide our journey with a fitting conclusion. In an Op-Ed published in *Newsweek* Magazine appearing July 23rd, Dr. Risch wrote:

"Since publication of my May 27th article, seven more studies have demonstrated similar benefit. In a lengthy follow-up letter, also published by AJE, I discuss these seven studies and renew my call for the immediate early use of hydroxychloroquine in high-risk patients.

These seven studies include: an additional 400 high-risk patients treated by Dr. Vladimir Zelenko, with zero deaths; four studies totaling almost 500 high-risk patients treated in nursing homes and clinics across the U.S., with no deaths; a controlled trial of more than 700 high-risk patients in Brazil, with significantly reduced risk of hospitalization and two deaths among 334 patients treated with hydroxychloroquine; and another study of 398 matched patients in France, also with significantly reduced hospitalization risk. Since my letter was published, even more doctors have reported to me their completely successful use."

He described two "natural experiments" in Brazil and Switzerland where HCQ use was associated with a substantial reduction in death rates. Both episodes suggest that a combination of hydroxychloroquine and its companion medications reduces mortality and should be immediately adopted as the new standard of care in high-risk patients.

Dr. Risch concludes that early use of HCQ is essential on both ethical and scientific grounds:

"In the future, I believe this misbegotten episode regarding hydroxychloroquine will be studied by sociologists of medicine as a classic example of how extra-scientific factors overrode clear-cut medical evidence. But for now, reality demands a clear, scientific eye on the evidence and where it points. For the sake of high-risk patients, for the sake of our parents and grandparents, for the sake of the unemployed, for our economy and for our polity, especially those disproportionally affected, we must start treating immediately."

The leading U.S. public health spokesman responded to a question about hydroxychloroquine with this answer,

"If you are talking about a medical question, listen to the medical experts – that's the advice – you will not get a conflicting message from the medical experts about things like hydroxychloroquine..."

However, nothing could be further from the truth. The problem is that we, the public, are bombarded daily with conflicting messages from leading authorities. Some say HCQ is dangerous and ineffective against COVID-19. Others say the opposite.

Dr. Risch is the associate editor of the *Journal of the National Cancer Institute*. He is on the editorial board of the *International Journal of Cancer*. He has authored over 300 peer-reviewed publications. He is considered one of the world's leading epidemiologists. He interprets the studies as showing support for the efficacy of hydroxychloroquine which is in direct conflict to the message given by his friends at the NIH.

For any readers who are under the illusion there is no conflict among experts on this, I would refer you to Appendix F entitled the Physician's Position. Their opinions mirrow mine and the majority of practicing physicians nationwide. This great silent majority agrees with Dr. Risch.

Some 25 specialties are represented, and most significantly, there were nine ICU specialists, six cardiologists, and seven ophthalmologists. The cardiologist don't feel a short course of HCQ is dangerous to the heart, and the eye specialists don't feel it harms the eyes. Why then does the public get fed this line of baloney?

Specialists Speak Out

Two cardiologist comments stand out. The first is by Dr. William Davis:

> "I am a cardiologist trained and experienced in electrophysiology. I have over 40 years of experience in arrhythmia analysis and treatment and have NEVER seen any arrhythmia related to the use of hydroxychloroquine."

Dr. Thomas Salvucci authored the second:

> "I am extremely troubled by the contamination of politics into the arena of science in general and medicine specifically. Which brings us to this article and the potential benefits of hydroxychloroquine. My criticism is this: reference to the dangers of hydroxychloroquine. The two references mentioned, ventricular arrhythmias and hepatic failure are so weak that this article in general cannot be taken seriously."

Two eye doctor comments are similarly noteworthy. Dr. James Hiatt, ophthalmologist, wrote,

> "Ignorant article. HCQ can be toxic when taken for years. No one has suggested a need for years of HCQ therapy for COVID-19."

Dr. Jeff Taylor also an ophthalmologist weighed in,

> "I can't believe that this article was actually written and posted in Medscape. The risk of macular (eye) toxicity is essentially zero when taking this drug at appropriate weight-based doses and for the length of time, it would be needed to treat the virus. When someone starts this for RA, I don't even do the first screening visit for retinal disease until six months and then yearly after that."

COMMENTS IN FAVOR OF HCQ TREATMENT
BY AREA OF SPECIALTY

- Anesthesiology   6
- Cardiologists: 5
- Intensive Care Specialists   9
- Emergency Room   2
- Allergy & Immunology   2
- Family Practice   11
- General Practice   8
- Endocrinology   3
- Gastroenterology   1
- Internal Medicine   5
- Pharmacist   9
- Orthopedic Surgery   4
- Rheumatology   2
- Pediatrics   3
- Psychiatry   4
- Opthalmology   7
- Dermatology   1
- Nephrology   1
- Ear Nose & Throat   1
- General Surgery   2
- Infectious Disease   2
- Oncology   3
- Physical Medicine   1
- Urology   1
- Medical Student   1

Rheumatology specialists have the most experience with HCQ because they treat those with rheumatoid arthritis and lupus. Both require HCQ. Many such patients take the drug twice a day for decades. Not only are these lupus patients rarely getting the heart and eye problems the media has alarmed everyone with, they somehow did not seem to get very ill with COVID-19 either.

For those who are skeptical, simply read the following comment by Dr. Olga Goodman, a practicing rheumatologist. She notes that none of her lupus patients needed hospitalization, while those few who got COVID-19 had only mild symptoms.

> "For huge local observation database, there are no single cases of hospital admission in our heavily affected area among patients compliant with HCQ therapy. Unfortunately some of them stopped it last few weeks after all these "publications" but still appear to be protected from severe disease. Despite being immunocompromised, elderly, having preexisting lung and heart issues, long-term steroids, etc. They still can catch coronavirus but the worst-case scenario just reported is as a 'bad cold'."

I was also struck by the number of physicians who would personally take HCQ for themselves, or prescribe it if a family member got sick. Earlier, I wrote about the famed physician-author Dr. Daniel Amen prescribing it for his parents who survived the disease.

Consider these comments. Dr. Maurice Valentini wrote,

> "In all the years of practicing optometry, I have never seen an actual case of Plaquenil retinopathy clinically, only in textbooks or online. If I had to choose between treatment with HCQ/Chloroquine and a full recovery or the remote possibility of visual impairment and death by drowning, it comes down to a no-brainer!"

Dr. G. Galindo said,

> "The French study of HCQ has great results. If I were to get
> sick with the Wuhan virus, I would take HCQ, because it has
> a lot of good reports on its effectiveness, and it is not
> expensive. There is nothing wrong with off-label meds for this
> virus."

Can 100 Specialists Be Wrong?

Do you believe all of these specialists are wrong? Ask yourself why
these comments have not been published by European or American
media. Ask why India has only a small fraction of the per-capita
COVID-19 death rate compared to Europe and the U.S. Why does
India mandates that all front-line health care workers take
hydroxychloroquine once per week?

Cardiologists writing in Appendix F feel HCQ is safe for your heart,
yet why does the health care establishment continue to warn and
frighten you? Why is it that the eye specialists feel HCQ is safe, yet
the health care establishment continues to keep people away from
it? Why exactly do the rheumatologists write that their lupus
patients who take HCQ are so protected from COVID-19? And why
is it that most practicing physicians would want HCQ for their
families or themselves if they were exposed to the virus?

The specialists writing in the Physician's Position have consistent
answers to these questions. Dr. Zeidan, a lung specialist offered his
opinion:

> "As long as there remains a marriage between science and
> politics, trouble will endure. Should we ask whether the cheap
> cost of hydroxychloroquine in comparison to let's say
> Remdesivir has something to do with everything else?"

Dr. James Ransom, Allergy and Clinical Immunology, writes:

> "Due to the "politicization "of this drug (a real shame for the
> medical profession), we are now told that Remdesivir is the
> real answer. This may be the way Big Pharma "kills" a cheap

generic drug that can be used "off-label" in early cases. Someday, maybe someone will tell us the truth about all this. In the meantime be skeptical of everything you read."

Dr. Alex Wonner, Surgeon:

"Very strange that Professor Raoult had better results with hydroxychloroquine by treating patients in the early phase and avoiding those going to the ICU, and suddenly this drug is discredited. But an American drug costing a fortune that has no real benefit in mortality is suddenly the standard of care!!!!

The power of money..."

Dr. Dinesh Ranjan, General Surgery,

"HCQ had two big factors working against it:

#1 It is exceedingly cheap (full course <$5, compared with Remdesivir $5000+)

#2 It was being proposed by Trump"

'You can't waste a crisis on something this cheap'

My colleagues clearly believe that Big Pharma, profits and politics are trumping science when it comes to the use of repurposed drugs. Since it is legal for doctors to prescribe them, these interests can use their influence to mislead the public. They drive a fear of repurposed drugs like HCQ.

In the old days we called this propaganda. Now it is termed "spin".

Either way, it involves lying to millions of people. Tragically, scientific studies can be run in such a way that interested parties can spin certain cheap drugs out of the running. This paves the way for approval of the expensive and patentable drug. It is similar to "fixing" a fight. The scientists force the disfavored drug to take the fall.

When I spoke with Dr. Ben Williams who has now survived his glioblastoma for over 25 years, he offered similar opinions. I told

Ben that the studies using HCQ at six times the normal dose (toxic) set it up for failure.

"Back when I was researching my cancer," he remarked, "I also saw studies that seemed designed to make certain drugs fail."

I would simply ask the reader to think critically and to read the raw, unedited, and unsolicited comments of the Physician's Position in Appendix F, and contrast them with the scripted, agenda-driven ones of the media. Making the correct decision here can save your life. Believing the wrong expert can kill you.

Dr. George Fareed

Dr. George Fareed, the hospitalist I spoke about in California's Imperial Valley, has treated over four hundred patients with the repurposed drug, HCQ, with great success. His local colleagues have treated thousands more also with success. In particular, Dr. Brian Tyson's account of curing 100% of his 1900 COVID-19 patients is contained in Appendix H. The Pandemic would end tomorrow if the nation adopted Tyson's and Fareed's treatment model. In an effort to accomplish this, Dr. Fareed wrote an "Open Letter to Dr. Anthony Fauci" which has since launched a Congressional Inquiry. See Appendix G..

Dr. Fareed comes from a generation of physicians who had to think on their feet during the AIDS crisis, which I might add was resolved with repurposed drug cocktails. Dr. Ben Williams credits the AIDS cocktails with providing him the insight to consider repurposed drugs for terminal cancer. He astutely observed that viruses and cancer are related through a similar set of evolutionary dynamics.

After all of the research spent in writing this book, reviewing the scientific literature, interviewing colleagues and survivors, I came to the inescapable conclusion that repurposed drugs must be used when all else has failed and when the benefits outweigh the risks. We did not need randomized placebo-controlled studies to implement penicillin or colchicine. We do not require them to save lives today.

We must employ good clinical judgment to save lives in this great pandemic. In terminal cancer or in a global pandemic as Dr. Jeff Colyer put it, "You must go with the army you have, not the one you wish you had." And as Dr. Ben Williams reminds us, "Because many of these drugs have been used for decades, their toxicities are well understood, as are their interactions with other drugs, thus ideal candidates for use in drug cocktails."

HCQ is one of the most studied and least toxic among them. It did not suddenly become dangerous overnight and should be used whenever a physician and patient together decide the benefits outweigh the risks.

Dr. Harvey Risch reflected upon the carnage wrought by this terrible pathogen, the loss of nearly one million souls, the reverberations to our economy, the seismic disruption to our way of life, and offered these words:

"For the sake of high-risk patients, for the sake of our parents and grandparents, for the sake of the unemployed, for our economy and for our polity, especially those disproportionally affected, we must start treating immediately."

In Flanders Fields

-John McCrae M.D., 1872-1918

"In Flanders fields the poppies blow
Between the crosses, row on row,
That mark our place; and in the sky
The larks, still bravely singing, fly
Scarce heard amid the guns below.

We are the Dead. Short days ago
We lived, felt dawn, saw sunset glow,
Loved and were loved, and now we lie
In Flanders fields.

Take up our quarrel with the foe:
To you from failing hands we throw

The torch; be yours to hold it high.
If ye break faith with us who die
We shall not sleep, though poppies grow
In Flanders fields."

REFERENCES

1. Aubrey, A. A Pinworm Medication is Being Tested as a Potential Anti-cancer Drug. *Shots Health News from NPR.* 2017 January 30.

2. Guerini, A., Triggiana, L., Maddallo, M., et al. Mebendazole is a Candidate for Drug Repurposing in Oncology: An Extensive Review of Current Literature. *Cancers (Basel).* 2019; 11(9):1284.

3. De Witt, M., Gamble, A., Hanson, D., et al. Repurposing Mebendazole as a Replacement for Vincristine for the Treatment of Brain Tumors. *Mol Med.* 2017; 23:50-56.

4. McLelland, J. *How to Starve Cancer… without starving yourself.* Agenor Publishing. 2018 United Kingdom.

5. Pantziarka, P., Bouche, G., Meheus, L., et al. Repurposing Drugs in Your Medicine Cabinet: Untapped Opportunities for Cancer Therapy? *Future Oncol.* 2015;11(2):181-184.

6. Agrawal, S., Vamadevan, P., Mazibuko, N., et al. A New Method for Ethical and Efficient Evidence Generation for Off-Label Medication Use in Oncology (A Case Study in Glioblastoma). *Front Pharmacol.* 2019; 10:681.

7. Bai, R., Staedtke, V., Aprhys, C., et al. Antiparasitic mebendazole shows survival benefit in 2 preclinical models of glioblastoma multiforme. *Neuro Oncol.* 2011; 13(9):974-982.

8. Bai, R., Staedtke, V., Rudin, C., et al. Effective treatment of diverse medulloblastoma models with mebendazole and its impact on tumor angiogenesis. *Neuro Oncol.* 2015; 17(4):545-554.

9. Simbulan-Rosenthal, C., Dakshanamurthy, S., Gaur, A., et al. The repurposed anthelmintic mebendazole in combination with trametinib suppresses refractory $NRAS^{Q61K}$ melanoma. *Oncotarget.* 2017; 8(8): 12576-12595.

10. Zhang, L., Bochkur, Dratver M., Yazal, T., et al. Mebendazole Potentiates Radiation Therapy in Triple-Negative Breast Cancer. *Int J Radiat Oncol Biol Phys.* 2019; 103(1):195-207.

11. Williamson, T., Bai, R., Staedtke, V., et al. Mebendazole and a non-steroidal anti-inflammatory combined to reduce tumor initiation in a colon cancer preclinical model. *Oncotarget.* 2016; 7(42):68571-68584.

12.   Larsen, A., Bai, R., Chung, J., et al. Repurposing the antihelmintic mebendazole as a hedgehog inhibitor. *Mol Cancer Ther.* 2015; 14(1):3-13.

13.   Guerini, A., Triggianni, L., Maddalo, M., et al. Mebendazole as a Candidate for Drug Repurposing in Oncology: An Extensive Review of Current Literature. *Cancers (Basel).* 2019; 11(9):1284.

14.   Verbaanderd, C., Rooman, I., Meheus, L., et al. On-Label or Off-Label? Overcoming Regulatory and Financial Barriers to Bring Repurposed Medicines to Cancer Patients. *Front Pharmacol.* 2019; 10:1664.

15.   Hancock, F. Medicine already in use may help cancer treatments. *Stuff.com New Zealand.* 2019 May 20.

16.   How Professor Ben Williams beat his brain cancer. *Canceractive.com.* 2017 May 11.

17.   *Surviving Terminal Cancer.* Directed by Dominic Hill, Indigo Rebel Films on Vimeo, 2015.

18.   Wood, W., Igbavboa, U., Muller, W. et al. Statins, Bcl-2 and apoptosis: cell death or cell protection? *Mol Neurobiol.* 2013; 48(2):308-314.

19.   McLelland, J. *How to Starve Cancer... without starving yourself.* Agenor Publishing. 2018 United Kingdom.

20.   Kofron, C., Chapman, A. Breast Cancer with Brain Metastasis: Perspective from a Long-Term Survivor. *Integr Cancer Ther.* 2020; 19:1534735419890017.

21.   Wenner, C., Martzen, M., Lu, H., et al. Polysaccharide-K augments docetaxel-induced tumor suppression and antitumor response in an immunocompetent murine model of human prostate cancer. *Int J Oncol.* 2012; 40(4):905-913.

22.   Gossard, B. (ED). 2019 *Disease prevention and treatment.* Life Extension.

23.   Cufí, S., Vazquez-Martin, A., Oliveras-Ferraros, C., et al. The anti-malarial chloroquine overcomes primary resistance and restores sensitivity to trastuzumab in HER2-positive breast cancer. *Sci Rep.* 2013; 3:2469.

24.   Mason, J., Fu, M., Chen, J., et al. Flaxseed oil enhances the effectiveness of trastuzumab in reducing the growth of HER2-overexpressing human breast tumors (BT-474). *J Nutr Biochem.* 2015; 26(1):16-23.

25. Zhang, L., Xu, L., Zhang, F., et al. Doxycycline inhibits the cancer stem cell phenotype and epithelial-to-mesenchymal transition in breast cancer. *Cell Cycle.* 2017; 16(8):737-745.

26. Chen, W., Holmes, M. Role of Aspirin in Breast Cancer Survival. *Curr Oncol Rep.* 2017; 19(7):48.

27. Unwin, N. The metabolic syndrome. *J R. Soc Med.* 2006; 99(9):457-462.

28. Solomon, S., McMurray, J., Pfeffer, M., et al. Cardiovascular risk associated with celecoxib in a clinical trial for colorectal adenoma prevention. *N Engl J Med.* 2005; 352(11):1071-1080.

29. García-Rodríguez, L., Soriano-Gabarró, M., Bromley, S., et al. New use of low-dose aspirin and risk of colorectal cancer by stage at diagnosis: a nested case control study in UK general practice. *BMC Cancer.* 2017; 17(1):637.

30. Bibbins-Domingo, K. Aspirin Use for the Primary Prevention of Cardiovascular Disease and Colorectal Cancer: U.S. Preventive Services Task Force Recommendation Statement. *Ann Intern Med.* 2016; 164(12):836-845.

31. Evans, J., Donnelly, L., Emslie-Smith, A., et al. Metformin and reduced risk of cancer in diabetic patients. *BMJ* 2005; 330(7503):1304-1305.

32. Wang, A., Aragaki, A., Tang, J., et al. Statin use and all-cancer survival: prospective results from the Woman's Health Initiative. *Br J Cancer.* 2016; 115(1):129-135.

33. Nielsen, S., Nordestgaard, B., Bojesen, S. Statin use and reduced cancer-related mortality. *N Engl J Med.* 2013; 367(19):1792-1802.

34. Bathaie, S., Ashrafi, M., Azizian, M., et al. Mevalonate Pathway and Human Cancers. *Curr Mol Pharmacol.* 2017; 10(2):77-85.

35. Nayak, A., Hayen, A., Zhu, L., et al. Legacy effects of statins on cardiovascular and all-cause mortality: a meta-analysis. *BMJ Open.* 2018; 8(9):e020584.

36. Moyad, M., Vogelzang, N. Heart healthy equals prostate healthy and statins, aspirin, and/or metformin (SAM) are the ideal recommendations for prostate cancer prevention. *Asian J Androl.* 2015; 17(5):783-791.

37. Moyad, M. Preventing Aggressive Prostate Cancer with Proven Cardiovascular Disease Preventive Methods. *Asian J Androl.* 2015; 17(6):874-877.

38. Pantziarka, P. Li Fraumeni syndrome, cancer and senescence: a new hypothesis. *Cancer Cell Int.* 2013; 13(1):35.
39. Cousins, S. Repurposing drugs to fight cancer. *New York Times.* 2020, February 25.
40. Pantziarka, P., Bouche, G., Meheus, L., et al. The Repurposing Drugs in Oncology (ReDO) Project. *Ecancermedicalscience.* 2014; 8:442.
41. Pantziarka, P, Bouche, G., Sukhatme, V., et al. Repurposing Drugs in Oncology (ReDo)-Propranalol as an anti-cancer agent. *Ecancermedicalscience.* 2016; 10:680.
42. Pantziarka, P., Verbaanderd, C., Sukhatme, V., et al. ReDO_DB: the repurposing drugs in oncology database. *Ecancermedicalscience.* 2018; 12:886.
43. Hodgson, H. Consultation and informed opinion. *Clin Med (Lond).* 2015; 15(1):3-4.
44. Van Norman, G. Expanding Patient Access to Investigational Drugs: Single Patient Investigational New Drug and the "Right to Try." *JACC Basic Transl Sci.* 2018; 3(2):280-293.
45. Gyawali, B., Pantziarka, P., Crispino, S., et al. Does the oncology community have a rejection bias when it comes to repurposed drugs? *Ecancermedicalscience.* 2018; 12:ed76.
46. Pantziarka, P. Primed for cancer: Li Fraumeni Syndrome and the pre-cancerous niche. *Ecancermedicalscience.* 2015; 9:541.
47. Steele, C., Thomas, C., Henley, S., et al. Vital Signs: Trends un Incidence of Cancers Associated with Overweight and Obesity- United States, 2005-2014. *MMWR Morb Mortal Wkly Rep.* 2017; 66(39):1052-1058.
48. Wulaningsih, W., Garmo, H., Holmberg, L., et al. Serum Lipids and the Risk of Gastrointestinal Malignancies in the Swedish AMORIS Study. *J Cancer Epidemiol.* 2012; 2012:792034.
49. Sun, H., Huang, X., Wang, Z., et al. Triglyceride-to-high Density Lipoprotein Cholesterol Ratio Predicts Clinical Outcomes in Patients with Gastric Cancer. *J Cancer.* 2019; 10(27):6829-6836.
50. Dai, D., Chen, B., Wang, B., et al. *J Cancer* 2016; 7(12):1747-1754.
51. Mignone, L., Wu, T., Horowitz, M., et al. Whey protein: The "whey" forward for treatment of type 2 diabetes? *World J Diabetes.* 2015; 6(14):1274-1284.
52. Hope, J. *The Coffee Cure Diet: Live Longer and Look Younger.* Hope Pressworks International LLC. 2019 Redding, CA.

53. Longo, V., Fontana, L. Calorie restriction and cancer prevention: metabolic and molecular mechanisms. *Trends Pharmacol Sci.* 2010; 31(2):89-98.

54. Longo, V., Mattson, M. Fasting: molecular mechanisms and clinical applications. *Cell Metab.* 2014; 19(2):181-192.

55. Williamson, T., Bai, R., Staedtke, V., et al. Mebendazole and a non-steroidal anti-inflammatory combined to reduce tumor initiation in a colon cancer preclinical model. *Oncotarget.* 2016; 7(42):68571-68584.

56. Saraei, P., Asadi, I., Kakar, M., et al. The beneficial effects of metformin on cancer prevention and therapy: a comprehensive review of recent advances. *Cancer Manag Res.* 2019; 11:3295-3313.

57. Mahmood, K., Naeem, M., Rahimnajjad, N. Metformin: The Hidden Chronicles of a Magic Drug. *Eur J Intern Med.* 2013; 24(1):20-26.

58. Heckman-Stoddard, B., DeCensi, A., Sahasrabuddhe, V., et al. Repurposing metformin for the prevention of cancer and cancer recurrence. *Diabetologia.* 2017; 60(9):1639-1647.

59. Lee, J., Kang, M., Byun, W., et al. Metformin overcomes resistance to cisplatin in triple-negative breast cancer (TNBC) cells by targeting RAD51. *Breast Cancer Res.* 2019; 21(1):115.

60. Song, C., Lee, H., Dings, R., et al. Metformin kills and radiosensitizes cancer cells and preferentially kills cancer stem cells. *Sci Rep.* 2012; 2:362.

61. Voltan, R., Rimondi, E., Melloni, E., et al. Metformin combined with sodium dichloroacetate promotes B-leukemic cell death by suppressing anti-apoptotic protein Mcl-1. *Oncotarget.* 2016; 7(14):18965-18977.

62. Tong, D., Liu, Q., Liu, G., et al. Metformin inhibits castration-induced EMT in prostate cancer by repressing COX2/PGE2/STAT3 axis. *Cancer Lett.* 2017; 389:23-32.

63. Gandini, S., Puntoni, M., Heckman-Stoddard, B., et al. Metformin and Cancer Risk and Mortality: A Systematic Review and Meta-Analysis Taking Into Account Biases and Confounders. *Cancer Prev Res.* 2014; 7(9):867-885.

64. Kamarudin, M., Sarker, M., Zhou, J., et al. Metformin in Colorectal Cancer: Molecular Mechanism, Preclinical and Clinical Aspects. *J Exp Clin Cancer Res.* 2019; 38(491):10.1186/s13046-019-1495-2.

65. Xu, H., Aldrich, M., Chen, Q., et al. Validating Drug Repurposing Signals Using Electronic Health Records: A Case Study of Metformin Associated with Reduced Cancer Mortality. *J Am Med Inform Assoc.* 2015; 22(1):179-191.

66. Decensi, A., Putoni, M., Goodwin, P., et al. Metformin and cancer risk in diabetic patients: a systemic review and meta-analysis. *Cancer Prev Res (Phila).* 2010; 3(11):1451-1461.

67. Tseng, C. Metformin reduces ovarian cancer risk in Taiwanese women with type 2 diabetes mellitus. *Diabetes Metab Res Rev.* 2015; 31(6):619-626.

68. Tseng, C. Metformin significantly reduces incident prostate cancer risk in Taiwanese men with type 2 diabetes mellitus. *Eur J Cancer.* 2014; 50(16):2831-2837.

69. Tseng, C. Metformin may reduce bladder cancer risk in Taiwanese patients with type 2 diabetes. *Acta Diabetol.* 2014; 51(2):295-303.

70. Bannister, C., Holden, S., Jenkins-Jones, S., et al. Can people with type 2 diabetes live longer than those without? A comparison of mortality in people initiated with metformin or sulphonylurea monotherapy and matched, non-diabetic controls. *Diabetes Obes Metab.* 2014; 16(11):1165-1173.

71. Campbell, J., Bellman, S., Stephenson, M. et al. Metformin reduces all-cause mortality in diseases of ageing independent of its effect on diabetes control: A systematic review meta-analysis. *Ageing Res Rev.* 2017; 40:31-44.

72. Ambe, C., Mahipal, A., Fulp, J., et al. Effect of Metformin Use on Survival in Resectable Pancreatic Cancer: A Single-Institution Experience and Review of the Literature. *PLoS One.* 2016; 11(3):e0151632.

73. Sadeghi, N., Abbruzzese, J., Yeung, S., et al. Metformin use is associated with better survival of diabetic patients with pancreatic cancer. *Clin Cancer Res.* 2012; 18(10):2905-2912.

74. Shi, P., Liu, W., Wang, H., et al. Metformin suppresses triple-negative breast cancer stem cells by targeting KLF5 for degradation. *Cell Discov.* 2017; 3:17010.

75. Barriére, G., Tartary, M., Rigaud, M. Metformin: a rising star to fight the epithelial mesenchymal transition in oncology. *Anticancer Agents Med Chem.* 2013; 13(2):333-340.

76. Anisimov, V., Berstein, L., Popovich, I., et al. If started early in life, metformin treatment increases life span and postpones

tumors in female SHR mice. *Aging (Albany NY)* 2011; 3(2):148-157.

77.   Madeo, F., Carmona-Gutierrez, D., Hofer, S., et al. Caloric Restriction Mimetics against Age-Associated Disease: Targets, Mechanisms, and Therapeutic Potential. *Cell Metab.* 2019; 29(3):592-610.

78.   Anisimov, V., Berstein, L., Egormin, P., et al. Metformin slows down aging and extends life span of female SHR mice. *Cell Cycle.* 2008; 7(17):2769-2773.

79.   Cătoi, A., Andreicut, A., Vodnar, D., et al. Metformin Modulates the Mechanisms of Ageing. *Intech Open.* 2019; 89431

80.   Trinkley, K., Anderson, H., Nair, K., et al. Assessing the incidence of acidosis in patients receiving metformin with and without risk factors for lactic acidosis. *Ther Adv Chronic Dis.* 2018; 9(9):179-190.

81.   Dillon, J. "Don't think of cancer as a "Superman." *Yale Medicine Magazine.* Spring 2012.

82.   Yoshida, G. Therapeutic strategies of drug repositioning targeting autophagy to induce cancer cell death: from pathophysiology to treatment. *J. Hematol Oncol.* 2017; 10:67.

83.   Cluntun, A., Lukey, M., Cerione, R., et al. Glutamine Metabolism in Cancer: Understanding the Heterogeneity. *Trends Cancer.* 2017; 3(3):169-180.

84.   Ferrara, N., Hillan, K., Novotny, W. Bevacizumab (Avastin), a humanized anti-VEGF monoclonal antibody for cancer therapy. *Biochem Biophys Res Commun.* 2005; 333(2):328-335.

85.   McLelland, J. *How to Starve Cancer… without starving yourself.* Agenor Publishing. 2018 United Kingdom.

86.   Wojtukiewicz, M., Hempel, D., Sierko, E., et al. Antiplatelet agents for cancer treatment: a real perspective or just an echo from the past? *Cancer Metastasis Rev.* 2017; 36(2):305-329.

87.   Hope, J. *The Coffee Cure Diet: Live Longer Look Younger.* Hope Pressworks International LLC. 2019 Redding, CA.

88.   Lee, C., Raffaghello, L., Brandhorst, S., et al. Fasting cycles retard growth of tumors and sensitize a range of cancer cell types to chemotherapy. *Sci Transl Med.* 2012; 4(124):124ra27.

89.   Prokesch, A., Graef, F., Madl, T., et al. Liver p53 is stabilized upon starvation and required for amino acid catabolism and gluconeogenesis. *FASEB J.* 2017; 31(2):732-742.

90.   Takebe, N., Miele, L., Harris, P., et al. Targeting Notch, Hedgehog, and Wnt pathways in cancer stem cells: clinical update. *Nat Rev Clin Oncol.* 2015; 12(8):445-464.

91.   Takebe, N., Harris, P., Warren, R., et al. Targeting cancer stem cells by inhibiting Wnt, Notch, and Hedgehog pathways. *Nat Rev Clin Oncol.* 2011; 8(2):97-106.

92.   Yang, J., Wang, C., Zhang, Z., et al. Curcumin inhibits the survival and metastasis of prostate cancer cells via the Notch-1 signaling pathway. *APMIS.* 2017; 125(2):134-140.

93.   Naujokat, C., McKee, D. The "Big Five" Phytochemicals Targeting Cancer Cells: Curcumin EGCG, Sulforaphane, Resveratrol, and Genistein. *Curr Med Chem.* 2020: 32107991.

94.   Zhou, P., Wang, C., Hu, Z., et al. Genistein induces apoptosis of colon cancer cells by reversal of epithelial-to-mesenchymal via a Notch1/NF-kB/slug/E-cadherin pathway. *BMC Cancer.* 2017; 17(1):813.

95.   Kumar, G., Farooqui, M., Rao, C. Role of Dietary Cancer-Preventive Phytochemicals in Pancreatic Cancer Stem Cells. *Curr Pharmacol Rep.* 2018; 4(4):326-335.

96.   Radhakrishnan, P., Bryant, V., Blowers, E., et al. Targeting the NF-kB and mTOR pathways with quinoxalin urea analog that inhibits IKKß for pancreas cancer therapy. *Clin Cancer Res.* 2013; 19(8):2025-2035.

97.   Harris, D., Li, L., Chen, M., et al. Diverse mechanisms of growth inhibition by luteolin resveratrol, and quercetin in MIA PaCa-2 cells: a comparative glucose tracer study with the fatty acid synthase inhibitor C75. *Metabolomics.* 2012; 8(2):201-210.

98.   Li, Y., Li, P., Roberts, M., et al. Multi-targeted therapy of cancer by niclosamide: A new application for an old drug. *Cancer Lett.* 2014; 349(1):8-14.

99.   Li, F., Zhou, K., Gao, L., et al. Radiation induces the generation of cancer stem cells: A novel mechanism for cancer radioresistance. *Oncol Lett.* 2016; 12(5):3059-3065.

100.   Schulz, A., Meyer, F., Dubrovska, A., et al. Cancer Stem Cells and Radioresistance: DNA Repair and Beyond. *Cancers (Basel).* 2019; 11(6):862.

101.   Xu, X, Su, B, Xie, C., et al. Sonic hedgehog-Gli1 signaling pathway regulates the epithelial, mesenchymal, transition (EMT) by mediating a new target gene, S100A4, in pancreatic cancer cells. *PLoS One.* 2014; 9(7):e96441.

102. Najifi, M., Farhood, B., Mortezaee, K., Cancer stem Cells (CSCs) in cancer progression and therapy. *J Cell Physiol.* 2019; 234(6):8381-8395.

103. Bariwal, J., Kumar, V., Dong, Y., et al. Design of Hedgehog pathway inhibitors for cancer treatment. *Med Res Rev.* 2019; 39(3):1137-1204.

104. Yu, Y., Cheng, L., Yan, B., et al. Overexpression of Gremlin 1 by sonic hedgehog signaling promotes pancreatic cancer progression. *Int J Oncol.* 2018; 53(6):2445-2457.

105. Feldmann, G., Dhara, S., Fendrich, B., et al. Blockade of hedgehog signaling inhibits pancreatic cancer invasion and metastases: a new paradigm for combination therapy in solid cancers. *Cancer Res.* 2007; 67(5):2187-2196.

106. Sun, X, Liu, X., Huang, D. Curcumin reverses the epithelial-mesenchymal transition of pancreatic cancer cells by inhibiting the Hedgehog signaling pathway. *Oncol Rep.* 2013; 29(6):2401-2407.

107. Rodova, M., Fu, J., Watkins, D., et al. Sonic hedgehog signaling inhibition provides opportunities for targeted therapy by sulforaphane in regulating pancreatic cancer stem cell self-renewal. *PLoS One.* 2012; 7(9):e46083.

108. Li, W., Zhao, Y., Tao, B., et al. Effects of quercetin on hedgehog signaling in chronic myeloid leukemia KBM7 cells. *Chin J Integr Med.* 2014; 20(10):776-781.

109. Pantziarka, P., Bouche, G., Meheus, L., et al. Repurposing Drugs in Oncology (ReDO)-mebenadazole as an anti-cancer agent. *Ecancermedicalscience* 2014; 8:443.

110. Schulten, H. Pleiotrophic Effects of Metformin on Cancer. *Int J Mol Sci.* 2018; 19(10):2850.

111. Zheng, M., Jiang, Y., Chen, W., et al. Snail and Slug collaborate on EMT and tumor metastasis through miR-101-mediated EZH2 axis in oral tongue squamous cell carcinoma. *Oncotarget.* 2015; 6(9):6794-6810.

112. Krump, N., You, J. Molecular mechanisms of viral oncogenesis in humans. *Nat Rev Microbiol.* 2018; 16(11):684-698.

113. Esposito, M., Mondal, N., Greco, D., et al. Bone vascular niche E-selectin induces mesenchymal-epithelial transition in Wnt activation in cancer cells to promote bone metastasis. *Nat Cell Biol.* 2019; 21(5):627-639.

114.   Hao, Y., Lafita-Navarro, M., Zacharias, L., et al. Induction of LEF1 by MYC activates the WNT pathway and maintains cell proliferation. *Cell Commun Signal.* 2019; 17(1):129.

115.   Zhou, E., Cheng, S., Yang, R., et al. Combination of chemoprevention: future direction of colorectal cancer prevention. *Eur J Cancer Prev.* 2012; 21(3):231-240.

116.   Pan, J., Ding, K., Wang, C. Niclosamide, an old antihelminthic agent, demonstrates antitumor activity by blocking multiple signaling pathways of cancer stem cells. *Chin J Cancer.* 2012; 31(4):178-184.

117.   Fabregat, I., Fernando, J., Mainez, J., et al. TGF-beta signaling in cancer treatment. *Curr Pharm Des.* 2014; 20(17):2934-2947.

118.   Zhang, R., Tao, F., Ruan, S., et al. The TGFß1-FOXM1-HMGA1-TGFß1 positive feedback loop increases the cisplatin resistance of non-small cell lung cancer by inducing G6PD expression. *Am J Transl Res.* 2019; 11(11):6860-6876.

119.   Dancea, H., Shareef, M., Ahmed, M. Role of Radiation-induced TGF-beta Signaling in Cancer Therapy. *Mol Cell Pharmacol.* 2009; 1(1):44-56.

120.   Li, Z., Zhou, W., Zang, Y., et al. ERK Regulates HIF1α-Mediated Platinum Resistance by Directly Targeting PHD2 in Ovarian Cancer. *Clin Cancer Res.* 2019; DOI: 10.1158/1078-0432. CCR-18-4145.

121.   Zhao, Y., Cao, J., Melamed, A., et al. Losartan Enhances Chemotherapy Efficacy and Reduces Ascites in Ovarian Cancer Models by Normalizing the Tumor Stroma. *PNAS.* 2019; 116(6): 2210-2219.

122.   Wakabayashi, H., Oda, H., Yamauchi, K., et al. Lactoferrin for prevention of common viral infections. *J Infect Chemother.* 2014; 20(11):666-671.

123.   Wendt, M., Allington, T., Schiemann, W., Mechanisms of the epithelial mesenchymal transition by TGF-beta. *Future Oncol.* 2009; 5(8):1145-1168.

124.   Katsuno, Y., Meyer, D., Zhang, Z., et al. Chronic TGF-ß Exposure Drives Stabilized EMT, Tumor Stemness, and Cancer Drug Resistance with Vulnerability to Bitopic. mTOR Inhibition. *Sci Signal* 2019; 12(570):eaau8544.

125.   Yin, J., Xing, H., Ye, J. Efficacy of Berberine in Patients with Type II Diabetes Mellitus. *Metabolism.* 2008; 57(5):712-717.

126. Kondo, A., Takeda, T., Li, B., et al. Epigallocatechin-3-gallate Potentiates Curcumin's Ability to Suppress Uterine Leiomyosarcoma Cell Growth and Induce Apoptosis. *Int J Clin Oncol.* 2013; 18(3):380-388.

127. Melnik, B. Dietary Intervention in Acne. *Dermatoendocrinol.* 2012; 4(1):20-32.

128. Vazquez-Martin, A., López-Bonetc, E., Cufí, S., et al. Repositioning chloroquine and metformin to eliminate cancer stem cell traits in pre-malignant lesions. *Drug Resist Updat.* 2011; 14(0):212-223.

129. Tanaka, Y., Hirata, M., Shinome, S., et al. Distribution analysis of epertinib in brain metastasis of HER2-positive breast cancer by imaging mass spectrometry and prospect for antitumor activity. *Sci Rep.* 2018; 8(1):343.

130. Wojtukiewicz, M., Hempel, D., Sierko, E., et al. Antiplatelet Agents for Cancer Treatment: A real Perspective or Just an Echo from the Past? *Cancer Metastasis Rev.* 2017; 36(2):305-329.

131. Pantziarka, P, Bouche, G., Sukhatme, V., et al. Repurposing Drugs in Oncology (ReDo)-Propranolol as an anti-cancer agent. *Ecancermedicalscience.* 2016; 10:680.

132. Agrawal, S., Vamadevan, P., Mazibuko, N., et al. A New Method for Ethical and Efficient Evidence Generation for Off-Label Medication Use in Oncology (A Study in Glioblastoma). *Front Pharmacol.* 2019; 10:681.

133. Lecour, S., Lamont, K. Natural polyphenols and cardioprotection. *Mini Rev Med Chem.* 2011; 11(14):1191-1209.

134. Wan, L., Dong, H., Xu, H., et al. Aspirin, lysine, mifepristone, and doxycycline combined can effectively and safely prevent and treat cancer metastasis: prevent seeds from gemmating on soil. *Oncotarget.* 2015; 6(34):35157-35172.

135. Wang, J., Chen, J., Wan, L., et al. Synthesis, spectral characterization, and in vitro cellular activities of metapristone, a potential cancer metastatic chemopreventive agent derived from mifepristone (RU486). *AAPS J.* 2014; 16(2):289-298.

136. Liao, X., Lochhead, P., Nishihara, R., et al. Aspirin use, tumor PIK3CA mutation, and colorectal-cancer survival. *N Engl J Med.* 2012; 367(17):1596-1606.

137. Rothwell, P., Wilson, M., Price, J., et al. Effect of daily aspirin on risk of cancer metastasis: a study of incident cancers during

randomized controlled trials. *Lancet.* 2012; 379(9826):1591-1601.

138.   Duivenvoorden, W., Popović, S., Lhoták, S., et al.   Doxycycline decreases tumor burden in a bone metastasis model of human breast cancer. *Cancer Res.* 2002; 62(6):1588-1591.

139.   Ibrahim-Hashim, A., Wojtkowiak, J., Ribeiro, M., et al. Free Base Lysine Increases Survival and Reduces Metastasis in Prostate Cancer Model. *J Cancer Sci Ther.* 2011; Suppl 1(4):JCST-S1-004.

140.   Kast, R., Skuli, N., Karpel-Massler, G., et al. Blocking epithelial-to-mesenchymal transition in glioblastoma with a sextet of repurposed drugs: the EIS regimen. *Oncotarget.* 2017; 8(37):60727-60749.

141.   Anderson, A., Shifren, A., Nathan, S. A safety evaluation of pirfenidone for the treatment of idiopathic pulmonary fibrosis. *Expert Opin Drug Saf.* 2016; 15(7):975-982.

142.   Lopez-de la Mora, D., Sanchez-Roque, C., Montoya-Buelna, M., et al. Role and New Insights of Pirfenidone in Fibrotic Diseases. *Int J. Med Sci.* 2015; 12(11):840-847.

143.   Flores-Contereras, L., Sandoval-Rodríguez, A., Mena-Enriquez, M., et al. Treatment with pirfenidone for two years decreases fibrosis, cytokine levels and enhances CB2 gene expression in patients with chronic hepatitis C. *BMC Gastroenterol.* 2014; 14:131.

144.   Wang, H., Shen, W., Hu, X, et al.   Quetiapine inhibits osteoclastogenesis and prevents human breast cancer-induced bone loss through suppression of the RANKL-mediated MAPK, and NF-kB signaling pathways. *Breast Cancer Res Treat.* 2015; 149(3):705-714.

145.   Liu, Y, Wang, J., Ni, T., et al. CCL20 mediates RANK/RANKL-induced epithelial-mesenchymal transition in endometrial cancer cells. *Oncotarget.* 2016; 7(18):25328-25339.

146.   Kast, R., Skuli, N., Karpel-Massler, G., et al. Blocking epithelial-to-mesenchymal transition in glioblastoma with a sextet of repurposed drugs: the EIS regimen. *Oncotarget.* 2017; 8(37):60727-60749.

147.   Pace, J., DeBerardinis, A., Sail, V., et al.   Repurposing the Clinically Efficacious Antifungal Agent Itraconazole as an Anticancer Chemotherapeutic. *J Med Chem.* 2016; 59(8):3635-3649.

148. Kim, J., Tang, J., Gong, R., et al. Itraconazole, a commonly used antifungal that inhibits Hedgehog pathway activity and cancer growth. *Cancer Cell.* 2010; 17(4):388-399.

149. Barriére, G., Tartary, M., Rigaud, M., Metformin: a rising star to fight the epithelial mesenchymal transition in oncology. *Anticancer Agents Med Chem.* 2013; 13(2):333-340.

150. Lin, H., Li, N., He, H., et al. AMPK Inhibits the Stimulatory Effects of TGF-ß on Smad2/3 Activity, Cell Migration, and Epithelial-to-Mesenchymal Transition. *Mol Pharmacol.* 2015; 88(6):1062-1071.

151. Cheng, K., Hao, M. Metformin Inhibits TGF-ß1-Induced Epithelial-to-Mesenchymal Transition via PKM2 Relative-mTOR/p70s6k Signaling Pathway in Cervical Carcinoma Cells. *Int J Mol Sci.* 2016; 17(12).

152. Nakayama, A., Ninomiya, I., Harada, S., et al. Metformin inhibits the radiation-induced invasive phenotype of esophageal squamous cell carcinoma. *Int J Oncol.* 2016; 49(5):1890-1898.

153. Ippolito, L., Marini, A., Cavallini, L., et al. Metabolic shift toward oxidative phosphorylation in docetaxel resistant prostate cancer cells. *Oncotarget.* 2016; 7(38):61890-61904.

154. Kurimoto, R., Iwasawa, S., Ebata, T., et al. Drug resistance originating from a TGF-ß/FGF-2- driven epithelial-to mesenchymal transition and its reversion in human lung adenocarcinoma cell lines harboring an EGFR mutation. *Int J Oncol.* 2016; 48(5):1825-1836.

155. Wahdan-Alaswad, R., Harrell, J., Fan, Z., et al. Metformin attenuates transforming growth factor beta (TGF-ß) mediated oncogenesis in mesenchymal stem-like/claudin-low triple negative breast cancer. *Cell Cycle.* 2016; 15(8):1046-1059.

156. Liu, Z., Qi, S., Zhao, X, et al. Metformin inhibits 17ß-estradiol-induced epithelial-to-mesenchymal transition via ßKlotho-related ERK1/2 signaling and AMPKα signaling in endometrial adenocarcinoma cells. *Oncotarget.* 2016; 7(16):21315-21331.

157. Zhang, J., Shen, C., Wang, L., et al. Metformin inhibits epithelial-to-mesenchymal transition in prostate cancer cells: involvement of the tumor suppressor miR30a and its target gene SOX4. *Biochem Biphys Res Commun.* 2014; 452(3):746-752.

158. Liu, Y, He, C., Haung, X. Metformin partially reverses the carboplatin-resistance in NSCLC by inhibiting glucose metabolism. *Oncotarget.* 2017; 8(43):75206-75216.

159.   Sesen, J., Dahan, P., Scotland, S., et al. Metformin inhibits growth of human glioblastoma cells and enhances therapeutic response. *PLoS One.* 2015; 10(4):e0123721.

160.   Yang, S., Li, S., Lu, G., et al. Metformin treatment reduces temozolomide resistance of glioblastoma cells. *Oncotarget.* 2016; 7(48):78787-78803.

161.   Skaga, E., Skaga, I., Grieg, Z., et al. The efficacy of a coordinated pharmacological blockade in glioblastoma stem cells with nine repurposed drugs using the CUSP9 strategy. *J Cancer Res Clin Oncol.* 2019; 145(6):1495-1507.

162.   *Surviving Terminal Cancer.* Directed by Dominic Hill, Indigo Rebel Films on Vimeo, 2015.

163.   Cufí, S., Vazquez-Martin, A., Oliveras-Ferraros, C., et al. The anti-malarial chloroquine overcomes primary resistance and restores sensitivity to trastuzumab in HER2-positive breast cancer. *Sci Rep.* 2013; 3:2469(1-13).

164.   Li, J., Zhu, F., Lubet, R., et al. Quercetin-3-methyl ether inhibits lapatinib-sensitive and resistant breast cancer cell growth by inducing G2/M arrest and apoptosis. *Mol Carcinog.* 2013; 52(2):134-143.

165.   Mason, J., Fu, M., Chen, J., et al. Flaxseed oil enhances the effectiveness of trastuzumab in reducing the growth of HER2-overexpressing human breast tumors (BT-474). *J Nutr Biochem.* 2015; 26:16-23.

166.   Proietti, S., Cucina, A., D'Anselmi, F., et al. Melatonin and vitamin D3 synergistically down-regulate Akt and MDM2 leading to TGFß-1-dependent growth inhibition of breast cancer cells. *J Pineal Res.* 2011; 50:150-158.

167.   Reiter, R., Rosales-Corral, S., Tan, D., et al. Melatonin, a Full Service Anti-Agent: Inhibition of Initiation, Progression, and Metastasis. *Int J Mol Sci.* 2017; 18(4):843.

168.   Xing, F., Liu, Y., Sharma, S., et al. Pterostilbene (PTER) suppresses breast cancer brain metastasis by targeting a c-Met mediated inflammation network. *Cancer Res.* 2016; 76(14)suppl:abstract 905.

169.   Moyad, M., Lee, J. "The Supplement Handbook: A Trusted Experts Guide to What Works and what's Worthless for More Than 100 Conditions." *Rodale Books* 2014.

170. Sanchez, W., McGee, S., Connor, T., et al. Dichloroacetate inhibits aerobic glycolysis in multiple myeloma cells and increases sensitivity to bortezomib. *Br J Cancer.* 2013; 108(8):1624-1633.

171. Bazzan, A., Zabrecky, G., Wintering, M., et al. Retrospective Evaluation of Clinical Experience with Intravenous Ascorbic Acid in Patients with Cancer. *Integr Cancer Ther.* 2018; 17(3):912-920.

172. Knott, S., Wagenblast, E., Khan, S., et al. Asparagine Bioavailability Governs Metastasis in a Model of Breast Cancer. *Nature.* 2018; 554(7692):378-381.

173. Kuo, C., Ann, D. When fats commit crimes: fatty acid metabolism, cancer stemness and therapeutic resistance. *Cancer Commun (Lond).* 2018; 38(1):47.

174. Beloribi-Djefflia, S., Vasseur, S., Guillaumond, F., et al. Lipid metabolic reprogramming in cancer cells. *Oncogenesis.* 2016, January 25.

175. Simsek, C., Esin, E., Yalcin, S. Metronomic Chemotherapy: A Systematic Review of the Literature and Clinical Experience. *J Oncol.* 2019; 2019:5483791.

176. Gupte, P., Giramkar, S., Harke, S., et al. Evaluation of the Efficacy and Safety of Capsule Longvida ® Optimized Curcumin (Solid Lipid Curcumin Particles) in Knee Osteoarthritis: A Pilot Clinical Study. *J Inflamm Res.* 2019; 12:145-152.

177. Verbaanderd, C., Maes, H., Schaaf, M., et al. Repurposing Drugs in Oncology (ReDO)-chloroquine and hydroxychloroquine as anti-cancer agents. *Ecancermedicalscience.* 2017; 11:781.

178. Ellegaard, A., Dehlendorff, C., Vind, A., et al. Repurposing Cationic Amphiphilic Antihistamines for Cancer Treatment. *EBioMedicine.* 2016; 9:130-139.

179. Zhang, P., Lai, Z., Chen, H., et al. Curcumin Synergizes with 5-fluorouracil by Impairing AMPK/ULK1-dependent Autophagy, AKT Activity and Enhancing Apoptosis in Colon Cancer Cells with Tumor Growth Inhibition in Xenograft Mice. *J Exp Clin Cancer Res.* 2017; 36(1):190.

180. Nowak-Sliwinska, P., Scapozza, L., Altaba, A. Drug repurposing in oncology: Compounds, pathways, phenotypes, and computational approaches for colorectal cancer. *Biochim Biophys Acta Rev Cancer.* 2019; 1871(2):434-454.

181. Pantziarka, P., Bouche, G., Meheus, L., et al. Repurposing drugs in oncology (ReDO)-cimetidine as an anti-cancer agent. *Ecancermedicalscience.* 2014; 8:485.

182. Matsumoto, S., Imaeda, Y., Umemoto, S., et al. Cimetidine increases survival of colorectal cancer patients with high levels of sialyl Lewis-X and sialyl Lewis-A epitope expression on tumor cells. *Br J Cancer.* 2002; 86(2):161-167.

183. Tønnesen, H., Knigge, U., Bülow, S., et al. Effect of cimetidine on survival after gastric cancer. *Lancet.* 1988; 2(8618):990-992.

184. Pantziarka, P., Bouche, G., Sukhatme, V., et al. Repurposing Drugs in Oncology (ReDO)-Propranolol as an anti-cancer agent. *Ecancermedicalscience.* 2016; 10:680.

185. Choy, C., Raytis, J., Smith, D., et al. Inhibition of ß2-adrenergic Receptor Reduces Triple-Negative Breast Cancer Brain Metastases; The Potential Benefit of Perioperative ß-Blockade. *Oncol Rep.* 2016; 35(6):3135-3142.

186. Verbaanderd, C., Maes, H., Schaaf, M., et al. Repurposing Drugs in Oncology (ReDO)-chloroquine and hydroxychloroquine as anti-cancer agents. *Ecancermedicalscience.* 2017; 11:781.

187. Briceño, E., Reyes, S., Sotelo, J. Therapy of Glioblastoma Multiforme Improved by the Antimutagenic Chloroquine. *Neurosurg Focus.* 2003; 14(2):e3.

188. Sotelo, J., Briceño, E., López-González, M. Adding Chloroquine to Conventional Treatment for Glioblastoma Multiforme: A Randomized Double-Blind, Placebo-Controlled Trial. *Ann Intern Med.* 2006; 144(5):337-343.

189. Levy, J., Thompson, J., Griesinger, A., et al. Autophagy Inhibition Improves Chemosensitivity in BRAF (V600E) Brain Tumors. *Cancer Discov.* 2014; 4(7):773-780.

190. Montanari, F., Lu, M., Marcus, S., et al. A Phase II Trial of Chloroquine in Combination with Bortezomib and Cyclophosphamide in Patients with Relapsed and Refractory Multiple Myeloma. *Blood.* 2014; 124(21):57-75.

191. Boone, B., Bahary, N., Zureikat, A., et al. Safety and Biologic Response of Pre-operative Autophagy Inhibition in Combination with Gemcitabine in Patients with Pancreatic Adenocarcinoma. *Ann Surg Oncol.* 2014; 22(13):4402-4410.

192. Rosenfeldt, M., O'Prey, J., Morton, J., et al. p53 Status Determines the Role of Autophagy in Pancreatic Tumor Development. *Nature.* 2013; 504:296-300.

193. Jonckheere, N., Vincent, A., VanSeuningen, I. Of Autophagy and in Vivo Pancreatic Carcinogenesis: The p53 Status Matters! *Clin Res Hepatol Gastroenterol.* 2014; 38(4): 423-425.

194. Sukhatme, V., Bouche, G., Meheus, L., et al. Repurposing Drugs in Oncology (ReDO)-nitroglycerine as an anti-cancer agent. *Ecancermedicalscience.* 2015; 9:568.

195. Yasuda, H., Yamaya, M., Nakayama, K., et al. Randomized Phase II Trial Comparing Nitroglycerine Plus Vinorelbine and Cisplatin with Vinorelbine and Cisplatin Alone in Previously Untreated Stage IIIB/IV Non-Small-Cell Lung Cancer. *J Clin Oncol.* 2006; 24(4):688-694.

196. Yasuda, H., Nakayama K, Watanabe, M., et al. Nitroglycerine Treatment May Enhance Chemosensitivity to Docetaxel and Carboplatin in Patients with Lung Adenocarcinoma. *Clin Cancer Res.* 2006; 12(22):6748-6757.

197. Siemens, D., Heaton, J., Adams, M., et al. Phase II Study of Nitric Oxide Donor for Men with Increasing Prostate-Specific Antigen Level After Surgery or Radiotherapy for Prostate Cancer. <u>*Urology.*</u> 2009; 74(4):878-883.

198. Pantziarka, P., Sukhatme, V., Bouche, G., et al. Repurposing Drugs in Oncology (ReDO)-itraconazole as an anti-cancer agent. *Econcermedicalscience.* 2015; 9:521.

199. Vreugdenhil, G., Raemaekers, J., VanDijke, B., et al. Itraconazole and Multidrug Resistance: Possible Effects on Remission Rate and Disease-Free Survival in Acute Leukemia. *Ann Hematol.* 1993; 67(3):107-109.

200. Antonarakis, E., Heath, E., Smith, D. et al. Repurposing Itraconazole as a Treatment for Advanced Prostate Cancer: A Noncomparative Randomized Phase II Trial in Men with Metastatic Castration-Resistant Prostate Cancer. *Oncologist.* 2013; 18(2): 163-173.

201. Suzman, D., Antonarakis, E. High-dose Itraconazole as a Non-Castrating Therapy for a Patient with Biochemically Recurrent Prostate Cancer. *Clin Genitourin Cancer.* 2014; 12(2):e51-e53.

202. Rudin, C., Brahmer, J., Juergens, R., et al. Phase II Study of Pemetrexed and Itraconazole as Second-Line Therapy for Metastatic Nonsquamous, Non-Small-Cell Lung Cancer. *J Thorac Oncol.* 2013; 8(5):619-623.

203. Tsubamoto, H., Sonoda, T., Yamasaki, M., et al. Impact of Combination Chemotherapy with Itraconazole on Survival for

Patients with Recurrent or Persistent Ovarian Clear-Cell Carcinoma. *Anticancer Res.* 2014; 34(4):2007-2014.

204. Tsubamoto, H., Sonoda, T., Inoue, K., Impact of Itraconazole on the Survival of Heavily Pre-Treated Patients with Triple-Negative Breast Cancer. *Anticancer Res.* 2014; 34(7):3839-3844.

205. Lockhart, N., Waddell, J., Schrock, N. Itraconazole Therapy in a Pancreatic Adenocarcinoma Patient: A Case Report. *J Oncol Pharm Pract.* 2016; 22(3):528-532.

206. Fabian, D., Eibl, M., Alnahhas, I., et al. Treatment of Glioblastoma (GBM) with the Addition of Tumor-Treating Fields (TTF): A Review. *Cancers (Basel).* 2019; 11(2):174.

207. Chiocca, E., Aguilar, L., Bell, S. Phase IB Study of Gene-Mediated Cytotoxic Immunotherapy Adjuvant to Up-Front Surgery and Intensive Timing Radiation for Malignant Glioma. *J Clin Oncol.* 2011; 29(27):3611-3619.

208. Redmond, K., Mehta, M.   Stereotactic Radiosurgery for Glioblastoma. *Cureus.* 2015; 7(12):e413.

209. Wang, Z., Jensen, M., Zenklusen, J. A Practical Guide to The Cancer Genome Atlas (TCGA). *Methods Mol Biol.* 2016; 1418:111-141.

210. Mamula, K. LifeX startups face especially long odds in attacking some of medicine's biggest challenges. *Pittsburgh Post Gazette.* 2018, December 24.

211. Idrus, A. Notable Labs lands $40M to expand AI-based cancer treatment tech. *FierceBiotech.* 2019, July 16.

212. Mamula, K. Chasing big dreams at lifeX south side incubator filled with startups determined to conquer devastating medical challenges. *Pittsburgh Post Gazette.* 2018, December 24.

213. Fabian, D., Eibl, M., Alnahhas, I., et al. Treatment of Glioblastoma (GBM) with the Addition of Tumor-Treating Fields (TTF): A Review. *Cancers (Basel).* 2019; 11(2):e174.

214. *Surviving Terminal Cancer*. Directed by Dominic Hill, Indigo Rebel Films on Vimeo, 2015.

215. Roan, S. Beating Cancer—One Patient at a Time. *UCI News UCI magazine.* 2020, January 29.

216. Woolams, C. Repurposed old drugs as new and effective treatments. *Cancer Active.* 2018, May 13.

217. Lin, M., Coronavirus and COVID-19: The Basic Biology behind the Epidemic. YouTube. https://youtu.be/qOF5a3I7puQ 2020, March 23.

218. Khafaie, M., Rahim, F. Cross-Country Comparison of Case Fatality Rates of COVID-19/SARS-CoV-2. *Osong Public Health Res Perspect.* 2020; 11(2):74-80.

219. Lang, J., Yang, N., Deng, J., et al. Inhibition of SARS pseudovirus cell entry by lactoferrin binding to heparin sulfate proteoglycans. *PLoS One* 2011; 6(8):e23710.

220. teVelthuis, A., van den Worm, S., Sims, A., et al. Zn(2+) Inhibits Coronavirus and Arterivirus RNA Polymerase Activity in Vitro and Zinc Ionophores Block the Replication of These Viruses in Cell Culture. *PloS Pathog.* 2010; 6(11):e1001176.

221. Skalny, A., Rink, L., Ajsuvakova, O., et al. Zinc and Respiratory Tract Infections: Perspectives for COVID-19 (Review). *Int J Mol Med.* 2020; 46(1):17-26.

222. Seheult, R. Medical Videos and Lectures Explained Clearly. Available at http://www.Medcram.com. Accessed 2020, May 28.

223. Wu, J., Leung, K., Bushman, M., et al. Estimating clinical severity of COVID-19 from the transmission dynamics in Wuhan, China. *Nature Medicine* 2020; 26:506-510.

224. De Wilde, A., Jochmans, D., Posthuma, C., et al. Screening of an FDA-approved compound library identifies four small-molecule inhibitors of Middle East respiratory syndrome coronavirus replication in cell culture. *Antimicrob Agents Chemother.* 2014; 58(8):4875-4884.

225. Vincent, M., Bergeron, E., Benjannet, S., et al. Chloroquine is a potent inhibitor of SARS coronavirus infection and spread. *Virol J.* 2005; 2:69.

226. Wang, M., Cao R., Zhang, L., et al. Remdesivir and chloroquine effectively inhibit the recently emerged novel coronavirus (2019-nCoV) in vitro. *Cell Res.* 2020; 30(3):269-271.

227. Rolain, J., Colson, P., Raoult, D., et al. Recycling of chloroquine and its hydroxyl analogue to face bacterial, fungal, and viral infections in the 21st century. *Int J Antimicrob Agents* 2007; 30(4):297-308.

228. Devaux, C., Rolain, J., Colson, P., Raoult, D. New insights on the antiviral effects of chloroquine against coronavirus: what to expect for COVID-19? *Int J Antimicrob Agents.* 2020 March; 05938.

229. Savarino, A., Boelaert, J., Cassone, A., et al. Effects of chloroquine on viral infections: an old drug against today's diseases? *Lancet Infect Dis.* 2003; 3:722-727.

230.   Chu, C., Cheng, V., Hung, I., et al.   Role of lopinavir/ritonavir in the treatment of SARS: initial virological and clinical findings. *Thorax.* 2004; 59(3):252-256.

231.   Chan, K., Lai, S., Chu, C., et al.   Treatment of severe acute respiratory syndrome with lopinavir/ritonavir: a multicenter retrospective matched cohort study. *Hong Kong Med J.* 2003; 9(6):399-406.

232.   Park, S., Lee, J., Son, J., et al.   Post-exposure prophylaxis for Middle East respiratory syndrome in healthcare workers. *J Hosp Infect.* 2019; 101(1):42-46.

233.   Yan, A. Chinese expert who came down with Wuhan coronavirus after saying it was controllable thinks he was infected through his eyes. *South China Morning Post.* 2020 Jan 23.

234.   Ng, H., Narasaraju, T., Phoon, M., et al. Doxycycline Treatment Attenuates Acute Lung Injury in Mice Infected with Virulent Influenza H3N2 Virus: Involvement of Matrix Metalloproteinases. *Exp Mol Pathol.* 2012; 92(3):287-295.

235.   Hoffmann, M., Kleine-Weber, H, Schroeder, S., et al. SARS-CoV-2 Cell Entry Depends on ACE2 and TMPRSS2 and Is Blocked by a Clinically Proven Protease Inhibitor. *Cell.* 2020; 181(2):271-280.e8.

236.   TED Talk. The Next Outbreak? We're Not Ready-Bill Gates. YouTube. http://www.youtu.be/v=6Af6b_wyiwl. Published 2015, April 3.

237.   Cai, Q., Yang, M., Liu, D., et al. Experimental Treatment with Favipiravir for COVID-19: An Open-Label Control Study. 2020; 10.1016/J.eng.2020.03.007.

238.   Vincent, M., Bergeron, E., Benjannet, S., et al. Chloroquine is a potent inhibitor of SARS coronavirus infection and spread. *Virol J.* 2005; 2:69.

239.   Gautret, P., Lagier, J., Parola, P., et al. Hydroxychloroquine and azithromycin as a treatment of COVID-19: results of an open-label non-randomized clinical trial. *Int J. Antimicrob Agents.* 2020 March; 105949.

240.   Zhou, F., Yu, T., Du, R., et al. Clinical course and risk factors for mortality of adult inpatients with COVID-19 in Wuhan, China: a retrospective cohort study. *Lancet.* 2020 March: 30566-3.

241.   Monaco, K.   Could an Anti-Malarial Be an Adjunctive T2D Therapy? *Med Page Today.* 2019 April 27.

242. Kuanal, J. Coronavirus PandemicP: ICMR recommends use of 'hydroxychloroquine' for treatment of high risk cases. *Jagran English.* 2020 March 23.

243. Foster, J., Rachdi, R. Professor Raoult Shows Promising Results of His Study on 1,061 Patients 91% Recovered Against COVID-19 with Hydroxychloroquine. *United States Press Agency News.* 2020 April 12.

244. Whitely, J. 39 elderly Texans successfully complete hydroxychloroquine treatment for COVID-19, doctor says. *WFAA ABC 8.* 2020, April 14.

245. Retraction Watch Staff. Hydroxychloroquine for COVID-19 Study Did Not Meet 'Expected Standard.' *Medscape Perspective Commentary.* Comments. 2020 April 8.

246. Frellick, M. No hydroxychloroquine benefit in small randomized COVID-19 trial. *Messcape Medical News.* Comments 2020, April 16.

247. Melles, R., Marmor, M. The risk of toxic retinopathy in patients on long-term hydroxychloroquine therapy. *JAMA Ophthalmol.* 2014; 132(12):1453-1460.

248. "The cardiotoxicity of antimalarials." *World Health Organization-Malaria Policy Advisory Meeting.* 2017 March 22.

249. Zhou, F., Yu, T., Du, R., et al. Clinical course and risk factors for mortality of adult inpatients with COVID-19 in Wuhan, China: a retrospective cohort study. *Lancet.* 2020; 395(10229):p1054-1062.

250. Kesselheim, A., Franklin, J., Kim, S., et al. Reductions in Use of Colchicine after FDA Enforcement of Market Exclusivity in a Commercially Insured Population. *J Gen Intern Med.* 2015; 30(11):1633-1638.

251. Retraction Watch Staff. Hydroxychloroquine for COVID-19 Study Did Not Meet 'Expected Standard.' *Medscape Perspective.* Comments. 2020 April 8.

252. Biswas, J. What makes bats the perfect host for deadly coronaviruses? Scientists reveal. *International Business Times.* 2020 February 16.

253. Keyaerts, E., Vijgen, L., Maes, P., et al. In vitro inhibition of severe acute respiratory syndrome coronavirus by chloroquine. *Biochem Biophys Res Commun.* 2004; 323(1):264-268.

254. de Wilde, A., Jochmans, D., Posthuma, C., et al. Screening of an FDA-approved compound library identifies four small-molecule

inhibitors of Middle East respiratory syndrome coronavirus replication in cell culture. *Antimicrob Agents Chemother.* 2014; 58(8)4875-4884.

255.   Gautret, P., Lagier, J., Parola, P., et al. Hydroxychloroquine and azithromycin as a treatment of COVID-19: results of an open-label non-randomized clinical trial. *Int J Antimicrob Agents.* 2020 March 20:105949.

256.   Singh, A., Singh A., Shaikh, A., et al. Chloroquine and hydroxychloroquine in the treatment of COVID-19 with or without diabetes: A systemic search and a narrative review with a special reference to India and other developing countries. *Diabetes Metab Syndr.* 2020; 14(3):241-246.

257.   Colson, P., Rolain, J., Lagier, J., et al. Chloroquine and hydroxychloroquine as available weapons to fight COVID-19. *Int J Antimicrob Agents.* 2020 March; 4:105932.

258.   Vanhaver, A. COVID-19 Belgium update of April 17, 2020. *New York School of Regional Anesthesia News.* 2020 April 17.

259.   Raoult, D., Zumla, A., Locatelli, F., et al. Coronavirus infections: Epidemiological, clinical, and immunological features and hypotheses. *Cell Stress.* 2020; 4(4):66-75.

260.   Hui, D., Wong, K., Ko, F., et al. The 1-year impact of severe acute respiratory syndrome on pulmonary function, exercise capacity, and quality of life in a cohort of survivors. *Chest.* 2005; 128(4):2247-2261.

261.   Perkett, E., Oranatowski, W., Poschet, J., et al. Chloroquine normalizes aberrant transforming growth factor beta activity in cystic fibrosis bronchial epithelial cells. *Pediatr Pulmonol.* 2006; 41(8):771-778.

262.   Jang, C., Choi, J., Byun, M., et al. Chloroquine inhibits production of TNF-ά, IL-Iß and IL-6 from lipopolysaccharide-stimulated human monocytes/macrophages by different modes. *Rheumatology (Oxford).* 2006; 45(6):703-710.

263.   Ruiz-Irastorza, G., Egurbide, M., Pijoan, J., et al. Effect of antimalarials on thrombosis and survival in patients with systemic lupus erythematosus. *Lupus.* 2006; 15(9):577-583.

264.   Farias, K., Machado, P., de Almeida Jr., et al. Chloroquine Interferes with dengue-2 Virus Replication in U937 Cells. *Microbiol Immunol.* 2014; 58(6):318-326.

265.   Kakodkar, P., Kaka, N., Baig, M. A Comprehensive Literature Review on the Clinical Presentation, and Management of the

Pandemic Coronavirus Disease 2019 (COVID-19). *Cureus.* 2020; 12(4):e7560.

266. Curley, G., Laffey, J. Future Therapies for ARDS. *Intensive Care Med.* 2015; 41(2):322-326.

267. Esler, M., Esler, D. Can angiotensin receptor-blocking drugs perhaps be harmful in the COVID-19 pandemic? *J Hypertens.* 2020; 38(5):781-782.

268. Kow, C., Zaidi, S., Hasan, S. Cardiovascular Disease and Use of Renin-Angiotensin System Inhibitors in COVID-19. *Am j Cardiovasc Drugs.* 2020 April 13:1-5.

269. Walters, T., Kalman, J., Patel, S. et al. Angiotension converting enzyme 2 activity and human atrial fibrillation: increase plasma angiotensin converting enzyme 2 activity is associated with atrial fibrillation and more advanced left atrial structure remodelling. *E P Europace.* 2017; 19(8):1280-1287.

270. Ramchand, J., Patel, S., Srivastava, P., et al. Elevated plasma angiotensin converting enzyme 2 activity is an independent predictor of major adverse cardiac events in patients with obstructive coronary artery disease. *PLoS One.* 2018; 13(6):e0198144.

271. Slachta, A. Hypertension 'a key dangerous factor' in COVID-19 mortality. *Cardiovascular Business.* 2020 March 12.

272. Ebhardt, T., Remondini, C., Bertacche, M. 99% of Those Who Died From Virus Had Other Illness Italy Says. *Bloomberg World News.* 2020 March 18.

273. Henriques, M. Coronavirus: Why death and mortality rates differ. *BBC Future News.* 2020 April 1.

274. Hope, J. *The Coffee Cure Diet: Live Longer Look Younger.* Hope Pressworks International LLC. 2019 Redding, CA

275. Kuanal, J. Coronavirus Pandemic: ICMR recommends use of 'hydroxychloroquine' for treatment of high-risk cases. *Jagran English.* 2020 March 23.

276. Hoekstra, K. Opinion: Michigan's doctors fight coronavirus in governor's office. *The Detroit News.* 2020 March 26.

277. Mitchell, T. Don't wait for proof positive, give this combo a test in real world and real time. Editorial. *Los Vegas Tribune.* 2020 April 2.

278. Roose, K., Rosenburg, M. Touting Virus Cure, 'Simple Country Doctor' Becomes a Right-Wing Star. *The New York Times.* 2020 April 2.

279. Kuanal, J. Coronavirus Pandemic: ICMR recommends use of 'hydroxychloroquine' for treatment of high-risk cases. *Jagran English.* 2020 March 23.

280. Colson, P., Rolain, J., Raoult, D. Chloroquine for the 2019 novel coronavirus SARS-CoV-2. *Int J Antimicrob Agents* 2020; 55(3):105923.

281. Colyer, J., Hinthorn, D. These Drugs Are Helping Our Coronavirus Patients. *Wall Street Journal Opinion.* 2020 March 22.

282. Curated Content. COVID-19 patients go from 'very ill' to 'symptom-free' in 8 to 12 hours with hydroxychloroquine & zinc. *Accounting Weekly.* 2020, April 8.

283. Lambert, H. Oregon veteran recovers from COVID-19, celebrates 104th birthday. *Koin@6news.* 2020 April 1.

284. Selsky, A. Oregon relaxes new restrictions on drugs to fight coronavirus. *East Oregonian.* 2020 April 2.

285. Bascome, E. Following Oddo's push, Cuomo amends executive order affecting nursing homes. *Silive.com.* 2020 March 28.

286. Royal, D. Florida Doctors Cautiously Using Hydroxychloroquine to Fight Coronavirus. *WLRN News.* 2020 April 10.

287. Sharon, K. Elderly OC couple recovers from coronavirus, swears by hydroxychloroquine. *The Orange County Register.* 2020 April 16.

288. Rolain, J., Colson, P., Raoult, D. Recycling of chloroquine and its hydroxyl analogue to face bacterial, fungal, and viral infections in the 21st Century. *Int J Antimicrob Agents.* 2007; 30(4):297-308.

289. Fine, H. Soon-Shiong Sets Sights on Virus. *Los Angeles Business.* 2020, April 20.

290. LA Times. The Science Behind the Coronavirus, Series II. YouTube. http://www.Youtu.be/v=rRMkEDwJxbU. Published 2020, April 13.

291. Chen, J., Hu, C., Chen, L., et al. Clinical Study of Mesenchymal Stem Cell Treating Acute Respiratory Distress Syndrome Induced by Epidemic Influenza A (H7N9) Infection, a Hint for COVID-19 Treatment. *Engineering (Beijing).* 2020; 10.1016/j.eng.2020.02.006.

292. Leng, Z., Zhu, R., Hou, W., et al. Transplantation of ACE2 Mesenchymal Stem Cells Improves the Outcome of Patients with COVID-19 Pneumonia. *Aging and Disease.* 2020; 11(2):10.14336.

293. Mahmood, K., Naeem, M., Rahimnajjad, N., Metformin: The Hidden Chronicles of a Magic Drug. *Eur J Intern Med.* 2013; 24(1):20-26.

294. Alarcón, G., McGwin, G., Bertoli, A., et al. Effect of Hydroxychloroquine on the Survival of Patients with Systemic Lupus Erythematosus: Data from LUMINA a Multiethnic US Cohort (LUMINA L). *Ann Rheum Dis.* 2007; 66(9):1168-1172.

295. Forouzandeh, F., Salazar, G., Patrushev, N., et al. Metformin Beyond Diabetes: Pleiotrophic Benefits of Metformin in Attenuation of Atherosclerosis. *J Am Heart Assoc.* 2014; 3(6):e001202.

296. Liu, D., Li, X., Zhang, Y., et al. Chloroquine and Hydroxychloroquine Are Associated with Reduced Cardiovascular Risk: A Systematic Review and Meta-Analysis. *Drug Des Devel Ther.* 2018; 12:1685-1695.

297. Wang, J., Zhu, L., Hu, K., et al. Effects of Metformin Treatment on Serum Levels of C-reactive Protein and interleukin-6 in Women with Polycystic Ovary Syndrome: A Meta-Analysis: A PRISMA-compliant Article. *Medicine (Baltimore).* 2017; 96(39):e8183.

298. Sacre, K., Criswell, L., McCune, J. Hydroxychloroquine is Associated with Impaired Interferon-Alpha and Tumor Necrosis Factor Alpha Production by Plasmacytoid Dendritic Cells in Systemic Lupus Erythematosus. *Arthritis Res Ther.* 2012; 14(3):R155.

299. Kravvariti, E., Koutsogianni, A., Samoli, E., et al. The Effect of Hydroxychloroquine on Thrombosis Prevention and Antiphospholipid Antibody Levels in Primary Antiphospholipid Syndrome: A Pilot Open Label Randomized Prospective Study. *Autoimmune Rev.* 2020; 19(4):102491.

300. Gupta, A. Real-World Clinical Effectiveness and Intolerability of Hydroxychloroquine 400 Mg in Uncontrolled Type 2 Diabetes Subjects Who Are Not Willing to Initiate Insulin Therapy (HYQ-Real-World Study). *Curr Diabetes Rev.* 2019; 15(6):510-519.

301. Paital, B., Das, K., Parida, S. Inter Nation Social Lockdown versus Medical Care Against COVID-19, a Mild Environmental Insight with Special Reference to India. *Sci Total Environ.* 2020; 728:138914.

302.   Luft, D., Schmülling, R., Eggstein, M. Lactic Acidosis in Biguanide-Treated Diabetics: A Review of 330 Cases. *Diabetalogia.* 1978; 14(2):75-87.

303.   Chan, N., Brain, H., Feher, M. Metformin-Associated Lactic Acidosis: A Rare or Very Rare Clinical Entity? *Diabetes Care.* 2003; 26(8):2471-2472.

304.   Salpeter, S., Greyber, E., Pasternak, G., et al. Risk of Fatal and Nonfatal Lactic Acidosis with Metformin Use in Type 2 Diabetes Mellitus: Systematic Review and Meta-Analysis. *Arch Intern Med.* 2003; 163(21):2594-2602.

305.   Bouchaud, O., Imbert, P., Touze, J., et al. Fatal Cardiotoxicity Related to Halofantrine: A Review Based on a Worldwide Safety Database. *Malar J.* 2009; 8:289.

306.   Munro, R., Morrison, E., McDonald, A., et al. Effect of Disease Modifying Agents on the Lipid Profiles of Patients with Rheumatoid Arthritis. *Ann Rheum Dis.* 1997; 56(6):374-377.

307.   Floris, A., Piga, M., Mangoni, A., et al. Protective Effects of Hydroxychloroquine Against Accelerated Atherosclerosis in Systemic Lupus Erythematosus. *Mediators Inflamm.* 2018; 2018:3424136.

308.   Kohli, U., Altujjar, M., Sharma, R., et al. Wide Interindividual Variability in Cardiovascular Toxicity of Loperamide: A Case Report in Review of Literature. *Heartrhythm Case Rep.* 2019; 5(4):221-224.

309.   Mukarram, O., Hindi, Y., Catalasan, G., et al. Loperamide Induced Torsades De Pointes: A Case Report and Review of the Literature. *Case Rep Med.* 2016; 2016:4061980.

310.   Lu, Z., Yuan, J., Li, M., et al. Cardiac Risks Associated with Antibiotics: Azithromycin and Levofloxacin. *Expert Opin Drug Saf.* 2015; 14(2):295-303.

311.   Rao, G., Mann, J., Shoaibi, A., et al. Azithromycin and Levofloxacin Use and Increased Risk of Cardiac Arrhythmia and Death. *Ann Fam Med.* 2014; 12(2):121-127.

312.   Chou, H., Wang, J., Chang, C. et all. Risks of Cardiac Arrhythmia and Mortality among Patients Using New-Generation Macrolides, Fluoroquinolones, and ß-Lactamase Inhibitors: A Taiwanese Nationwide Study. *Clin Infect Dis.* 2015; 60(4):566-577.

313.   Wang, Y., Zhang, D., Du, G., et al. Remdesivir in adults with severe COVID-19: A randomized double-blind, placebo-

controlled, mulicentre trial. *Lancet.* 2020; 395(10236):1569-1578.

314. Gilead Press Release. Data on 53 Patients Treated with Investigational Antiviral Remdesivir through the Compassionate Use Program Published in *New England Journal of Medicine.* 2020, April 10. Available at http://www.Gilead.com Accessed 2020, May 28.

315. Gilead Press Release. Gilead Announces Results from Phase III Trial of Investigational Antiviral Remdesivir in Patients with Severe COVID-19. 2020, April 29. Available at http://www.Gilead.com. Accessed 2020, May 28.

316. Baker, P., Kolata, G., Weiland, N. Remdesivir Shows Modest Benefits in Coronavirus Trial. *The New York Times.* 2020, April 29.

317. De La Cretaz, B. What you should know about Remdesivir, the Potential COVID-19 Treatment. *Refinery 29.* 2020, April 30.

318. Vliet, E. Gilead Announces Results from Phase III Trial of Investigational Antiviral Remdesivir in Patients with Severe COVID-19. *AAPS.* 2020, May 7.

319. Klar, R. FDA Head: Taking Hydroxychloroquine "Ultimately a Decision between a Patient and their Doctor." *The Hill.* 2020, May 19.

320. Million M., Lagier, J., Gautret, P., et al. Early Treatment of COVID-19 Patients with Hydroxychloroquine and Azithromycin: A Retrospective Analysis of 1,061 Cases in Marseille, France. *Travel Med Infect Dis.* 2020; 101738.

321. Bigelsen, S. Evidenced-based complementary treatment of pancreatic cancer: a review of adjunct therapies including paricalcitol, hydroxychloroquine, intravenous vitamin C, statins, metformin, curcumin, and aspirin. *Cancer Manag Res.* 2018; 10:2003-2018.

322. Risch, H., Streicher S., Wang, J., et al. Aspirin Use and Reduced Risk of Pancreatic Cancer. *Cancer Epidemiol Biomarkers Prev.* 2017; 26(1): 68-74 doi:10.1158/1055-9965.

323. Risch, H. Early Outpatient Treatment of Symptomatic, High-Risk COVID-19 Patients that Should be Ramped-Up Immediately as Key to the Pandemic Crisis, Am J Epidemiol. Doi:10.1093/aje/kwaa093.

324.   Bigelsen, S. Taking a Different Approach to Pancreatic Cancer Treatment. *Lets Win! Pancreatic Cancer.* February 14, 2017. Available at http://www.letswinpc.org Accessed 2020, May 28.

325.   Kast R., Karpel-Massler, G., Halatsch, M., et al. CUSP9* treatment protocol for recurrent glioblastoma: aprepitant, artesunate, auranofin, captopril, celecoxib, disulfiram, itraconazole, ritonavir, sertraline augmenting continuous low dose temozolomide. *Oncotarget.* 2014; 5(18): 8052-8082.

326.   Kelland, K. UK halts trial of hydroxychloroquine as 'useless' for COVID-19 patients. *Reuters Health News.* June 5, 2020.

327.   Mehra, M., Desai, S., Ruschitzka, F., et al., Hydroxychloroquine or Chloroquine with or without a macrolide for treatment of COVID-19: a multinational registry analysis. *The Lancet.* 2020: doi: 10.1016/S0140-6736(20)31180-6.

328.   Carlucci, P., Ahuja, T., Petrilli, C., et al. Hydroxychloroquine and azithromycin plus zinc vs hydroxychloroquine and azithromycin alone: outcomes in hospitalized COVID-19 patients. medRxiv. Doi: 10.1101/2020.05.02.20080036.

329.   Chatterjee, P., Anand, T., Singh, K., et al. Healthcare workers & SARS-CoV-2 infection in India: A case-control investigation in the time of COVID-19. IJMR. 2020; 151(5): 459-467.

330.   Boulware, D., Pullen, M., Bangdiwala, et al., A Randomized Trial of Hydroxychloroquine as Postexposure Prophylaxis for COVID-19. *NEJM.* 2020: doi: 10.1056/MEJMoa2016638.

331.   Geleris, J., Sun, Y., Platt, J., et al., Observational study of hydroxychloroquine in hospitalized patients with COVID-19. *N Engl J Med.* 2020; doi: 10.1056/NEJMoa2012410.

332.   Magagnoli, J., Narendran, F., Cummings, T., et al., Outcomes of hydroxychloroquine usage in United States veterans hospitalized with COVID-19. Med (2020) doi: 10.1016/j.medj.2020.06.001.

333.   Rosenberg, E., Dufort, E., Udo, T., et al. "Association of Treatment with Hydroxychloroquine or Azithromycin with In-Hospital Mortality in Patient's with COVID-19 in New York State." *JAMA.* 2020: doi:10.1001/JAMA.2020.8630.

334.   Arshad, S., Kilgore, P., Chaudhry, Z., et al. Treatment with Hydroxychloroquine, Azithromycin, and Combination in Patients Hospitalized with COVID-19. *Int J of Infectious Dis.* 2020; doi: 10.1016/j.ijid.2020.06.099.

335.   Borba, M., Val, F., Sampaio, V., et al. Effect of High Doses of Chloroquine Diphosphate as Adjunctive Therapy for Patients

Hospitalized with Severe Acute Respiratory Syndrome Coronavirus 2 (SARS-CoV-2) Infection: A Randomized Clinical Trial. *JAMA Netw Open*. 2020;3(4):e208857.

336. Scholz, M., Derwand, R., Zelenko, V., et al. COVID-19 Outpatients – Early Risk-Stratified Treatment with Zinc Plus Low Dose Hydroxychloroquine and Azithromycin: A Retrospective Case Series Study. *Preprints*: 2020
Doi: 10.20944/preprints202007.0025.v1

337. Mohammad, S., Clowse, M., Eudy, A., et al. Examination of Hydroxychloroquine Use and Hemolytic Anemia in G6PDH-Deficient Patients. *Arthritis Care Res (Hoboken)*. 2018;70(3):481-485. Doi:10.1002/acr.23296.

338. Yao, X., Ye, F., Zhang, M., et al. In vitro antiviral activity and projection of optimized dosing design of hydroxychloroquine for the treatment of severe acute respiratory syndrome coronavirus 2 (SARS-CoV-2). *Clin Infect Dis*. 2020; doi: 10.1093/cid/ciaa237.

339. Sayare S. He was a science star. Then he promoted a questionable cure for COVID-19. *New York Times Magazine*. May 12, 2020.

340. Biancatelli, R., Berrill, M., Catravas, J., et al. Quercetin and Vitamin C: An Experimental, Synergistic Therapy for the Prevention and Treatment of SARS-CoV-2 Related Disease (COVID-19). *Front Immunol*. 2020; doi:10.3389/fimmu.2020.01451.

APPENDIX A

MYTHS AND MISCONCEPTIONS

1) **Cancer treatment, using standard of care as currently practiced in major medical centers, is my best chance for survival.** Our current cancer treatment model involves surgery, chemotherapy, and radiation therapy. Overall, about 60% survive for about five years. Of these, many are left with permanent debilitating side effects ranging from brain damage to painful peripheral neuropathy and high-risk for secondary cancers. Modifying the current standard of treatment with the addition of repurposed drugs, metronomic chemotherapy, and more precise lower dose radiation therapy can improve survival substantially as well as decrease complications.

2) **If repurposed drug combinations for cancer were truly effective, then major cancer centers would already be using them.** They are in the context of clinical trials through the GlobalCures project. There are monumental legal financial and regulatory obstacles to widespread use, even with the marketing of new and effective cancer treatments. Repurposed drugs are highly effective, especially in advanced cancer cases where the expected survival is less than five years.

3) **Doctors frown on prescribing repurposed drugs.** While it is still true that many oncologists will decline to prescribe these off-label medications to treat cancer, the majority of family practice or general practitioners will prescribe them if they are nontoxic and are requested.

4) **The stories of long-term cancer survival for those using repurposed drugs are anecdotal and do not prove anything.** On the contrary, there are increasing numbers of patients who enjoy long-term survival who also use repurposed drug cocktails. Many studies show strong anticancer effects along multiple known molecular pathways that have proven effects both in vitro and in vivo. Clinical trials with repurposed drug cocktails at Care Oncology Clinic and those studies sponsored by the

Anticancer Research fund are showing improved survival compared to standard treatment alone.

5) **Using combinations of repurposed drugs is dangerous as it can produce drug interactions and toxicity.** Repurposed drugs are generally much safer than standard chemotherapy and radiation therapy. These old drugs have been used for many years to control blood pressure, cholesterol, or blood sugar.

Even combinations of them (i.e., metformin + statin + doxycycline) at standard doses are usually quite safe. If they are all prescribed under the supervision of a physician, usually your general practitioner, any toxicities should be noticed with appropriate countermeasures taken.

6) **Using repurposed drug combinations are not scientific.** Retrospective studies and mechanistic studies established the scientific basis for the anticancer use; that is, metformin raises AMPK, which lowers mTOR, thereby reducing the risk for cancer. When a number of studies all agree on an antitumor effect, that molecular target can be successfully identified. If the drugs have been used in the past for many decades safely for other purposes, there is little risk and great potential reward. This is science at its best.

7) **The evidence for using aspirin, metformin, or statins to prevent cancer is lacking.** On the contrary, hundreds of scientific studies link aspirin, statins, and metformin to lower risks of cancer and cancer death rates. These drugs have been in use for decades, and their safety profile is well-established. The aspirin data are clear in its use as chemo-prevention for colon cancer in those high-risk groups aged 50-59 and at low-risk for GI bleeding.

We have enough data for metformin to support its use as a preventative for cancer in those with insulin resistance or at high-risk, such as those populations with diabetes. Dr. Mark Moyad, a Professor at the University at Michigan Medical Center, has published strong recommendations to use S.A.M. for the prevention of prostate cancer. We use many daily medications for the prevention of heart disease. The time has come to use them as well in the prevention of cancer.

8) **We already have great strategies for early cancer detection and treatment in the United States. We have the world's best medical care. Why do we need to add repurposed drugs?** The truth of the matter is that cancer incidence and mortality are not decreasing across the board. Yes, we have slightly lower colon cancer deaths through early detection and treatment, but we continue to lose some 600,000 people a year to cancer, and there is almost nothing to offer stage IV cancer patients such as those with glioblastoma or pancreatic cancer other than chemotherapy, radiation, and exorbitant six-figure medical bills. How about instead adding repurposed drugs immediately, both for prevention and treatment, to cut this number down by one-third and improve survival and quality of life?

9) **You are not going to cure cancer with cocktails of supplements and off-label medications.** Very few diseases are ever cured. High blood pressure and diabetes are managed. Today, AIDS, once a quick killer, is managed as HIV with a cocktail of supplements and drugs. Cancer can be managed the same way if we choose to open our minds and utilize all of the resources available, including repurposed drugs. AIDS patients marched on the Capital and changed the laws to fast track HIV cocktails. They were not forced through the usual slow, arduous, and political FDA process. Repurposed drug combinations could be similarly fast-tracked if enough people spoke up.

AIDS medication cocktails work by keeping the viral count low so that a person can live in spite of having an incurable disease. In the same way, we can keep cancer counts low to provide a person long-term survival without actually curing or killing all of the cancer cells. It is all about educating the public and using our current knowledge.

APPENDIX B

FREQUENTLY ASKED QUESTIONS

1) **If repurposed drugs are so effective against cancer, then why have other doctors not written about this?** They have. Predominately in the scientific literature. That is where evidence is shared with other scientists. The starting point is usually in vitro and test tube experiments, as well as animal experiments. Later, results in human trials are published. These include studies examining large numbers of patients who use the drug. The evidence for the anticancer effects of aspirin, statins, metformin, and chloroquine are clear. There is encouraging evidence by new studies showing massive benefits and relatively low-risk profile in mebendazole to multiple cancers.

Do all physicians keep up on all articles on PubMed? The answer is very few. I can tell you that in completing one hundred hours in CME recently, the required course work to keep up one's license, there was not one mention of repurposed drug use in cancer. Dr. Ben Williams was incensed when his oncologist never told him about Accutane's potential activity against brain cancer even though his oncologist was aware of the study. I believe in informed consent.

All terminal cancer patients MUST be informed about the potential benefits of adding repurposed drug cocktails to standard treatment. Let them make the decision. I believe with this book I am helping provide access to this vital information.

2) **Don't you think your book is giving people false hope?** My friend developed GBM. I would want him to have the same information that I do. The Care Oncology Clinic has a clinical trial showing that 95 patients using their protocol have nearly doubled their survival. I think he should know about it.

I think he should be informed. He should be able to make his own decision with the current information. He should not be in the dark. Is that giving him false hope? I think not. It is giving him realistic hope.

3)   **You are not an oncologist or cancer specialist. What makes you qualified to make recommendations on cancer care?** Fair question. My field of physical medicine and rehabilitation crosses many specialties: neurology, orthopedics, rheumatology. That is because we are not defined by an organ system.

Instead, our specialty strives to maximize the quality of life, despite having a terminal or chronic condition. We help people with paralysis get up and move about. We help people without limbs get artificial limbs to improve function. I feel that using repurposed drugs to lengthen survival and improve quality of life in cancer patients is precisely a part of my duty as a physical medicine specialist and physician.

4)   **Isn't it against the law to prescribe medications off-label?** Doctors prescribe off-label medications all the time. The prescribing of amoxicillin for pediatric ear infections is off-label. When it comes to chronic pain or infection, doctors aren't too concerned about prescribing off-label.

Cancer specialists, however, are very formal and concerned. They often will decline to prescribe off-label unless the patient is a scientist or VIP. Family practitioners, on the other hand, are more likely to prescribe, like Dr. Jennings of New Zealand. If you approach them with a reasonable request, backed by a copy of a published scientific study, they are likely to prescribe the medication, even for cancer. However, they may tell you, "I'm not sure this will do any good, but it can't hurt you."

5)   **What about targeted immunotherapy, the advances made in melanoma treatments, the United States drop in colon cancer, and mapping the human genome? Why would we allow people to just "guess" and add a bunch of dirty drugs that might not work when we can stick with our current FDA approval process in good science?** First, all colon cancer death rates are rising in the rest of the world. In the United States, due to early detection with colonoscopies and removing precancerous adenomatous polyps, we have enjoyed a small victory in a slight decline.

But let me ask you, if you were in Dr. Ben Williams' shoes, and had read good studies about Accutane, would you want to add it? Would you take Melatonin if you were in Dr. Angela Chapman's shoes and knew it could enhance your chemotherapy's effectiveness? Why wouldn't you want to include these with stage IV cancer or glioma in which you were essentially handed a death sentence unless you did something different?

6) **What role do you see repurposed drugs playing in the next ten years?** It can take 1.8 billion dollars and 15 years to get a new molecule to market as a cancer drug. There is a huge chance it will fail. The investment in cancer research is drying up. Very few new drugs are currently being developed for cancer. The last FDA-approved molecule for glioblastoma treatment was released 16 years ago in 2004 with TMZ. That's not nearly enough. Meanwhile, we continue to cut, burn, and poison people with surgery, radiation, and chemotherapy.

The expense continues to bankrupt entire families, and the patients lose the fight 40% of the time within five years. Some 2,000 drugs are currently FDA-approved as safe for their particular use. Three hundred ten of these block key pathways of cancer. Mining of these repositioned drugs will yield rich dividends as these can be fashioned into cocktails to increase survival in many patients. If you were stranded on a desert island like the character in *Cast Away*, I guarantee that you would repurpose every available and possible resource to further your survival. Why would we not make similar use of repurposed drugs in cancer treatments today?

APPENDIX C

INFORMED CONSENT FOR REPURPOSED DRUG(S)

Please take this book to your medical doctor when you ask for the addition of a repurposed drug cocktail. Allow him to verify the studies and science for himself. Then add this question: "If my cancer is terminal anyway, and the repurposed drug cocktail is relatively nontoxic, and there is evidence it can improve my survival, what is the harm in adding it?" Then show him the Informed Consent Form below. Tell him you will sign it to absolve him of any liability, and this should motivate him to prescribe.

Background: I have requested that my doctor prescribe a drug or combination of drugs for the purpose of treating my cancer. Each of these drugs has already been FDA-approved to treat at least one condition. However, each has not been approved to treat cancer. Since my cancer carries a poor prognosis, I, as the patient, have requested, based upon scientific studies that I have shown to my doctor, a prescription to obtain these drug(s).

Informed Consent: I am aware that sufficient Phase II and Phase III clinical trials have not yet been conducted and approved. There is no guarantee this drug or drug combination will improve my survival. Moreover, there is a possibility that the drug or drug combination could lead to the development of various toxicities, which may not be predictable to my heart, lung, liver, kidney, brain, bone marrow, or other organs or systems.

Good Faith: I understand that my doctor is acting in good faith, with his usual skill and knowledge, and is granting my request for access to these drugs for the purpose of helping me survive my cancer. I hereby agree, in return, to forever hold him harmless for any unintended or adverse consequences of these drugs. This informed consent shall remain in full force and effect unless it is revoked in writing.

General Recommendations: This doctor advises the patient to continue to receive all standard of care cancer treatment. At no time is this physician advising the patient to forego standard of care treatment.

Questions Answered: As the patient, I certify that I have initiated this request for repurposed drugs. I confirm that I have received satisfactory answers to all my questions. I sign this consent with the full understanding that I may encounter side effects or toxicities from these drugs.

Signed: (Patient)   Dated:

Signed: (Doctor)   Dated:

Signed: (Witness)   Dated:

APPENDIX D

ABBREVIATIONS GLOSSARY

5 FU	5 fluorouracil
A1C:	Glycated hemoglobin
AIDS:	Acquired immunodeficiency syndrome
ALL:	Acute lymphocytic leukemia
AMPK:	AMP-activated protein kinase: 5' adenosine monophosphate-activated protein kinase
ATP:	Adenosine triphosphate
BPTES:	Refers to a selective glutaminase inhibitor
BRAF V600E:	Refers to mutation of BRAF gene at amino acid 600
BRAF:	Refers to protein that codes for B-Raf
BRCA:	The Breast Cancer Gene
C3M3 pulse NSAID:	Refers to 12 to 14 drug combination
CA 15-3:	Cancer antigen 15-3
CA 19-9:	Carbohydrate antigen 19-9
CA-125:	Cancer antigen 125
CAF:	Cancer associated fibroblast
CCL-2:	C motif chemokine ligand 2
CEA:	Carcinoembryonic antigen
CIM:	Cimetidine
COC:	Care Oncology Clinic
COX:	Cyclooxygenase
CQ:	Chloroquine
CR:	Caloric restriction
CRP:	C-reactive protein
CSC:	Cancer stem cell
CT DNA:	ctDNA: Circulating tumor DNA
CTC:	Circulating tumor cell
CUSP-9:	9 drug combination: Aprepitant Artesunate Auranofin Captopril Celecoxib Disulfiram Itraconazole Ritonavir Sertraline.
CXCL:	Chemokine ligand 1
CXCR4:	Chemokine receptor type 4
EGF:	Epidermal growth factor
EGFR:	Epidermal growth factor receptor

EIS:	6 drug combination: itraconazole, metformin, naproxen, pirfenidone, quetiapine, and rifampin
EMT-1:	Type 1 epithelial-mesenchymal transition
EMT-2:	Type 2 epithelial-mesenchymal transition
EMT-3:	Type 3 epithelial-mesenchymal transition
EMT:	Epithelial-Mesenchymal Transition
ERK:	Extracellular regulated kinase
FAP:	Familial Adenomatous Polyposis
G6PDH:	Glucose-6-phosphate dehydrogenase
GBM:	Glioblastoma multiforme
GERD:	Gastro esophageal reflux
GI:	Gastro-intestinal
GP:	General practitioner
H. pylori:	Heliobacter Pylori
HAMPT:	Refers to combination of repurposed drugs
HCQ:	Hydroxychloroquine
HCV:	Hepatitis C virus
HDL:	High density lipoprotein
Hep C:	Hepatitis C virus
HER2+:	Human epidermal growth factor receptor 2 positive
Hh:	Hedgehog signaling pathway
HIF:	Hypoxia-inducible factor
HNPCC:	Hereditary No-polyposis Colorectal Cancer
HPV:	Human Papilloma Virus
IGF:	Insulin-like growth factor
IL 1b:	Interleukin 1 beta
IL-6:	Interleukin 6
IR :	Insulin resistance
ITZ:	Itraconazole
KRAS:	Kirsten rat sarcoma viral oncogene homolog
RAS:	Refers to gene involved in RAS/MAPK pathway
LFS:	Li Fraumeni Syndrome
LDL:	Low-density lipoprotein
MAPK:	Mitogen activated protein kinase

MBZ:	Mebendazole
MET:	Mesenchymal-Epithelial Transition
MMP-2,3,7,9:	Refers to various matrix metalloproteinases
MMP:	Matrix metalloproteinase
mTOR:	The mammalian target of rapamycin
MYC:	MYC proto-Oncogene
NFkB:	Nuclear factor kappa-light-chain-enhancer of activated B Cells
RANK:	Receptor activator nuclear factor
NOTCH-1:	Refers to ligand activated receptor involved in NOTCH signaling
NOTCH-2:	Refers to ligand activated receptor involved in NOTCH signaling
NOTCH-3:	Refers to ligand activated receptor involved in NOTCH signaling
NOTCH-4:	Refers to ligand activated receptor involved in NOTCH signaling
NOTCH:	Refers to cell signaling pathway (derived from notched wings of fruit fly)
NSAID:	Non-Steroidal Anti-inflammatory Drug
NSCLC:	Non-small-cell lung carcinoma
NTG:	Nitroglycerin
OS:	Overall survival
OXPHOS:	Oxidative phosphorylation
P13k/AKT/mTOR:	Phosphatidylinositol-3-kinase(P13K)/AKT/MTOR pathway.
P53:	TP53: The p53 tumor suppressor gene
PCR:	Polymerase chain reaction
PDGF:	Platelet-derived growth factor
PFS:	Progression-free survival
POMP:	Refers to combination chemotherapy for leukemia
PSA:	Prostate-specific antigen
PSADT:	PSA doubling time
PSK:	Polysaccharide K
PTCH:	Refers to receptor for Hedgehog protein
RAF:	Refers to kinases that are part of the MAPK cascade
RAS:	Related to rat sarcoma oncogene GTPase family

ReDO:	Repurposed drugs in oncology project
S.A.D:	Refers to three drug combination: statin, aspirin, dipyridamole
S.A.M:	Refers to three drug combination: statin, aspirin, metformin
SHARE:	Refers to data base collected by Global Cures program
SLUG:	Also known as SNAIL-2: refers to downstream ligand of WnT signaling
SNAIL-1:	Refers to downstream ligand of WnT signaling
SNAIL-2:	Also known as SLUG: refers to downstream ligand of WnT signaling
STAT 3:	Signal transducer and activator of transcription 3
T1459:	Refers to specific resistant GBM cancer cell colony
T1506:	Refers to specific resistant GBM cancer cell colony
TAM:	Tumor activated macrophages
TG:	Triglyceride
TGF beta:	Transforming growth factor beta
TLR-9:	Toll-like receptor 9
TMZ:	Temozolomide
TNBC:	Triple negative breast cancer
TRE:	Time-restricted eating
VEGF:	Vascular endothelial growth factor
WnT:	Wingless Int-1 signaling pathway

APPENDIX E: ReDO DATA BASE[42]

Main Indications	WHO	Off-Patent	Vitro	Vivo	Cases	Obs.	Trials	Human	Date Update	Links
Acetaminophen	Paracetamol	Analgesia	Yes	Yes	Yes	Yes	Yes	Yes	Yes	Yes
Acetazolamide		Glaucoma, diuretic, epilepsy	Yes	Yes	Yes	Yes	No	No	Yes	Yes
Acetylsalicylic acid	**Aspirin**	Analgesia, swelling, prophylaxis of venous embolism and further heart attacks or strokes	Yes	Yes	Yes	Yes	No	Yes	Yes	Yes
Adapalene		Acne	No	Yes	Yes	Yes	No	No	No	No
Ademetionine	AdoMet, S-Adenosylmethionine	Liver disease	No	Yes	Yes	Yes	No	No	Yes	Yes
Agomelatine		Insomnia	No	No	Yes	No	No	No	No	No
Albendazole		Parasitic infection	Yes	Yes	Yes	Yes	Yes	No	Yes	Yes
Alendronic Acid	Alendronate	Osteoporosis	No	Yes	Yes	Yes	Yes	No	Yes	Yes
Aliskiren		Essential hypertension	No	No	Yes	No	No	No	No	No
Allopurinol		Gout	Yes	Yes	Yes	Yes	No	No	Yes	Yes
Alpha-Lipoic Acid	Thioctic Acid, Lipoic Acid	Diabetic neuropathy (Germany)	No	Yes	Yes	Yes	Yes	No	Yes	Yes
Amantadine		Parkinson's Disease, Influenza A	No	Yes	Yes	No	No	No	No	No
Amiloride		In congestive heart failure or hypertension treated with thiazides, to conserve potassium	Yes	Yes	Yes	Yes	No	No	No	No
Aminophylline		Asthma, chronic bronchitis	No	Yes	Yes	Yes	No	No	Yes	Yes
Amiodarone		Ventricular tachycardia/fibrillation	Yes	Yes	Yes	Yes	No	No	Yes	Yes
Amitriptyline		Depression	Yes	Yes	Yes	Yes	No	No	No	No
Amlodipine		Hypertension	Yes	Yes	Yes	Yes	No	No	No	No
Amodiaquine		Malaria	Yes	Yes	Yes	No	No	No	No	No
Anagrelide		Essential thrombocythemia	No	No	Yes	Yes	No	No	No	No
Anakinra		RA, NOMID, CAPS	No	No	Yes	Yes	Yes	No	Yes	Yes
Aprepitant		Nausea, vomiting	Yes	Yes	Yes	Yes	No	No	No	No
Aprotinin		Perioperative blood loss	No	No	Yes	Yes	No	No	Yes	Yes
Argatroban		Heparin-induced thrombocytopenia	No	Yes	Yes	Yes	No	No	No	No
Aripiprazole		Bipolar disorder, major depressive disorder, autistic disorder	No	Yes	Yes	No	No	No	No	No
Artesunate		Malaria	Yes	Yes	Yes	Yes	Yes	No	Yes	Yes
Ascorbic acid	**Ascorbate, Vitamin C**	Scurvy	Yes	Yes	Yes	Yes	Yes	No	Yes	Yes
Atenolol		Hypertension, angina pectoris	No	Yes	Yes	No	No	No	No	No
Atorvastatin		Coronary heart disease, acute coronary syndrome	No	Yes	Yes	Yes	No	Yes	Yes	Yes
Atovaquone		Pneumocystis carinii pneumonia, toxoplasmose	No	Yes	Yes	Yes	No	Yes	Yes	Yes
Atrial Natriuretic Peptide	Carperitide	Heart failure	No	No	Yes	Yes	No	Yes	Yes	Yes
Auranofin		RA	No	Yes	Yes	Yes	No	No	Yes	Yes
Azelastine		Allergies	No	Yes	Yes	No	No	No	No	No
Azithromycin		Bacterial infection, CAP, PID	Yes	Yes	Yes	Yes	No	No	Yes	Yes

Main Indications	WHO	Off-Patent	Vitro	Vivo	Cases	Obs.	Trials	Human	Date Update	Links
Bazedoxifene		Osteoporosis	No	No	Yes	Yes	No	No	Yes	Yes
Bedaquiline		Tuberculosis	Yes	No	Yes	No	No	No	No	No
Bemiparin		Venous thromboembolism, myocardial infarction	No	No	Yes	Yes	No	No	Yes	Yes
Benserazide		Parkinson's Disease	No	Yes	Yes	Yes	No	No	No	No
Benzatropine	Benztropine	Parkinson's Disease	No	Yes	Yes	Yes	No	No	No	No
Bepridil		Hypertension and chronic stable angina	No	Yes	Yes	Yes	No	No	No	No
Bezafibrate		Hyperlipidemia	No	Yes	Yes	Yes	No	No	Yes	Yes
Biperiden		Parkinson's Disease	Yes	Yes	Yes	Yes	No	No	No	No
Bosentan		PAH	No	Yes	Yes	Yes	No	No	Yes	Yes
Brexpiprazole		Schizophrenia, major depressive disorder	No	No	Yes	Yes	No	No	No	No
Bromocriptine		Parkinson's Disease, prevention of lactation	No	Yes	Yes	Yes	No	No	Yes	Yes
Cabergoline		Hyperprolactinemia	No	Yes	Yes	Yes	No	No	Yes	Yes
Caffeine		Newborn apnea	No	Yes	Yes	Yes	Yes	No	Yes	Yes
Calcipotriol	Vitamin D3	Psoriasis	No	Yes	Yes	Yes	Yes	No	Yes	Yes
Calcitriol	Vitamin D3	Vitamin D deficiency	No	Yes	Yes	Yes	Yes	No	Yes	Yes
Canagliflozin		Diabetes	No	No	Yes	Yes	No	No	No	No
Candesartan		Hypertension	No	Yes	Yes	Yes	No	No	Yes	Yes
Captopril		Hypertension	No	Yes	Yes	Yes	No	No	Yes	Yes
Carbimazole		Hyperthyroidism	No	Yes	Yes	No	No	No	No	No
Carglumic Acid		Hyperammonaemia in N-acetylglutamate synthase deficiency	No	No	Yes	Yes	No	No	No	No
Carvedilol		Hypertension	No	Yes	Yes	Yes	No	No	Yes	Yes
Celecoxib		OA, RA, JRA, AS, acute pain, primary dysmenorrhea	No	Yes	Yes	Yes	Yes	No	Yes	Yes
Cephalexin		Bacterial infections	No	Yes	Yes	Yes	No	No	Yes	Yes
Chloramphenicol		Superficial eye infections, typhoid fever	Yes	Yes	Yes	No	Yes	No	No	Yes
Chloroquine		Malaria, Extraintestinal Amebiasis	Yes	Yes	Yes	Yes	No	No	Yes	Yes
Chlorpromazine		Psychotic disorders, nausea and vomiting, anxiety, hiccups	Yes	Yes	Yes	Yes	No	No	Yes	Yes
Cholecalciferol	Colecalciferol, Vitamin D3	Vitamin D deficiency	Yes	Yes	Yes	Yes	Yes	No	Yes	Yes
Cholera Vaccine		Cholera	Yes	Yes	No	Yes	No	Yes	No	Yes
Ciclopirox		Athlete's foot, ringworm	No	Yes	Yes	Yes	No	No	Yes	Yes
Cidofovir		CMV-retinitis in AIDS	No	Yes	Yes	Yes	No	No	Yes	Yes
Cilnidipine		Hypertension	No	Yes	Yes	Yes	No	No	No	No
Cimetidine		Duodenal/gastric ulcers, GERD, pathological hypersecretory conditions	No	Yes	Yes	Yes	Yes	No	Yes	Yes
Ciprofloxacin		Antibiotic	Yes	Yes	Yes	Yes	No	No	Yes	Yes
Citalopram		Depression	No	Yes	Yes	Yes	No	No	Yes	Yes
Clarithromycin		Bacterial infections	Yes	Yes	Yes	Yes	Yes	No	Yes	Yes
Clemastine		Allergies	No	Yes	Yes	No	No	No	No	No

Main indications	WHO	Off-Patent	Vitro	Vivo	Cases	Obs.	Trials	Human	Date Update	Links
Clodronic acid	Clodronate	Osteolytic lesions, hypercalcaemia and bone pain associated with skeletal metastases in patients with breast cancer or multiple myeloma	No	Yes	Yes	Yes	Yes	No	Yes	Yes
Clofazimine		Leprosy	Yes	Yes	Yes	Yes	No	No	Yes	Yes
Clofoctol		Bacterial infections	No	Yes	Yes	Yes	No	No	No	No
Clomifene		Ovulatory dysfunction	Yes	Yes	Yes	Yes	No	No	Yes	Yes
Clomipramine		Obsessive Compulsive Disorder	Yes	Yes	Yes	Yes	No	No	No	No
Clopidogrel		Stroke, post-myocardial infarction	Yes	Yes	Yes	Yes	No	No	Yes	Yes
Clotrimazole		Fungal infections	Yes	Yes	Yes	Yes	No	No	No	No
Colchicine		Gout	No	Yes	Yes	Yes	No	No	Yes	Yes
Cyproheptadine		Allergies	No	Yes	Yes	Yes	Yes	Yes	Yes	Yes
Dalteparin		DVT (prophylaxis), unstable angina/non-Q-wave myocardial infarction	No	Yes	Yes	Yes	Yes	No	Yes	Yes
Danazol		Endometriosis, fibrocystic breast disease, hereditary angioedema	No	Yes	Yes	Yes	No	No	Yes	Yes
Dapsone		Dermatitis herpetiformis, leprosy	Yes	Yes	Yes	Yes	No	No	Yes	Yes
Deferasirox		Acute iron intoxication, chronic iron overload	No	No	Yes	Yes	No	No	Yes	Yes
Deferiprone		Iron overload in thalassemia major	No	No	Yes	Yes	No	No	No	No
Deferoxamine	Desferrioxamine	Acute iron intoxication, chronic iron overload	Yes	Yes	Yes	Yes	No	No	Yes	Yes
Desmopressin		Diabetes Insipidus, bedwetting, hemophilia A, von Willebrand's disease	Yes	Yes	Yes	Yes	No	No	Yes	Yes
Diazoxide		Chronic intractable hypoglycaemia, acute hypertension	Yes	Yes	Yes	Yes	Yes	No	Yes	Yes
Diclofenac		OA, RA, AS	No	Yes	Yes	Yes	Yes	No	Yes	Yes
Diflunisal		OA, RA, mild to moderate pain	No	Yes	Yes	Yes	No	No	No	No
Digitoxin		Congestive HF, atrial fibrillation, atrial flutter, PAT, cardiogenic shock	No	Yes	Yes	Yes	No	No	Yes	Yes
Digoxin		Heart failure, atrial fibrillation	Yes	Yes	Yes	Yes	No	No	Yes	Yes
Dimethyl Fumarate		Psoriasis, Multiple Sclerosis	No	Yes	Yes	Yes	No	No	Yes	Yes
Dipyridamole		Thromboembolism Prophylaxis Post-Cardiac Valve Replacement	No	Yes	Yes	Yes	No	No	Yes	Yes
Disulfiram		Chronic alcoholism	No	Yes	Yes	Yes	No	No	Yes	Yes
Donepezil		Alzheimer's Disease	No	Yes	Yes	Yes	No	No	Yes	Yes
Doxazosin		Hypertension, benign prostatic hyperplasia	No	Yes	Yes	Yes	No	No	No	No
Doxycycline		Respiratory/urinary tract/3phthalmic infection	Yes	Yes	Yes	Yes	Yes	No	Yes	Yes
Dronedarone		Paroxysmal or	No	Yes	Yes	Yes	No	No	No	No

Main Indications	WHO	Off-Patent	Vitro	Vivo	Cases	Obs.	Trials	Human	Date Update	Links
		persistent atrial fibrillation								
Dutasteride		Benign prostatic hyperplasia	No	Yes	Yes	Yes	Yes	No	Yes	Yes
Ebastine		Allergies	No	Yes	Yes	Yes	No	No	No	No
Efavirenz		Anti-retroviral	Yes	Yes	Yes	Yes	No	No	Yes	Yes
Eflornithine	DFMO	Adjunct to laser therapy for facial hirsutism in women, African trypanosomiasis	Yes	Yes	Yes	Yes	Yes	No	Yes	Yes
Emetine		Amoebiasis	No	Yes	Yes	Yes	No	No	No	No
Enalapril		Hypertension	Yes	Yes	Yes	Yes	No	No	Yes	Yes
Enoxaparin		Prophylaxis of venous thromboembolism	Yes	Yes	Yes	Yes	No	No	Yes	Yes
Epalrestat		Diabetes	No	Yes	Yes	Yes	No	No	Yes	Yes
Esomeprazole		Antacid	No	Yes	Yes	Yes	Yes	Yes	Yes	Yes
Ethacrynic Acid	Etacrynic acid	Diuretic	No	Yes	Yes	Yes	Yes	No	No	Yes
Etodolac		Analgesia	No	Yes	Yes	Yes	Yes	No	Yes	Yes
Etoricoxib		OA, RA, AS	No	Yes	Yes	Yes	No	No	Yes	Yes
Famotidine		Antacid	No	Yes	Yes	Yes	No	No	Yes	Yes
Fasudil		Vasodilator	No	Unclear	Yes	Yes	No	No	No	No
Felodipine		Hypertension	No	Yes	Yes	Yes	No	No	No	No
Fenofibrate		Hyperlipidemia	No	Yes	Yes	Yes	Yes	No	Yes	Yes
Fenoldopam		Acute hypertension	No	Yes	Yes	Yes	No	No	No	No
Finasteride		Benign prostatic hyperplasia	No	Yes	Yes	Yes	Yes	Yes	Yes	Yes
Fingolimod		Multiple Sclerosis	No	No	Yes	Yes	No	No	Yes	Yes
Flubendazole		Parasitic infection	No	Yes	Yes	Yes	No	No	No	No
Flucytosine	5-Fluorocytosine	Candida and/or Cryptococcus	Yes	Yes	Yes	Yes	No	No	Yes	Yes
Flunarizine		Migraine	No	Yes	Yes	Yes	No	No	No	No
Fluoxetine	Prozac	Depression	Yes	Yes	Yes	Yes	No	No	No	No
Fluphenazine		Psychotic disorders	Yes	Yes	Yes	Yes	No	No	Yes	Yes
Flurbiprofen		Analgesia	No	Yes	Yes	Yes	No	Yes	Yes	Yes
Fluspirilene		Psychotic disorders	No	Yes	Yes	Yes	No	No	No	No
Fluvastatin		Hyperlipidemia	No	Yes	Yes	Yes	Yes	Yes	Yes	Yes
Fluvoxamine		Depression	No	Yes	Yes	Yes	Yes	No	No	Yes
Ganciclovir		Anti-viral	No	Yes	Yes	Yes	Yes	No	Yes	Yes
Glibenclamide	Glyburide	Diabetes	No	Yes	Yes	Yes	No	No	No	No
Glipizide		Diabetes	No	Yes	Yes	Yes	No	No	No	No
Griseofulvin		Fungal infections	Yes	Yes	Yes	Yes	Yes	No	No	Yes
Haloperidol		Psychotic disorders	Yes	Yes	Yes	Yes	No	No	No	No
Hydralazine		Hypertension	Yes	Yes	Yes	Yes	No	No	Yes	Yes
Hydroxychloroquine		Malaria	Yes	Yes	Yes	Yes	Yes	No	Yes	Yes
Hymecromone		Antispasmodic	No	Yes	Yes	Yes	No	No	Yes	Yes
Ibandronic acid	Ibandronate	Osteoporosis	No	Yes	Yes	Yes	Yes	No	Yes	Yes
Ibudilast		Multiple sclerosis, asthma, cerebrovascular disease	No	Yes	Yes	Yes	No	No	Yes	Yes

Main Indications	WHO	Off-Patent	Vitro	Vivo	Cases	Obs.	Trials	Human	Date Update	Links
Ibuprofen		Analgesia	Yes	Yes	Yes	Yes	No	No	Yes	Yes
Idebenone		Leber's Hereditary Optic Neuropathy	No	No	Yes	No	No	No	No	No
Imipramine		Depression	No	Yes	Yes	Yes	No	No	Yes	Yes
Indomethacin	Indometacin	Analgesia	No	Yes	Yes	Yes	Yes	No	Yes	Yes
Irbesartan		Hypertension	No	Yes	Yes	Yes	Yes	Yes	No	Yes
Itraconazole		Fungal infections	Yes	Yes	Yes	Yes	Yes	Yes	Yes	Yes
Ivermectin		Parasitic infection	Yes	Yes	Yes	Yes	No	No	Yes	Yes
Ketamine		Anesthetic	Yes	Yes	Yes	Yes	No	No	Yes	Yes
Ketoconazole		Fungal infections	No	Yes	Yes	Yes	Yes	Yes	Yes	Yes
Ketoprofen		Analgesia	No	Yes	Yes	Yes	No	No	No	No
Ketorolac		Post-operative analgesia	No	Yes	Yes	Yes	Yes	Yes	Yes	Yes
L-Arginine		Nutraceutical	No	Yes	Yes	Yes	No	No	Yes	Yes
L-Glutamine		Nutraceutical	No	Yes	Yes	Yes	No	No	Yes	Yes
Lamotrigine		Epilepsy	Yes	Yes	Yes	Yes	No	No	No	No
Lansoprazole		Antacid	No	Yes	Yes	Yes	No	Yes	Yes	Yes
Leflunomide		Arthritis	No	Yes	Yes	Yes	No	No	Yes	Yes
Levamisole		Parasitic infection	Yes	Yes	Yes	Yes	Yes	No	Yes	Yes
Levetiracetam		Epilepsy	No	Yes	Yes	No	Yes	Yes	Yes	Yes
Levofloxacin		Antibiotic	Yes	Yes	Yes	Yes	Yes	No	No	Yes
Levonorgestrel		Contraceptive	Yes	Yes	Yes	Yes	Yes	Yes	Yes	Yes
Lidocaine		Anesthetic	Yes	Yes	Yes	Yes	No	No	Yes	Yes
Liraglutide		Diabetes	No	No	Yes	No	No	No	No	No
Lithium		Bipolar disorders	Yes	Yes	Yes	Yes	Yes	No	Yes	Yes
Loperamide		Diarrhea	Yes	Yes	Yes	No	No	No	No	No
Lopinavir		Anti-retroviral	Yes	Yes	Yes	Yes	No	No	Yes	Yes
Loratadine		Allergies	Yes	Yes	Yes	No	No	Yes	No	Yes
Losartan		Hypertension	Yes	Yes	Yes	Yes	No	Yes	Yes	Yes
Lovastatin		Hyperlipidemia	No	Yes	Yes	Yes	Yes	No	Yes	Yes
Loxoprofen		Analgesia	No	Yes	Yes	Yes	Yes	Yes	No	Yes
Macitentan		Pulmonary arterial hypertension	No	No	Yes	Yes	No	No	Yes	Yes
Manidipine		Hypertension	No	Yes	Yes	Yes	No	No	No	No
Maraviroc		Anti-retroviral	No	No	Yes	Yes	No	No	Yes	Yes
Mebendazole		Parasitic infection	Yes	Yes	Yes	Yes	Yes	No	Yes	Yes
Meclizine	Meclozine	Antiemetic	No	Yes	Yes	No	No	No	Yes	Yes
Meclofenamate	Meclofenamic acid	Analgesia	No	Yes	Yes	Yes	No	No	Yes	Yes
Mefloquine		Malaria	Yes	Yes	Yes	Yes	No	No	Yes	Yes
Megestrol Acetate		Hormone	No	Yes	Yes	Yes	Yes	Yes	Yes	Yes
Melatonin		Insomnia	No	Yes	Yes	Yes	Yes	No	Yes	Yes
Meloxicam		Analgesia	No	Yes	Yes	Yes	Yes	No	Yes	Yes
Memantine		Alzheimer's Disease	No	Yes	Yes	No	No	No	Yes	Yes
Mepacrine	Quinacrine	Parasitic infection	No	Yes	Yes	Yes	No	No	Yes	Yes
Mepyramine		Allergies	No	Yes	Yes	Yes	No	No	No	No
Mesalazine	Mesalamine, 5-aminosalicylic acid	Inflammatory bowel disease	No	Yes	Yes	Yes	No	No	No	No

Main Indications	WHO	Off-Patent	Vitro	Vivo	Cases	Obs.	Trials	Human	Date Update	Links
Metformin		Diabetes	Yes	Yes	Yes	Yes	Yes	Yes	Yes	Yes
Methazolamide		Antiglaucoma, diuretic	No	Yes	No	No	No	No	Yes	Yes
Methimazole	Thiamazole	Hyperthyroidism	Yes	Yes	No	No	Yes	No	Yes	Yes
Methylene blue	Methylthioninium chloride	Methemoglobinemia, cyanide toxicity	Yes	Yes	Yes	Yes	No	No	Yes	Yes
Methylnaltrexone		Opioid-induced constipation	No	No	Yes	Yes	No	Yes	No	Yes
Metoclopramide		Anti-emesis	Yes	Yes	Yes	Yes	No	No	Yes	Yes
Miconazole		Fungal infections	Yes	Yes	Yes	Yes	No	No	Yes	Yes
Midazolam		Sedation	Yes	Yes	Yes	Yes	No	No	No	No
Mifepristone		Abortifacient	Yes	Yes	Yes	Yes	Yes	No	Yes	Yes
Miltefosine	Hexadecylphosphocholine	Leishmaniasis	Yes	Yes	Yes	Yes	Yes	No	Yes	Yes
Minocycline		Antibiotic	No	Yes	Yes	Yes	No	No	Yes	Yes
Mirtazapine		Depression	No	Yes	Yes	Yes	No	No	No	No
Mometasone	Mometasone furoate	Asthma prophylaxis	No	Yes	Yes	No	No	No	No	No
Montelukast		Allergies	No	Yes	Yes	Yes	No	No	No	No
Mycophenolate	Mycophenolic acid	Immunosuppressant	No	Yes	Yes	Yes	Yes	No	No	Yes
Nadroparin		Prophylaxis of venous thromboembolism	No	Yes	Yes	Yes	No	Yes	Yes	Yes
Naftopidil		Benign prostatic hyperplasia	No	Unclear	Yes	Yes	Yes	Yes	Yes	Yes
Naltrexone		Opioid receptor antagonist	No	Yes	Yes	Yes	Yes	No	Yes	Yes
Naproxen		Analgesia	No	Yes	Yes	Yes	Yes	No	Yes	Yes
Nelfinavir		Anti-retroviral	No	No	Yes	Yes	No	No	Yes	Yes
Niclosamide		Parasitic infection	Yes	Yes	Yes	Yes	No	No	Yes	Yes
Nicotinamide	Niacinamide	Niacin Deficiency, Skin cancer chemoprevention	Yes	Yes	Yes	Yes	No	No	Yes	Yes
Nifedipine		Hypertension	Yes	Yes	Yes	Yes	Yes	No	Yes	Yes
Nifuroxazide		Colitis, acute diarrhea	No	Yes	Yes	Yes	No	No	No	No
Nifurtimox		Chagas disease, African sleeping sickness	Yes	Unclear	Yes	Yes	Yes	No	Yes	Yes
Nimesulide		Analgesia	No	Yes	Yes	Yes	No	No	Yes	Yes
Nimodipine		Hypertension	No	Yes	Yes	Yes	No	No	No	No
Nisoldipine		Hypertension	No	Yes	Yes	Yes	No	No	No	No
Nitazoxanide		Anti-protozoal	No	Yes	Yes	Yes	No	No	No	No
Nitisinone		Hereditary tyrosinemia type 1	No	No	No	No	Yes	No	No	Yes
Nitroglycerin	Glyceryl trinitrate	Nitro-vasodilator	Yes	Yes	Yes	Yes	Yes	No	Yes	Yes
Nitroxoline		Antibiotic	No	Yes	Yes	Yes	No	No	Yes	Yes
Norethandrolone		Aplastic anemia	No	Yes	Yes	Yes	No	No	Yes	Yes
Noscapine		Anti-tussive	No	Yes	Yes	Yes	No	No	Yes	Yes
Obeticholic acid		Primary biliary cholangitis	No	No	Yes	Yes	No	No	No	No
Olanzapine		Psychotic disorders	No	Yes	Yes	Yes	No	No	No	No
Olmesartan		Hypertension	No	Yes	Yes	Yes	No	No	No	No
Olsalazine		Rheumatoid arthritis; ulcerative colitis; active Crohn's Disease.	No	Yes	Yes	Yes	No	No	No	No
Omega 3	Lovaza, Fish Oil, Omacor,	Hyperlipidemia	No	Unclear	Yes	Yes	Yes	Yes	Yes	Yes

Main Indications	WHO	Off-Patent	Vitro	Vivo	Cases	Obs.	Trials	Human	Date Update	Links
	eicosapentaenoic acid, docosahexaenoic acid									
Omeprazole		Antacid	Yes	Yes	Yes	Yes	Yes	No	Yes	Yes
Orlistat		Obesity	No	Yes	Yes	Yes	No	No	No	No
Ormeloxifene		Contraceptive	No	Yes	Yes	Yes	No	No	No	No
Oseltamivir		Anti-viral	Yes	Yes	Yes	Yes	No	No	No	No
Ouabain		Cardiac arrhythmia	No	Yes	Yes	Yes	No	No	No	No
Oxcarbazepine		Epilepsy	No	Yes	Yes	No	No	Yes	No	Yes
Pamidronic acid	Pamidronate	Osteoporosis	No	Yes	Yes	Yes	Yes	No	Yes	Yes
Pantoprazole		Antacid	No	Yes	Yes	Yes	Yes	Yes	Yes	Yes
Parecoxib		Post-operative analgesia	No	Yes	Yes	Yes	No	No	Yes	Yes
Paricalcitol	Vitamin D2	Hyperparathyroidism	No	Yes	Yes	Yes	Yes	No	Yes	Yes
Paroxetine		Depression	No	Yes	Yes	Yes	No	No	No	No
Penfluridol		Psychotic disorders	No	Yes	Yes	Yes	No	No	No	No
Pentamidine		Parasitic infection	Yes	Yes	Yes	Yes	No	No	Yes	Yes
Pentoxifylline		Peripheral artery disease	No	Yes	Yes	Yes	No	No	Yes	Yes
Perphenazine		Psychotic disorders	No	Yes	Yes	Yes	No	No	No	No
Phenoxybenzamine		Pheochromocytoma	No	Yes	Yes	Yes	No	No	No	No
Phentolamine		Vasodilator	No	Yes	Yes	Yes	No	No	No	No
Phenylbutyrate	Glycerol Phenylbutyrate	Urea cycle disorders	No	Unclear	Yes	Yes	Yes	No	Yes	Yes
Phenytoin		Epilepsy	Yes	Yes	Yes	Yes	No	No	No	No
Pimozide		Psychotic disorders	No	Yes	Yes	Yes	Yes	No	No	Yes
Pioglitazone		Diabetes	No	Yes	Yes	Yes	Yes	No	Yes	Yes
Pirfenidone		Anti-fibrotic	No	No	Yes	Yes	No	No	Yes	Yes
Piroxicam		Analgesia	No	Yes	Yes	Yes	Yes	No	Yes	Yes
Plerixafor	AMD3100	Autologous HSCT	No	No	Yes	Yes	No	No	Yes	Yes
Posaconazole		Fungal infections	No	Yes	Yes	Yes	No	No	Yes	Yes
Pravastatin		Hyperlipidemia	No	Yes	Yes	Yes	No	Yes	Yes	Yes
Prazosin		Hypertension	No	Yes	Yes	Yes	No	No	No	No
Prochlorperazine	Prochlorperazine dimaleate	Psychotic disorders	No	Yes	Yes	Yes	No	No	Yes	Yes
Promethazine		Psychotic disorders	No	Yes	Yes	Yes	No	No	No	No
Propafenone		Anti-arryhtmic	No	Yes	Yes	Yes	No	No	No	No
<u>Propranolol</u>		Hypertension	Yes	Yes	Yes	Yes	Yes	Yes	Yes	Yes
Pyridoxine	Vitamin B6	Vitamin B6 deficiency	Yes	Yes	Yes	Yes	No	No	Yes	Yes
Pyrimethamine		Parasitic infection	Yes	Yes	Yes	Yes	Yes	No	Yes	Yes
Pyrvinium Pamoate	Pyrvinium	Parasitic infection	No	Yes	Yes	Yes	No	No	No	No
Quetiapine		Psychotic disorders	No	Yes	Yes	No	No	No	No	No
Rabeprazole		Antacid	No	Yes	Yes	Yes	No	No	Yes	Yes
Ranitidine		Antacid	Yes	Yes	Yes	Yes	Yes	No	Yes	Yes
Ranolazine		Anti-angina	No	No	Yes	Yes	No	No	No	No
Repaglinide		Diabetes	No	No	Yes	Yes	No	No	No	No
Reserpine		Hypertension, anti-psychotic	No	Yes	Yes	Yes	No	No	No	No
Ribavirin		Anti-viral	Yes	Yes	Yes	Yes	Yes	No	Yes	Yes

Main Indications	WHO	Off-Patent	Vitro	Vivo	Cases	Obs.	Trials	Human	Date Update	Links
Rifabutin		Antibiotic	Yes	Yes	Yes	No	No	No	No	No
Rifampicin	Rifampin	Tuberculosis	Yes	Yes	Yes	Yes	Yes	No	No	Yes
Riluzole		ALS	No	Yes	Yes	Yes	No	No	Yes	Yes
Risedronic acid	Risedronate	Osteoporosis, prophylaxis of skeletal fractures, Paget's disease	No	Yes	Yes	Yes	No	No	Yes	Yes
Risperidone		Psychotic disorders	Yes	Yes	Yes	Yes	No	No	No	No
Ritonavir		Anti-retroviral	Yes	No	Yes	Yes	Yes	No	Yes	Yes
Roflumilast		COPD	No	No	Yes	Yes	No	No	Yes	Yes
Rosuvastatin		Hyperlipidemia	No	Yes	Yes	Yes	No	No	Yes	Yes
Roxatidine		Antacid	No	Yes	Yes	Yes	No	No	No	No
Roxithromycin		Bacterial infections	No	Yes	Yes	Yes	Yes	No	No	Yes
Sertraline		Depression	No	Yes	Yes	Yes	No	No	Yes	Yes
Sildenafil		Erectile dysfunction	No	Yes	Yes	Yes	Yes	No	Yes	Yes
Simvastatin		Hyperlipidemia	Yes	Yes	Yes	No	Yes	Yes	Yes	Yes
Sirolim	Rapamycin	Inhibit organ transplant rejection	No	Yes	Yes	Yes	Yes	No	Yes	Yes
Sodium Aurothiomalate		Active progressive rheumatoid arthritis	No	Yes	Yes	Yes	No	No	Yes	Yes
Sodium Bicarbonate		Relief of wind and griping pains	Yes	Yes	Yes	Yes	Yes	No	Yes	Yes
Spironolactone		Congestive cardiac failure, Hepatic cirrhosis with ascites and oedema, Malignant ascites, Nephrotic syndrome, Diagnosis and treatment of primary aldosteronism.	Yes	Yes	Yes	Yes	No	No	Yes	Yes
Sulfasalazine		Rheumatoid arthritis; ulcerative colitis; active Crohn's Disease.	Yes	Yes	Yes	Yes	Yes	No	Yes	Yes
Sulindac		Relief of signs and symptoms of osteoarthritis, rheumatoid arthritis, ankylosing spondylitis, acute painful shoulder (acute subacromial bursitis/supraspinatus tendinitis), and acute gouty arthritis.	No	Yes	Yes	Yes	No	Yes	Yes	Yes
Suramin		African sleeping sickness	No	Unclear	Yes	Yes	Yes	No	Yes	Yes
Tadalafil		Erectile dysfunction	No	Yes	Yes	Yes	No	No	Yes	Yes
Telmisartan		Hypertension, cardiovascular prevention	Yes	Yes	Yes	Yes	No	Yes	No	Yes
Terbinafine		Treatment of tinea pedis (athlete's foot), tinea cruris (dhobie (jock) itch) and tinea corporis (ringworm)	Yes	Yes	Yes	Yes	No	No	Yes	Yes
Teriflunomide		Relapsing multiple sclerosis	No	Yes	Yes	Yes	No	No	No	No
Thiabendazole		Parasitic infection	No	Unclear	Yes	Yes	No	No	No	No
Thioridazine		Psychotic disorders	No	Yes	Yes	Yes	Yes	No	Yes	Yes
Ticagrelor		Prevention of atherothrombotic events in combo with ASA	No	No	Yes	Yes	No	No	Yes	Yes
Ticlopidine		Prevent strokes, blood loss	No	Yes	Yes	Yes	Yes	No	Yes	Yes

Main Indications	WHO	Off-Patent	Vitro	Vivo	Cases	Obs.	Trials	Human	Date Update	Links
Tigecycline		Infections	No	No	Yes	Yes	No	No	Yes	Yes
Timolol		Hypertension, ischemic heart disease, migraine	Yes	Yes	No	No	Yes	Yes	Yes	Yes
Tinzaparin		Prophylaxis of venous thromboembolism	No	No	Yes	Yes	No	No	Yes	Yes
Tioconazole		Parasitic infection	No	Yes	Yes	Yes	No	No	No	No
Tocilizumab		Rheumatoid arthritis	No	No	Yes	Yes	No	No	Yes	Yes
Tofacitinib		Rheumatoid arthritis	No	No	Yes	Yes	Yes	No	No	Yes
Tolfenamic Acid	Tolfenamate	Migraine	No	Yes	Yes	Yes	No	No	No	No
Topiramate		Epilepsy (tonic clonic seizure)	No	Yes	Yes	Yes	No	No	No	No
Tranexamic Acid		Blood loss - fibrinolysis	Yes	Yes	Yes	Yes	No	No	Yes	Yes
Trazodone		Depression, anxiety	No	No	Yes	Yes	No	No	No	No
Triamterene		Diuretic, oedema in cardiac failure, cirrhosis of the liver or the nephrotic syndrome, and in that associated with corticosteroid treatment	No	Yes	Yes	Yes	No	No	No	No
Trifluoperazine		Psychotic disorders	No	No	Yes	Yes	No	No	Yes	Yes
Trimetazidine		Angina pectoris	No	Yes	Yes	Yes	No	No	Yes	Yes
Ulinastatin		Severe sepsis & pancreatitis	No	Unclear	Yes	Yes	No	No	Yes	Yes
Ursodeoxycholic acid	UCDA, Ursodiol	Gallstones, primary biliary cirrhosis	No	Yes	Yes	Yes	No	Yes	Yes	Yes
Valproic Acid	Valproate	Epilepsy	Yes	Yes	Yes	Yes	Yes	Yes	Yes	Yes
Valsartan		Hypertension, myocardial infarction, heart failure	No	Yes	Yes	Yes	No	Yes	No	Yes
Vardenafil		Erectile dysfunction	No	No	Yes	Yes	No	No	Yes	Yes
Verapamil		Hypertension, angina pectoris	Yes	Yes	Yes	Yes	Yes	No	Yes	Yes
Verteporfin		Exudative age-related macular degeneration	No	No	Yes	Yes	Yes	No	Yes	Yes
Warfarin		Prophylaxis of systemic embolism, of venous thrombosis and pulmonary embolism.	Yes	Yes	Yes	Yes	No	Yes	Yes	Yes
Zidovudine	Azidothymidine	Anti-retroviral	Yes	Yes	Yes	Yes	Yes	No	Yes	Yes
Zileuton		Asthma prophylaxis	No	Yes	Yes	Yes	No	No	Yes	Yes
Zoledronic Acid	Zoledronate	Osteoporosis, prophylaxis of skeletal fractures and treat hypercalcemia of malignancy, treat pain from bone metastases	Yes	Yes	Yes	Yes	Yes	Yes	Yes	Yes

Important note for patients: This list identifies drugs that, based on their scientific properties, warrant further scientific investigation. In most cases the existing scientific evidence for their effects on cancer is very limited. Further scientific and clinical research is needed before any statements regarding their anti-cancer activity can be made. This list is not intended to be used as a source for possible treatment options for patients.

APPENDIX F

THE PHYSICIANS' POSITION:

100 POINTS OF VIEW

The following are various physicians' comments regarding various publications.

I.   Geleris, J., Sun, Y., Platt, J., et al., Observational study of hydroxychloroquine in hospitalized patients with COVID-19. *N Engl J Med.* 2020; doi: 10.1056/NEJMoa2012410

<u>*Medpage Today* Comment Section</u> [Walker, M. HCQ in Hospitalized COVID-19 Patients: No Better, No Worse? *Medpage Today.* May 7, 2020]

May 8, 2020

Dr. John H. Abeles, distinguished physician, HIV researcher, cancer pioneer and founder of BryoLogyx:

> "I cannot understand why the NEJM would publish such a study and the authors concluding what they did with such a poor retrospective observation of clearly imbalanced groups - where the hydroxychloroquine treated group is so much more ill.
>
> Do the editors and authors have a political agenda to discredit a real potential therapy, a trend that is disturbingly common in normal reliable medical areas?"

Dr. John H. Abeles:

> "Many active oral antivirals - against influenza, e.g., oseltamivir and herpes, e.g., valacyclovir are optimally effective when given early in the disease. The same likely applies to the oral regimen of hydroxychloroquine plus zinc and added either azithromycin or doxycycline.
>
> By the time the majority of COVID-19 patients are hospitalized, they have well passed the peak of viral titers and are now suffering from the ravages of the cytokine storm hyper-inflammation - with alveolar exudates, haemocoagulation (anti-phospholipid antibodies and endothelitis are probable factors), possibly a haemoglobinopathy and other widespread autoimmune damage.
>
> This could explain the somewhat disappointing results with the pure and potent antiviral Remdesivir also. The fairest trial of any oral antiviral - and many extant drugs are in study - is in the outpatient/home setting. Hospital trials are bound to disappoint, in my view."

May 8, 2020

Michael Bernhardt, M.D:

> "Doesn't prove anything, just more anecdotal evidence. The HCQ was started when the patient was sicker. Start them on HCQ when they were first diagnosed, then follow them through and compare them to a control group. Simple science. Given there is no other proven treatment that is safe, it is a treatment that shouldn't be ignored."

May 8, 2020

Dr. G. Galindo:

> "The French study of HCQ has great results. It is peer reviewed now and does not show the same detriments the New England study shows. If I were to get sick with the Wuhan virus, I would take HCQ, because it has a lot of good reports on its effectiveness, and it is not expensive. There is nothing wrong with off-label meds for this virus."

May 8, 2020

Dr. Iraj Akhvan, Internist in New York:

> "Politics and politics, again and again, COVID-19 kills, but hydroxychloroquine doesn't. Shame on NEJM for allowing and participating in this level of low level non-scientific reporting. They selected the sickest group of the people, which at best according to the recent studies had less than a 3% of survival; if they were admitted to ICU and ended up intubated and treated with hydroxychloroquine, and came out with such a report.
>
> For our patient's sakes, leave the politics and the money out of the medicine, leave the sick to the medical community. You need, like any study, to take into consideration the number of the patients who have been treated with these combinations as outpatients by their practicing physicians, and did well, did not end up going to the hospitals, having complications such as ARDS, intravascular coagulation, and increased chance of mortality. Your article at best is on a level of someone who is going to jump off of a bridge and took an aspirin before he jumped, so the argument is that aspirin should not be used."

II.   Magagnoli, J., Narendran, F., Cummings, T., et al., Outcomes of hydroxychloroquine usage in United States veterans hospitalized with COVID-19. Med (2020) doi: 10.1016/j.medj.2020.06.001

Conflict of Interest Disclosure:

Disclosure forms provided by the authors are available with the NEJM. JA is a co-founder of iVeena Holdings, iVeena Delivery Systems and Inflammasome Therapeutics, and has received consultancy fees from Allergan, Biogen, Boehringer Ingelheim, Immunovant, Janssen, Olix Pharmaceuticals, Retinal Solutions, and Saksin LifeSciences, all unrelated to this work.

JA is named as an inventor on a patent application filed by the University of Virginia relating to COVID-19 but unrelated to this work. SSS has received research grants from Boehringer Ingelheim, Gilead Sciences, Portola Pharmaceuticals, and United Therapeutics, all unrelated to this work. The other authors declare no competing interests.

A.   *Medpage Today* Comment Section: [Walker, M. HCQ Tied to Increased Mortality in Male Vets   with Severe COVID-19. *Medpage Today*. April 21, 2020.]

April 22, 2020

Dr. Barry Levine:

> "It is more likely that chloroquine or hydroxychloroquine will be useful either as prophylactics or as mitigating early stages of infection, than when given as a last ditch

intervention. Some in vivo data supports this. For example, all mice survived that were given chloroquine two hours BEFORE inoculation and then received it daily. The coronavirus in question was otherwise fatal in untreated mice."

https://www.ncbi.nlm.nih.gov/pmc/articles/PMC7114176/

April 22, 2020

Davester, PhD., Biostatistician:

"Good comments. Jewells expresses some of my concern with this study. This was a retrospective observational study that attempted to adjust for naturally occurring differences with propensity scores. A weak design, in my opinion, when it comes to making decisions about drug efficacy. Also propensity scores are not a great cure-all for studies lacking adequate controls and randomization. There's plenty of criticism surrounding propensity scores right now, ranging from they are not effective at balancing group differences to they are misleading. Until more rigorous studies are forthcoming, I would accept clinician judgement over the results of this study."

B.   *Medscape* Comment Section: [Frellick, M. Hydroxychloroquine Ineffective for COVID-19, VA Study Suggests. *Medscape.* April 23, 2020.]

April 28, 2020

Idana Merrick, Pharmacist:

"I have been a pharmacist for over 40 years. This VA "study" is an embarrassment to the medical literature. It is an anecdotal politically motivated hit job. From what I have read hydroxychloroquine with zinc and azithromycin is useful in less critical patients started very early in the progression of COVID-19. It reminds me of Tamiflu in that if Tamiflu is not started within 24-48 hours of onset of flu symptoms, it is not effective. Even when it is effective it only shortens symptoms by 18 hours or so.

The real problem with hydroxychloroquine and azithromycin is that no pharmaceutical company can make billions of dollars. I hope the double blind study helps clarify the issue. Finally, hydroxychloroquine is like every drug known to man, it has a plethora of side effects; some severe, some not so severe. If it were half as toxic as a biased media insinuates, thousands of people would have died of HCQ, but that is not the case.

Medscape, shame on you for implying this is a valid study vilifying a drug without a properly designed study--matched groups, etc. You never compare patients with multiple morbidities on ventilators with less ill patients not on ventilators. I expect higher ethics from Medscape editors."

April 25, 2020

Dr. Stephen Smith, Infectious Disease Physician:

"Just after the article was posted, I e-mailed Drs. Sutton and Ambati and asked what HCQ dosing regimens were used. I have yet to receive a response. It is unheard to say any drug doesn't work without providing closing dosing data. Days of HCQ, dose per day, total dose. None of those data are in the "study.""

Surviving Cancer, Covid 19, & Disease

Notice, no one from UVAs ID section participated.

Dr. Ambati is a research ophthalmologist at UVA. Dr. Narendran, and Dr. Pereira are not US-licensed physicians; they work in Dr. Ambati's retina lab.

This thing cannot be called a study in any way. It is some sort of publicity stunt. None of the authors is an infectious disease physician. None could have taken care of a single COVID patient, not one."

April 24, 2020

Dr. Jeffrey Taylor, Ophthalmologist:

"We can't say that hydroxychloroquine works unless we have a randomized clinical trial, but we can use a retrospective review to say it doesn't work.... Medscape is embarrassing."

April 24, 2020

Dr. Jimmy Chang, Family Medicine:

"If the study population is the hospitalized patients, please forget about it. It will be a negative trial. HCQ has to be given early, upon diagnosis, to those high risk groups."

April 24, 2020

Dr. Olga Bukarov, General Practitice:

"We sell chemo and radiation ($500 profit/patient) that has a success rate of 3% and we think it is successful. But HCQ ($10/patient) is not?"

April 24, 2020

Dr. Monique Martin, Internist:

"Publishing this conclusion without a peer review is irresponsible. The p-value shows that the patients not receiving Plaquenil were not nearly as sick and therefore the lower death rate in that group makes sense. The title is sensationalist and just plain irresponsible. I expect a higher standard."

April 24, 2020

Dr. Mustafa Serri, Anesthesiologist:

"I think the main purpose for HCQ is to reduce the viral load by blocking virus replication not to kill the virus as mentioned above. Therefore, it is crucial to be taken at early stages to avoid high viral load in triggering damaging immune response (cytokines wave/HLH picture) that lead to mechanical ventilation or MOF.

Recently I noticed all studies against HCQ treatment for COVID-19 used in patients with high viral load which reflects two probabilities; either not understanding the principle behind using the HCQ or in support of propaganda against HCQ treatment."

April 24, 2020

Dr. Kurt Kilpatrick:

> "Clearly a propaganda piece. Politics should be kept out of science and medicine, but it is an election year. Using only late stage disease progression in the HCQ group is a major tip off. It gets worse the more you look at the design and sample selections."

April 24, 2020

Dr. Albert Tartini, Nephrologist states:

> "Absolutely useless study. Early intervention has been the key to successfully treating COVID-19 with Plaquenil. The patients that I have used it on early all improved by the third dose. The authors, the NIH guidelines for Covid need themselves to be reviewed."

> C. *Medscape* Comment Section: [Kincaid, E. COVID-19 Daily: VA Hydroxychloroquine Study, Relief Funds. *Medscape Today*. April 23, 2020]

April 24, 2020

Dr. Jose Rodriguez, Pharmacist:

> "The study design is flawed. The patient population is as follows; the analysis examined 97 patients treated with hydroxychloroquine alone, 113 treated with a combination of hydroxychloroquine and azithromycin, and the rest with neither drug.

> Part of the problem is that the patient entry into the study was not well managed so disease progression in the different arms was not equally weighted. The reader should look at the analysis provided by Dr. Gautret in France.

> I would suggest that the authors revisit the study conclusions and provide us additional insights on the various patient outcomes."

April 23, 2020

Dr. James Hall, Oncologist:

> "Recent article may be in Medscape about a husband and wife, couple of attending at mass general discussed that the husband was hospitalized and quite sick. He was in a study that it appeared that part of the standard arm was hydroxychloroquine and azithromycin. Yes, the VA study was not worthy of being labeled as science."

April 23, 2020

Dr. David Rogers, Internist:

> "The higher mortality in this "study" had nothing to do with the use of the drug. The treatment group had more risk factors for higher mortality than the "control group." Very poor design. I also have questions about the integrity of the "study" coming out of China and call this state propaganda until proven otherwise."

April 23, 2020

Dr. Johnny Peet, OB/GYN:

> "Terrible study. Do we wait to start antibiotics for community acquired pneumonia until the patient is intubated? If we did, antibiotics would not work well at all. Medscape should not even cover this study."

April 23, 2020

Dr. Earl Morgan, Emergency Medicine:

> "I couldn't agree with Dr. Rethman more strongly. We do need research regarding all aspects of the coronavirus; however, it needs to be quality research. Poorly conducted studies have the potential to do more harm than no research at all. Thank you for the opportunity to allow my comments."

April 24, 2020

Dr. Thomas Cowan, Orthopedic Surgeon:

> "Horribly done and horribly reported retrospective "survey." The sickest patients received HCQ or HCQ/AZ and succumbed usually on a ventilator. Most of these patients were lymphopenic and close to cytokine storm. All patients were on supplemental O2, and elderly. This garbage report is not a study, and no peer review journal will publish it. Shame on Medscape for giving it the light of day."

III.   Gautret, P., Lagier, J., Parola, P., et al., Hydroxychloroquine and azithromycin as a treatment of COVID-19: results of an open-label non-randomized clinical trial. *Int J Antimicrob Agents.* (prepress) doi: 10.1016./j.ijantimicag.2020.105949

    A.   *Medscape* Comments: [Retraction Watch Staff. Hydroxychloroquine for COVID-19 Study Did Not Meet Expected Standard. *Medscape.* April 8, 2020]

April 23, 2020

Dr. Douglas Robinson, General Surgeon:

> "Did anyone actually look at the VA study? Totally flawed. Treatments were on ventilated patients who have poor outcomes regardless. Some patients in the non-hydroxychloroquine group actually got Zithromax. Politics have totally ruined this discussion and Medscape seems to be a part of the politics."

April 14, 2020

Dr. Thomas Kaye, Pharmacist:

> "With the expanded use of hydroxychloroquine in the pandemic that has been used on numerous patients recently, the outcome should be correlated as a meta-study to evaluate the effectiveness. I suspect that there is adequate number of medical records to evaluate and allocate results to outcomes. Scientific principle is useful if you have the time to perform a well-controlled study, but COVID-19 is demanding for a current treatment or prevention.

The FDA and NIH are part of a very large bureaucracy which moves like a sloth. It is time to evaluate these departments and wash out the ruinous regulations and the painful dialogue coming from them."

April 14, 2020

Dr. Susan Happell-Opsomer:

"If this drug works who cares what the study results conclude; certainly not the patient whose life has been saved. If everyone would just stop this political nonsense, maybe something of value could be accomplished. Good grief. I have never seen so many immature got-to-have-the-last-word ridiculous people."

April 13, 2020

Dr. Richard Sadler, Critical Care/Intensive Care:

"We are not going to have the luxury of all kinds of time to look at this drug combination for months and months. It is go-time now. We can intelligently try this, watch it, and make a decision on its effectiveness while we wait for the studies to be completed. I understand protocol, but at some point, we have to use logic and evidence instead of slow motion analysis in certain cases. I see a lot of promise for hydroxychloroquine, potentially with Z-pak and zinc. I have treated over 300 patients so far with excellent results. This is an opinion article, not facts. We don't need partisan misuse of information at this point."

April 10, 2020

Dr. Daniel Weiss, Endocrinologist:

"I agree with Dr. McCarthy. And now the French group (Raoult and colleagues) have treated over 1,000 patients with excellent results (soon to be published). Their large case series is compelling enough data along with data from others in the US (Medscape deleted my last post with that site URL). We can do RCTs and still treat patients with a very safe combination of medications while awaiting RCT results.

Penicillin and sulfonamides were rapidly deployed in the battlefields well before widespread RCTs with these agents! Sadly, the objection to the use of hydroxychloroquine has become politicized."

April 10, 2020

Dr. Karen McCarthy, Family Medicine:

"Yes, I think it is negligence on our part for not offering hydroxychloroquine and zinc (and possibly Z-pack) treatment to our patients that are COVID-19 positive. If we offer this treatment early on, it will decrease hospitalizations, morbidity, and mortality and carrier states!

Rheumatologists and internists (like myself) have prescribed Plaquenil for years with no side effects. I have also used hydroxychloroquine in Africa and Haiti for years to treat their malaria. Again, I have not seen any significant side effects. Malaria is a terrible disease and it would be malpractice to not offer hydroxychloroquine to these patients.

For patients with this horrific COVID-19 infection, I believe it is negligent on our part not to offer this treatment. It is sad, but I do think some doctors in leadership positions are more concerned about being politically correct instead of caring about the health of our patients. And just a reminder, we should hold the WHO accountable for suppressing the information that this virus was being transferred from human to human as they knew about this information in late December. Thank you."

B. *Medscape* Comments: [Mock, J. Hospitals Update Hydroxychloroquine Protocols after FDA Warning. *Medscape*. April 28, 2020]

May 1, 2020

Dr. James Ransom, Allergy and Clinical Immunology:

"Nobody has studied the possibility that HCQ use has been one reason for the decrease in ventilator cases. It is being widely used for early cases and this may be one reason for fewer ICU patients. Of course, due to the "politicization" of this drug (a real shame for the medical profession), we are now told that Remdesivir is the real answer. This may be the way Big Pharma "kills" a cheap generic drug that can be used "off-label" in early cases.

Someday, maybe someone will tell us the truth about all this. In the meantime be skeptical of everything you read."

May 5, 2020

Robert Biles, Other healthcare provider:

"Maybe Medscape will get the drift after all the postings below that so many obviously forced political articles (shrouded in the name of medical information) are not welcome. It is legitimate to publicize FDA warnings, but the constant harangue of HCQ negative articles is both tiring and counterproductive. Please Medscape editors put the hammer down that you continue to use against this administration in the name of medical information."

May 1, 2020

Bill Rhodes, Other healthcare provider:

From the WHOs own 2017 Monograph on: The cardiotoxicity of antimalarials.

"Despite hundreds of millions of doses administered in the treatment of malaria, there have been no reports of sudden unexplained death associated with quinine, chloroquine, or amodiaquine, although each drug causes QT/QTc interval prolongation."

May 1, 2020

Dr. Chi Truong, Pediatrics:

"Please use hydroxychloroquine (HCQ) early to save COVID-19 patients. Please do not conclude that HCQ fails after you only give it to the very late and severe hospitalized cases. Our professional responsibility is look for the best time frame to get its highest efficacy in COVID-19."

April 30, 2020

Dr. Michael Rosenblatt, DPM:

"I have never really seen a truly politicized medication like this in my 77-years with the exception of Oxycontin which is genuinely dangerous. The Big Pharma pushed this to the hilt. It caused irreparable damage. It is hard to post anything remotely political here so I will try to keep away from it. In my opinion, COVID-19 will be like any other viral infection. Each treatment will have to be tailored to the needs of the particular patient you are treating. This will be no different for a patient who needs stents for cardiac vessels. Patients will vary.

There are few substitutes for HCQ that can help prevent cytokine storms. One example might be Quercetin. Blood filtering devices have been successfully used, but they are expensive and require enormous staff support. Probably a congressional representative would get it, but not you or me, and certainly not your dad even if he was a US combat veteran. This study is not very encouraging. It looks like your best bet so far is still HCQ. Like it or not, we are stuck with it.

Dr. Fauci is very enthusiastic about Gilead pharmaceutical product, Remdesivir, which NIH brought to testing by its support. It is not nearly as good as ordinary ivermectin and vastly more expensive. Plus it has a lot of side effects ivermectin does not have. Thank God President Trump said nothing about ivermectin! There is no indication that Remdesivir prevents cytokine storms. I would respectfully ask Dr. Fauci, since he is gaga over this, if it does. Azithromycin can cause arrhythmias. A possible substitute would be doxycycline and it lowers pleural and alveolar inflammation which is very good, but has no antiviral effects like azithromycin or zinc.

I am not certain how we can get out of this political fix that we are in. I have to come to the conclusion that if you have elderly patients and are a prescriber, you should get some HCQ and put it in a desk drawer and save it if you are over 60. It may become illegal for licensed physicians to prescribe. It already is in Nevada unless you are hospitalized or in the ER.

Everyone knows that a correct dose of HCQ is quite safe. I am not completely sure about azithromycin. Please consult a cardiologist if you aren't either. I hope those who politicize medicine realize what a fix they are getting us into. Medscape editors, I am trying my best to stay apolitical."

April 29, 2020

Dr. Vladimir Groysman, Anesthesiology:

"The drug is working, you need to start earlier, not at a time when patients are intubated and crashing. Agree with Dr. Badolato. It is a political shame. All the world uses hydroxychloroquine."

April 29, 2020

Dr. Joseph Badolato, Family Practice:

> "I never thought that I would see the day when a potential lifesaving drug was either summarily dismissed or marginalized due to "safety issue" simply because it was mentioned by our President. How truly despicable."

April 29, 2020

Dr. John Wuertz, Psychiatry:

> "So the study the FDA based the recommendations on stated it was possibly killing more people being treated who were very ill with the coronavirus. Other study showed the hydroxychloroquine worked best when given early. The recommendations are not to give it as an outpatient, but to use it in sicker patients in the hospital? If doctors abide by this, then I guess if it is later discovered that lives were lost that could have been saved, the doctors will be held harmless and not be sued?"

April 29, 2020

Dr. Boutros Zeidan, Pulmonology:

> "Just a couple of hypothetical/comments:
>
> If you were one of the FDA personnel issuing that warning, how would you act if a close relative or loved one who tested positive for COVID-19 seeking your advice because of a lingering fever, cough, and some dyspnea, but declined to go to a hospital in the area with no active medical trials, asked about COVID-19 treatment?
>
> I presume that, "Do no harm" applies to not only harmful acts, but also harms from lack of action.
>
> As long as there remains a marriage between science and politics, trouble will endure. Although, I am certainly not a fan of the current President, who for whatever strange reason decided to endorse hydroxychloroquine, my observations tell me that if his predecessor had done the exact same thing; the very same drug would have universally been accepted as the miracle drug.
>
> Should we ask whether the cheap cost of hydroxychloroquine in comparison to let's say Remdesivir has something to do with everything else?"

April 28, 2020

Dr. Sam Gallo, Ophthalmology:

> "Since I'm a pharmacist and a medical doctor (ophthalmologist), please explain this to me like I'm a 3 year-old. Why isn't a baseline EKG recommended in the hydroxychloroquine package insert, but an ophthalmic exam is? Why do my rheumatology colleagues routinely prescribe it in an outpatient setting without getting and EKG and with no hesitation? Something to ponder."

April 28, 2020

Dr. Victor Forys, Internist:

"You ask a leading question, the answer to which you most certainly know. It is a political issue. Before it became a political issue, there were no concerns related to cardiac arrhythmia with HCQ treatment.

Ophthalmic issues were addressed by annual or semi-annual visual field testing. After the medication became politicized the issues concerning sudden blindness and cardiac death became paramount. Some people were upset about a possible treatment modality. It is not hard to understand, just hard to believe."

April 28, 2020

Pat Riley, Other Healthcare Provider:

"Why the push against the triple therapy when so many have been cured with it? How can a physician not treat a patient with this option when he has nothing else to offer that might save a patient's life? Case in point...a healthy young man 24 years of age got COVID-19.

He was put on a ventilator, coded three days later, and physical compressions revived him where he remained in a medically induced coma for two weeks. The family was told to expect that he would be gone.

The patient was given the zinc, Azithromycin, and hydroxychloroquine and he recovered in two days and was discharged two days later. He is doing well and owes his life to this treatment."

April 28, 2020

Dr. Nosa Aigbe Lebarty, Family Medicine:

"I would hope that everyone understands that these drugs have been used for years...for malaria, lupus, etc, etc... There are folks still taking these drugs on a daily basis so we just realize that the side effects are such that we cannot administer these medicines outside of the hospital??"

April 28, 2020

Dr. Linda Harrison, Family Medicine:

"I totally agree. Many of us who actually treat patients are also where the viral infections respond best when treatment is instituted immediately at the first signs of illness, for example; Tamiflu with influenza, and Valtrex with shingles or cold sores.

I have patients who have been taking 400 mg daily for ten years with MCTD and Sjogren's with multiple organ diagnosis, multiple other diagnoses, including diabetes and hypertension. Did anyone else see the article published last year about the benefits of hydroxychloroquine in type II diabetes associated with weight loss and controlled blood sugars? Come on people! Let physicians decide appropriate treatments."

C. *Medscape* Comments: [Hughes, S. Remdesivir Now 'Standard of Care' for COVID-19, Fauci Says. *Medscape*. April 29, 2020]

May 5, 2020

Dr. Alex Wonner, Surgeon:

"Very strange that Professor Raoult had better results with hydroxychloroquine by treating patients in the early phase and avoiding those going to the ICU and suddenly this drug is discredited. But an American drug costing a fortune that has no real benefit in mortality is suddenly the standard of care!!!!

The power of money..."

May 1, 2020

Bill Rhoades, Other Healthcare Provider:

"Fauci's own NIAID Remdesivir study: Changed multiple parameters on the fly, expanding the size (twice) in an effort to achieve statistical significance for mortality. When this failed, they changed mortality from a primary endpoint to a secondary observation to avoid failure of the final result. When they ran out of masked placebo (due to the trial expansion) the managers said, "just use unmasked saline". When it was pointed out an unmasked placebo was pointless, they dropped the placebo altogether.

Early Data from Gilead's Compassionate Use of Remdesivir for COVID-19: 25% of patients receiving it have severe side effects, including multiple-organ dysfunction syndrome, septic shock, and acute kidney injury. Another 23% demonstrated evidence of liver damage on lab tests."

May 1, 2020

Bill Rhoades, Other Health Care Provider:

"The VA study that effectively killed HCQ use in the United States was quite the sham-show, and Fauci surely knew this. Unknown doses of HCQ were given only to the sickest patients, typically shortly before they were put on a vent (which we now know can hasten death).

Almost all of the patients given HCQ were elderly black males, which statistically are the racial, gender & age group most likely to have a poor outcome with advanced Covid. There was no peer review, though all who have looked at the details have torn this trial to shreds. It would be laughable if the consequences were not so devastating to the fight to contain this plague."

D. *Medscape* Comments: [Hobbs, B., Osmotherly, K. Hydroxychloroquine: Possible COVID Drug Can be Toxic to Retinas. *Medscape*. April 2, 2020]

April 8, 2020

Dr. Sanjay Agarwal, Ophthalmology:

"I am a retina specialist and screen patients on hydroxychloroquine routinely. We monitor these patients on a yearly basis and retinal toxicity is rare even after years of usage. To suggest that retinal toxicity is somehow a risk for Covid patients for a 10 day course is completely ridiculous and irresponsible. I'm amazed this article was even written. Let's discuss (appropriately) if the drug is effective against Covid and other possible side effects. NOT retinal toxicity during a 10 day course."

April 8, 2020

Dr. Daniel Quistorff, General Practice:

"Headline should read: 'Hydroxychloroquine does NOT cause retinal damage during a 5-day course.'"

April 8, 2020

Dr. Navin Mehta, Family Practice:

"I am appalled at the level of thinking of some of the administrative medical people.

Some of them have not had much experience at medical practice and real-life decision making for a patient with symptoms and disease.

I was taught to make a presumptive diagnosis based on symptoms. I was trained to use drugs that were reasonably safe and tried, without waiting for "tests". I was also taught that if the illness is life threatening, there is no harm in trying a "newer" or alternative drug which has minimal side effects.

Based on this above training and experience, I find it totally unjustified for the administrators sitting in high chairs, particularly in England, to even suggest NOT using one drug or another. In particular, we should NOT have to wait for a double-blind clinical trial to use suggested drugs like Chloroquine/hydroxychloroquine, zinc, broad spectrum antibiotics (nobody seems to emphasize secondary bacterial invasion in many viral respiratory infections), and even Vitamin C and/or D. Each one of these have well-defined side effects and contraindications, which the front-line physician is well aware of when he prescribes it, and all GPs are sensible enough to check and recheck development of side effects or harm to patients.

The underlying urgency of the situation is not fully understood by the statistics oriented administrator physician or non-physician, in a way it is so well understood by the doctor treating his patient.

I think it is imperative that we give these high placed administrative persons a retirement package and put real doctors in charge."

April 7, 2020

Dr. H. Stamboliu, Internist:

> "This is ridiculous! It is not going to affect the retina in the 10 days of treatment. My wife is a rheumatologist and has a lot of experience using the drug. FDA indicates to check the eyes after 5 years of using the Plaquenil at the appropriate dose but every patient goes actually each year."

April 7, 2020

Dr. Bob Dick, Internist states:

> "Why would you write this article?
>
> Even the title is misleading.
>
> There is no toxicity of this drug given for a week.
>
> For Covid that is worth 2 sentences. That especially applies to retinal problems. It's because of irresponsible and irrational statements by doctors, politicians, and media that US has lowest percentage of usage by physicians (23%) of HCQ amongst 30 countries with Large Covid problems.
>
> That translates to thousands of additional hospital stays and hundreds more deaths based on both double blind studies and thousands of case reports.
>
> Not a cure but a highly effective drug and the only drug that's available, and cheap and proven safe. FDA should have approved this for Covid two weeks ago."

April 9, 2020

Dr. Lee Angioletti, Ophthalmology:

> "What is the high risk of death taking HCQ that has safety data for 55 years? Increased QT? Also, he said it may have a mild to no effect is better than watching someone slip into ARDS with no treatment. HC needs to be taken EARLY at the very start of symptoms and in fact should be given as a prophylaxis to healthcare workers the same way our Marines took HCQ to prevent malaria."

April 7, 2020

Dr. James Hiatt, Ophthalmology:

> "Ignorant article. HCQ can be toxic when taken for years. No one has suggested a need for years of HCQ therapy for COVID-19."

April 6, 2020

Dr. Samuel Zuckerman, Pediatrics:

> "The title totally is misleading. You need to arrive deep into the article to find that the dosing and longevity of treatment for Covid make this an unlikely complication. POLITICS!!!"

April 6, 2020

Dr. James Wassum, Oncologist:

> "Our hospital system had a COVID-19 conference call for retired physicians. The ophthalmologist who cares for all RA and other disease patients treated with hydroxchloroquine spoke to retinal toxicity. In his experience he has not seen this even in patients treated for 4 or more years."

April 4, 2020

Dr. Jeff Taylor, Ophthalmology:

> "I can't believe that this article was actually written and posted in Medscape. The risk of macular toxicity is essentially zero when taking this drug at appropriate weight based doses and for the length of time it would be needed to treat the virus. When someone starts this for RA, I don't even do the first screening visit for retinal disease until six months and then yearly after that."

April 3, 2020

Dr. Emilio Gonzalez, Rheumatology:

> "Not toxic at all if taken for just a short period of time. It may be potentially toxic to the retina if the dose exceeds 5 mg per kilo per day, taken over 5 years, usually longer than 10 years, and even then. That's not the case at all in treating COVID-19, Come on!"

April 3, 2020

Dr. John Wendt, Pharmacist:

> "This is amazing that during a health crisis the "professionals" in charge of the CDC and FDA are not trying anything on the treatment side for these patients. The CDC dropped the ball after H1N1 and in their report they say they will learn from that pandemic and prepare for the next pandemic. 60,000,000 infected and 30,000 deaths... no vaccine, same situation we have today. Hydroxychloroquine and azithromycin clears the virus in 5 days. Therapy of 10 to 14 days would hardly cause any of these so called toxicities or side effects and would likely save 99% of lives... I think patients would be willing to "risk" the odds of side effects vs. a cure. Ludicrous."

April 3, 2020

Dr. Maurice Valentini, Optometry:

> "In all the years of practicing optometry I have never seen an actual case of Plaquenil retinopathy clinically, only in textbooks or online. The usual dose is 400 mg/day and many patients I see have been on it for years. Most patients, without other retinal or ocular media issues, usually show normal visual fields and fundus exams, and are at the 20/20 level of vision in both eyes.
>
> I feel comfortable saying that for the short duration COVID-19 patients on HCQ or Chloroquine the levels are well below toxic to cause maculopathy and most of the anecdotal evidence shows it is very effective both as a front-line treatment and prophylaxis to the virus.

If I had to choose between treatment with HCQ/Chloroquine and a full recovery or the remote possibility of visual impairment and death by drowning, it comes down to a no-brainer!"

April 3, 2020

Dr. Homin Lim, Orthopedic Surgery:

"Absolutely no reason for this article to appear anywhere during this crisis. It just spreads unnecessary anxiety amongst the general public who don't understand that the risk is almost nil. Shame on you for the 'alert'."

April 3, 2020

Dr. David Fraser, Rheumatology:

"As a rheumatologist who has prescribed Plaquenil to many many patients, it is one of the safest drugs we have for inflammatory arthritis. The eye side effects are only seen with chronic use. In addition, to recommend dosing based on body weight blood levels can be obtained to monitor therapy.

As all rheumatologists are used to doing, no patient is started on chronic therapy without a baseline eye exam. I do not refill this medication if a patient does not have their yearly (used to be 6 month) eye exam.

After 35 years in practice I have only seen eye or GI or skin complications as consistent albeit uncommon problems. Since the proposed use in COVID-19 is short term, and the possibility of eye complications is so remote the need for a prerequisite eye exam should not be an issue."

E.   *Medscape* Comments: [Duqueroy, V. COVID-19: More Hydroxychloroquine Data from France, More Questions. *Medscape*. March 30, 2020]

April 21, 2020

Dr. Fady Haddad, Internal Medicine:

"We used Didier Raoult's protocol in our center in Lebanon and in a remote hospital. We had obtained the same rate of death at 0.5%... There is lots of rational of using the dose of 600 mg for 10 days and not less regarding dose and time of treatment. Medicine is not only evidence based but it is also THE BEST AVAILABLE EVIDENCE."

April 15, 2020

Dr. Ali Tas, Internal Medicine:

"Hydroxychloroquine is a critical medicine in viral diseases especially Ebola and coronavirus. It is frequently used in malaria. In countries using this drug such as India, the incidence of COVID infection seems to be lower."

April 5, 2020

Dr. Cynthia Williams, Dentist:

"I don't understand the negativity about the use of HCQ for "compassionate use' until proper trials are completed. Millions have taken hydroxychloroquine as an anti-malarial, or for lupus and rheumatoid arthritis without "controlled" studies.

I have taken it myself many times while working in Africa as an anti-malarial.

No doctors seem to be concerned about medical problems or side effects as they write thousands of prescriptions for tourists, travelers, and ex-patriots as they travel to malaria country. I never had an EKG before my prescriptions and vaccinations were prescribed! Why now all the fuss? FDA has approved its use in this pandemic emergency. What IS the problem? Politics? Terrible thing for the medical community!"

April 1, 2020

Dr. William Neglia, Oncologist:

"Update from France 1,524 patients treated with hydroxychloroquine and azithromycin and one death." **https://www.mediterranee-infection.com/COVID-19/**

April 1, 2020

Dr. David Keller, Internist:

"This pandemic demands a quick, credible trial of hydroxychloroquine [HCQ] plus azithromycin [AZM] for treating COVID-19 infections. Our patients cannot wait for a large, perfect trial that reports its results in weeks. Thousands are dying daily, and rising. We need a trial that is fast and good, not slow and perfect.

How fast? One week, which is 1 day longer than the French trial took to show complete viral clearance in 100% of COVID-19 patients treated with HCQ plus AZM. Either HCQ plus AZM works, or it does not. The French trial took 6 days; we should be able to confirm it within a week."

   F.   *Medscape* Comments: [Swift, D. Off-Label Drug Use Linked to More Adverse Events. *Medscape*. November 10, 2015]

November 12, 2015

Marcelle Praetorius, Nurse Practitioner:

"Forcing all off-label uses of drugs to have clinical trials and FDA approval is bound to create new forms of patent only medications which will drastically increase medicine costs without increasing patient safety."

November 13, 2015

Dr. Cindy Smith, Dermatologist:

"I would love solid evidence-based data for everything I do. Unfortunately, it isn't available. I have been fighting a prior authorization battle for a patient for nearly one year in order to continue the use of dapsone and mycophenolate mofetil for severe benign mucosal (cicatricial) pemphigoid with ocular scarring.

Insurance has denied payment for MMF, stating that it's not FDA approved for this use. The problem is there are NO FDA approved medications for CP, so under that argument there are no treatment options for the patient who was in danger of blindness, could barely sit for the pain, and struggled to eat, thus complicating his diabetes. (Ironically, they are not challenging the dapsone, which has no FDA approval for this disease either.)

Hours of research (including extensive Medicare compendia review), multiple hoops, and an administrative law judge hearing finally achieved coverage but they've appealed the decision. This article is very useful but I fear insurance companies, including Medicare will use it to further complicate prescribing and create more prior authorization hoops.

There is no incentive for drug companies to study medications for rare diseases; there is no profit to be had. Until we have on-label options don't take away our off-label options; our patients need us to do the best we can for them when solutions are imperfect."

November 11, 2015

Dr. Jeffrey Gabel, OB/GYN:

"Starting back about 15 to 20 years ago, or more, not sure, there has been a concerted effort by the FDA to take away the right of doctors to use medications how they see fit as per literature or experience.

Many residency programs bowed to the pressure and began to stop the off-label use.

One example is the use of Cytotec, a prostaglandin oral medication for ulcer prevention in NSAID users but now commonly used in Obstetrics. In my area of the woods the University of Washington in Seattle refused to use the medication off-label, which is VERY cheap, and insisted on using only the extremely expensive preparations "approved".

I look at this issue as just one more attempt to reign in doctors and take away their autonomy and authority.

In my oh so humble opinion, doctors need to stop letting these groups and egomaniacs delve further and further into authoritarian, cookbook medicine and leave us to our own interpretation of the literature and our knowledge based on experience and training with INPUT from the committees in these Specialty Colleges. They do NOT know everything and are NOT the authority in medicine."

November 11, 2015

Lisa Miller, RN, Nurse:

"My doctors told me, and I happen to strongly agree, that patient treatment needs to be individualized. Medicine is not "one size fits (or works for) all." I wear a low-dose fentanyl patch for my severe fibromyalgia pain, even though fibro is RARELY treated that way; however, the University of Wisconsin Pain & Research Clinic agreed with my doctor doing that. The patch helped me go from pain so severe I couldn't be out of bed more than 20 minutes, was so depressed that I couldn't eat, and ended up being tube-fed for months!! After having narcotic pain meds I was soon able to safely and pretty comfortably return to work as an RN. Am also on Provigil to help my energy, because between the insomnia, fatigue and NO motivation to even leave my house, I needed the help it afforded me. Yes, MD's may use medications off-label not always carefully. Having said that, it's not like they don't know the drugs they're prescribing are off-label!"

G. *Medscape* Comments: [O'Rourke, K. Oncologists' Off-Label Prescribing Pits Access against Reimbursement. *Medscape.* October 15, 2018]

October 17, 2018

Dr. Denis Franklin, Psychiatrist:

"I couldn't bear to read this whole article, it made me so sad and angry. I'll offer a brief comment from an 84-year-old Family Doctor, Occupational Physician and Addiction and Forensic Psychiatrist. The author of the article quotes: "Clinicians should be following evidence-based medicine, said Zon, and for that, they rely on the US Food and Drug Administration (FDA)."

BUT, the FDA — DOES NOT REGULATE MEDICAL PRACTICE! It is not designed to do so and its processes will always be too cumbersome to track closely the advances in the science of evidence-based therapy. The whole pejorative concept of "off-label" was invented by malpractice lawyers who, when they had no other case to offer, began pretending that for a physician to prescribe differently from the medication label was a dereliction of the standards of medical practice. This was an intentional lie. The FDA governs only what manufacturers may claim on the label of an "ethical" medication. For this, they require expensive and prolonged clinical trials to prove efficacy and safety for specific uses. Manufacturers typically did a trial or two to get the drug on the market with whatever indications had been demonstrated.

After which they relied upon physicians to evaluate and follow the latest research pertaining to the actual practice of medicine, and to select and use medications on the basis of evolving clinical research as it became available. Most medications were prescribed for uses never included on the label.

But once a sufficient number of malpractice lawyers had falsely impugned the use of medications "off-label," the insurers leapt upon that excuse to not pay for those uses, calling them "experimental."

The problem here is that this fallacious but pernicious reasoning has now led to medical policies being determined by lawyers, and insurance corporations, sometimes driven by the unconscionable profiteering of pharmaceutical corporations and the failure of the government to control their pricing and profit margin.

It appears that government's self-fulfilling prophecy, that doctors, and what used to be called MEDICAL practice, needed to be managed by lawyers and businessmen, is now about to bear fruit — in the form of some form of socialized medicine. Now, in an ironic twist, it is being realized that lawyers and businessmen need to be managed by the government. Remember Eric Severeid's Law: All problems are created by solutions."

October 17, 2018

Dr. Paula Sparti, Family Medicine:

"I agree that ideally physicians should read and understand the medical literature related to a drug and use drugs according to the available literature and presented data. The burden of off-label prescribing is higher because of the astronomical costs of certain drugs. There usually is a clause in most insurance policies that "off-label" use of any FDA approved drug is allowed if the medical peer reviewed literature shows efficacy."

Dr. Sparti further stated, "In prescribing off-label drugs for a cancer, the oncologist has the responsibility to evaluate biomarkers that have evidence of predicting a response. The cost and toxicity of checkpoint inhibitors, for example, must be outweighed by the published evidence of efficacy. The additional work must be done to justify off-label immunotherapy and other cancer therapies."

H. *Medscape* Comments: [[Caplan, A. It's Too Dangerous to Prescribe Off-Label Drugs for COVID-19. *Medscape.* April 21, 2020]

April 29, 2020

Barry Creighton, Other Healthcare Provider:

"Ummm, is there a reason WHY Chloroquine is CONSISTENTLY NOT mentioned for use WITH ZINC? There have been a couple of studies that show in increases intracellular zinc in vitro because it is a zinc ionophore, and I think one was done in an animal model, and MedCram does a nice review. And yet, it is beginning to seem like that particular combo is actively avoided.

By the way, if I think I'm sick enough to need to go to a hospital, I'm calling ahead. If all they offer is a ventilator, I'm headed for another hospital or a HBOT chamber as fast as I can.

By the way, HOW many medications are used off label all the time? And, how many times do physicians have to actively experiment with medications on their patients until they figure out the one that works best?

Please, STOP with the nonsense."

April 29,2020

Dr. James McAllister, Pharmacist:

"At the time the President made that statement, physicians were already widely using that drug combination and there was no treatment other than supportive care.

I think the vast majority of physicians would perform their due diligence and choose what they thought was the best treatment; not because a layperson elected official recommended it. Also, since the statistics so far show that a majority of COVID-19 patients who end up on a ventilator perish, I would want to do all I could to keep them off one."

April 28, 2020

Dr. Gene Vialle, Anesthesiology:

> "I am a retired anesthesiologist and pharmacist. If I get coronavirus, I certainly plan to take hydroxychloroquine. It has been used by military, travelers, missionaries and autoimmune patients for decades. Silly politics."

April 27, 2020

Dr. Joel Spaulding, Pharmacist:

> "Since there is no "on label" drug with FDA approved indications for treatment of COVID-19 we are left ONLY with considering off-label meds that have a potential to mitigate symptoms or possibly decrease viral load.
>
> As have others have mentioned there are literally hundreds if not thousands of meds in use every day for off label indications many are quite effective and as time has shown, reasonably safe."

April 26, 2020

Dr. Eric Stocker, Cardiology:

> "I am intrigued by Dr. Vladimir Zev Zelenko's success (heard about him and tracked him down on YouTube). He is an FP who has treated 1450 patients in NYC with COVID as of a week or so ago with the following regimen: Hydroxychloroquine [HCQ] 200 mg bid, Azithromycin (AZ) 500 mg qd and Zinc sulfate 220 mg qd---all three for 5 consecutive days. He explains that HCQ is an ionophore that facilitates Zinc's entry into the cell. It is the Zinc that interferes with viral replication. AZ is preventing secondary bacterial infection.
>
> Studies using the above regimen are currently ongoing in several countries. I am wary of interpreting study results of HCQ without the concomitant use of Zinc.
>
> If I am heading south fast, I'll take invasive BiPAP before mechanical ventilation, COVID-19 convalescent plasma and ECMO---all have saved lives. However, long before then, I will take my chances with the above regimen if my baseline QTc interval is well below 500 msec and I do not have long QT syndrome, Brugada, RV dysplasia or a family history of sudden cardiac death. If I did, give me another EKG on Day 2 and 4."

Aril 26, 2020

Dr. Robert Silvetz, Oncology:

> "First, the mechanism of action IS understood. It is a zinc ionophore and we have more than 40 years of papers on the function of zinc as an antiviral. Not to mention 60 years on quinine derivatives.
>
> Second, I never want to read again about any doctor anywhere having his judgment over-ruled in an emergency by politicians, peer groups, medical directorates or others, on the basis of "it's not evidence based".

For Fauci, who supported the HCQ in SARS only to hypocritically ignore it now, going to the wall is not good enough. Plus, if you knew just how bad evidence-based medicine is in general, you would never read a study again. And contrary to assertions, HCQ is all over the Chinese literature in positive use. Cherry picking the negative results is just poor science. Incidentally, indomethacin works well too The Italian study from years ago is accurate even though it didn't get to human testing against SARS.

Third, once you know that zinc is an essential co-factor, why are we designing studies WITHOUT checking for zinc status? And are we aware that 50% of Chinese folks are utterly zinc deficient.? Do you think that would have a bearing on equivocal studies? And their rate of illness? Of course their data is manufactured and has no bearing with reality, so who knows what really happened in Wuhan...

In my entourage several went down with this COVID. Of those 4 suffered desaturations. They were all zinc primed, placed on HCQ and Z-pack. 8 hours later each was breathing normally again and made full recoveries.

This is mirrored by colleagues who ignored the WHO CDC NIH (they can no longer be trusted) using Vitamin C 50 gr IV to short-circuit impending cytokine storms, zinc primed them, and did HCQ+Zpack. Blinding fast recovery, one person pushing 72 years of age with a O2 sat of 65% who refused hospitalization."

April 29, 2020

Dr. Robert Petersen, Otolaryngology:

"If HCQ is so dangerous then how do the rheumatologists get away with giving it to thousands of patients? millions have taken it for malaria. Zinc is said to be required and the FDA seems not to know that in their studies.

One VA study shunted the worse cases to the HCQ patients so they didn't do as well. Women handle zinc better than men so more deaths in men. 1/5 of the population is said to be deficient in zinc. Why don't we have a survey of rheumatologists to see how many of their patients are coming down with the corona virus?"

April 22 through April 26, 2020

Bill Rhoades, Other Health Care Professional:

"If HCQ is truly quite dangerous, might it not be wise to advise it be pulled off the market?

RA is painful and debilitating, but not particularly fatal, & lupus patients aren't going to die in 30 days without this dangerous med. These patients are on HCQ for decades at a time! The typical course for COVID is 5-10 days.

It's a pandemic, old darlings. Not a time for wringing of hands and fatalistic caution. The case curve has been flattened, but is plateauing rather than falling off. Vaccine is a year away at best, & the economy is already foundering. Reports from China indicate a second wave may be rising in the short time since they've re-opened. How many times can we shut down in 2020, & for how long? Risk vs Reward. Is risk of a total economic collapse even part of the equation under consideration?"

"Doctors in the field bravely prescribing hydroxychloroquine EARLY in the disease are reporting good results, while clinical trials of HCQ on hospitalized patients (essentially salvage attempts) are reporting poor results.

So the "Best Medicine" is to tell the doctors in the field to STOP healing their patients, while failed salvage trials with HCQ undergo peer review.

We live in interesting times!"

"Bravery is properly considering risk vs potential reward and taking action while others are paralyzed with fear.

Hydroxychloroquine: Widely used generic for over half a century. FDA approved Safe and Effective for Malaria, Lupus and Rheumatoid Arthritis. Blocked viral entry of original SARS-CoV into cells (in vitro) & lowers inflammatory cascade.

Remdesivir: Failed at treating Ebola, failed at treating SARS, failed at treating MERS; yet the darling of Big Pharm & their pals at the NIH.

If one of these two forlorn hopes doesn't work, it's game-over for the entire economy and deaths of despair may come to equal death from COVID. The truly brave will take a gamble with treatment rather than standing like a deer caught in headlights."

April 22, 2020

Dr. Jane Chene:

"How ethical is it to tell a patient who has high risk of dying or is dying that you won't use your brain and the scientific data to help them with something new, because you are waiting for a "scientific" study. Many of the newer drugs studied and approved are pulled off the market because they end up harming people even though studied.

These old drugs have been around a long time and have low toxicity which has been way overblown by the purveyors of medical literature and "news" channels that are supported by drug companies."

April 26, 2020

Dr. Katherine Murray-Leisure, Infectious Disease:

"The VA study authors included an ophthalmology venture capitalist (Retina) and one with a patent on CoVid19; no impartial infectious diseases folks. VA study was done with late stage CoVid19 patients.

They were older hospitalized veterans, 68% of whom were black. We know that CoVid19 has poorer outcomes with Afro Americans regardless of therapies. VA study authors were engaged with the major pharmaceutical firms, who might have hopes for alternative therapeutics for CoVid19. Sorry, follow the money."

April 26, 2020

Dr. Francis Fazzano, Ob/Gyn:

"The political bias prevalent in Medscape coverage of this epidemic has become so obvious!"

April 26, 2020

Dr. Marsha Snyder, Family Medicine:

"The VA study was a highly flawed study. The main problem is that the treated group of patients had a much lower white blood cell count before treatment, compared to the non-treated group of patients. The two groups were not equal at the start. Covid 19 patients who have leukopenia while ill have a much worse prognosis.

In the VA study the patients that got the hydroxychloroquine had a much worse prognosis to start."

April 22, 2020

Dr. Allison Russo, Pharmacist:

"Many doctors are using this off label in patients who qualify. There is absolute no reason not to in the absence of contraindications."

April 21, 2020

MM Denver, Psychologist:

"There is a very large body of research from China from 2002 - to right now concerning SARS-CoVs. Hydroxychloroquine + zpak is one of the accepted treatment (and prophylactic) protocols. There are many, many others.

It is detrimentally western-centric to think the only valid medical knowledge originates with the US pharmo-medical industry. To improve outcomes more research in process and treatment is necessary, including real time paradigm altering discussion."

April 26, 2020

Dr. Mary Andrew:

"It's very funny that the media are so concerned about prescribing Z'paks, when millions of patients have taken it for (viral) bronchitis."

I.   *Medscape* Comments: [Frellick, M. No Hydroxychloroquine Benefit in Small Randomized COVID-19 Trial. *Medscape*. April 16, 2020]

April 22, 2020

Dr. Rick Hess, Internal Medicine:

"Apparently HCQ prevents infection by lowering the ph required for transfer of viral RNA from a human cell membrane vacuole into the human cell. If this is the case, we might expect it to have little effect on the later stages of infection after transfer has occurred.

Although there may be benefit from an anti-inflammatory effect. Dr. Wharton's suggestion seems spot on as HCQ might be more effective in prevention than in cure. I agree that the coding data would be a fast way to look at this question."

April 21, 2020

Dr. Robert Scoyni, Gastroenterology:

> "Why is there no mention of the study by Gautret in Medscape if you're going to cite a study with a small and unrandomized sample? I am credentialed at 4 hospitals and all of them utilize hydroxychloroquine in their protocols for Covid. Why even cite this study except for the fact that anything with the word Covid in it gets printed?"

April 19, 2020

Reni H, Clinical Nurse Specialist:

> "I just can't believe this article headline will be this if the bulk of the article does not even show conclusive data to support it. I am not political but people should really publish something that is factual rather than 3rd rate, inconclusive, data that has not really been subjected to rigorous study. In attempt to save life in desperate situations, it is one's personal decision to use something that could save their life, in face of possible death. I wish this article provided more facts than opinion."

April 18, 2020

Dr. Victor Forys, Internal Medicine:

> "The headline is "No Benefit". The investigators report that the study shows some decrease in symptoms and in biomarkers. Apparently, there seems to be a a bias in reporting any information related to hydroxychloroquine or any therapeutics for the treatment of COVID. Depending on the objectivity of the news media even the medical press is no longer possible.

> It's disappointing that the medical press has been infected with the same virus infecting the news media in general. Everyone has a right to their own opinion. The editor or whoever wrote the headline is unfortunately is putting out their opinion while ignoring the facts."

> "There are anecdotal reports that several drugs and therapies are beneficial in the treatment of COVID19. No definitive studies have been published on any one of the treatments being used.

> "Better to use common sense and treat where treatment is appropriate and safe. Antivirals have been a safe class of drugs in past and hydroxychloroquine is known to be safe and effective in the treatment of RA, plasma has a fairly good track record. Until we know for sure I believe we should use all the tools in the toolbox.

> People are sick and are dying. We should not just stand by with our hands in our pockets. We should use common sense and act."

April 21, 2020

Dr. Daniel Quistorff, General Practice:

> "Politics has nothing to do with this. HCQ has 4 mechanisms of action:

> 1. It binds the GBD of the spike protein preventing binding with the ACE-2 receptor

> https://www.sciencedirect.com/science/article/pii/S0924857920301102

2. It is known to block virus infection by increasing endosomal pH required for virus/cell fusion

   https://www.nature.com/articles/s41422-020-0282-0?fbclid=IwAR3c5iy9h65X1cnkrL6i6fJcWwi0ygN1LtI67SkcgREM4DyxxAcPauRuf5w

3. It has an anti-inflammatory effect which is protective against cytokine storm

   https://europepmc.org/article/med/8336306

4. It is a zinc ionophore allowing for higher levels of zinc to enter the cell which inhibits RNA polymerase.

   https://www.ncbi.nlm.nih.gov/pmc/articles/PMC4182877/

   https://www.ncbi.nlm.nih.gov/pmc/articles/PMC2973827/

And preliminary data from France, India, even South Dakota are showing the benefit."

J. *Medscape* Comments: [Kincaid, E. COVID-19 Daily: Fauci Testifies. HCQ Trials Lack ECG. Medscape. May 12, 2020]

May 13, 2020

Dr. Ben Geslani, Internal Medicine:

"Would anyone comment on the following pre-print regarding zinc and HCQ? It looks like this combo is better than plain HCQ or HCQ + AZT.

Hydroxychloroquine and azithromycin plus zinc vs hydroxychloroquine and azithromycin alone: outcomes in hospitalized COVID-19 patients **https://www.medrxiv.org/content/10.1101/2020.05.02.20080036v1#disqus_thread**"

May 12, 2020

Dr. Jesse Epps, Anesthesiology:

"I doubt this study by Novartis will "put the issue to rest". Multiple studies already show minimal benefit in HOSPITALIZED patients, which this study examines. I would expect adverse events in patients given a med that potentially prolongs QT after those patients already have the cytokine release and NET formation with the potential for inducing myocarditis.

I am amazed that no researchers are looking at HCQ at SYMPTOM ONSET, diagnosis as a way to limit disease progression.

The anecdotal studies in nursing homes in New York and Texas that kept residents out of the hospital and decreased mortality to about 2% seem significant enough to investigate to me. It is cheaper to keep people out of the hospital than build all of the surge facilities. So we know Covid causes cytokine release and NET formation(which results in vasculitis, thrombosis and potentially myocarditis).

We also know HCQ inhibits release of these cytokines and NET formation. We know that millions of patients take HCQ daily without adverse effects. Dr. Goodman has pointed out below that patients chronically on HCQ are having better outcomes after Covid infection in their Chicago registry, in spite of higher comorbidities.

It has also become obvious that the morbidity and mortality from this disease is not due to viral overload of some kind, but to the out of control immune response to the disease. So whether or not the in vitro viral inhibition with HCQ translates in vivo is likely irrelevant, when we know so much about the action of this drug on the immune response. Much of this research from peer reviewed journals is over a decade old and is very extensive.

The Trillion dollar question is why not these studies on the ability of HCQ to limit severity? Maybe it's too cheap of a drug to get the funding compared to an anti-viral that will cost $30,000."

May 12, 2020

Jose Hilario, Other Healthcare Provider:

"I just read the title; if it interests me, and I skip reading the article then just jump right in the comments and discussions section where I get better information and understanding of the topic. I find it very interesting to get a better picture of the truth from practitioners in the field than from those sitting in their cubicles, but that should not surprise anyone."

May 12, 2020

Dr. James Ransom, Allergy & Clinical Immunology:

"The anti-HCQ tilt of most new reports, usually quoting Dr. Fauci, are extremely odd. Dr. Goodman and others anecdotally point out that this is a drug of long usage and very rare cardiac abnormalities. I think we should follow the money to understand why this drug gets no respect.

Using it for HCQ is "off label," not popular with the FDA but also not against the law.

Big Pharma is striving to find a better drug. If found, it will sell for hundreds (thousands?) per course of treatment: how likely are they to support testing for HCQ efficacy, as it is generic and cheap?

Has any reporter examined whether Dr. Fauci has any consultancy contracts with any company working on vaccines or drugs for Covid 19? It would be nice to know about this, one way or the other."

May 12, 2020

Dr. Alton Thomson, Ob/Gyn:

"It's becoming obvious that no one wants the Hydrochloroquine trial to even be done much less succeed."

May 12, 2020

Dr. Olga Goodman, Rheumatologist:

"Yes as a rheumatologist, I can tell this is the safest drug unless significantly overdosed."

Dr. Wallace Gasiewicz, Internal Medicine:

"The WHO says Hydroxychloroquine is safe:

QUOTE:

Apart from halofantrine, antimalarial medicines that prolong the QT/QTc interval, such as quinine, chloroquine, artesunate-amodiaquine and dihydroartemisinin-piperaquine, have been associated with a low risk of cardiotoxicity.

https://www.who.int/malaria/mpac/mpac-mar2017-erg-cardiotoxicity-report-session2.pdf

Should everyone around the world being treated with Hydroxychloroquine be monitored for Long QT? Since azithromycin also causes prolonged QT, should we not monitor all patients on Z pack therapy?"

May 13, 2020

Marianne Schaffer, Health Business/Administration:

"More than 1000 front-line healthcare workers around the world have died from COVID-19. And that's in just a few months.

I bet it if was more than 1000 politicians we'd see appropriate actions being taken. YOU, physicians, are the experts. Speak out. Support one another."

IV.   Gupta, S., Nayak, R., "Off-Label Use of Medicine: Perspective of Physicians, Patients, Pharmaceutical Companies Regulatory Authorities." *J Pharmacol Pharmacother.* 2014; 5(2):88-92.

Comments by author:

"There have always been attempts from pharmaceutical companies to increase the use of their drug. Because of the financial aspects involved it is highly impractical to expect the pharmaceutical companies will restrict or stop off-label promotion, whereas, the regulatory agencies should always try to balance the need for rapid access to drugs for new indications against the limited information on the risk/benefit ratio.

On the other end of this paradigm off-labeled use gives freedoms to physicians to apply new therapeutic options based on the latest evidence. In fact, physicians may lawfully prescribe approved drugs for any use consistent with available scientific data and proper medical practice.

Sometimes patients suffering from terminal illness demand new approach or new treatment and if their logical demands are rejected it will definitely not benefit other new patients.

It has been recommended that the attempt should be to strike a balance in the best interest of the patient. Off-labeled use might be compared to a double-edged sword which the one end might be very useful for some patients while it can also expose them to unrestricted experimentation.

It has been recommended that proper off-label prescribing should only be encouraged by the distribution of truthful and non-misleading information. If off-label prescribing is disallowed, many new therapies and evidences will not come into the forefront because the incentive for pharmaceutical companies get the regulatory approval for new uses of old drugs by clinical testing is very less."

V.   Gazarian, M., Kelly, M., McPhee, J., et al. "Off-Label Use of Medicines: Consensus Recommendations for Evaluating Appropriateness" *Med J Aust* 2006; 185(10):544-548.

Comments by author:

"Off-label prescribing is the prescription of a registered medicine for a use that is not included in the product information. The practice is common, with rates up to 40% in adults and up to 90% in pediatric patients.

Off-label prescribing is not illegal and may sometimes be clinically appropriate, but is associated with a number of clinical safety and ethical issues. To date, no explicit guidance has been available to help clinicians assess appropriateness in off-label prescribing. We describe the development of a guide for clinicians, policymakers, and funders of health care in evaluating the appropriateness of medicines proposed for off-label use.

- Three broad categories of appropriate off-label use are identified:

- off-label use justified by high-quality evidence; use within the context of a formal research proposal;

- exceptional use justified by individual clinical circumstances.

An appropriate process for informed consent is proposed for each category. If there is no high-quality evidence supporting off-label use, and the medicine is not suitable for exceptional or research indicators, its use is generally not recommended.

This will reduce inappropriate use, enhance patient safety by reducing exposure to unnecessary risk, and may stimulate more clinically relevant medicine research."

VI.   Lerose, R., Musto, P., Aieta, P., et al. "Off-Label Use of Anti-Cancer Drugs Between Clinical Practice and Research: The Italian Experience." *Eur J Clin Pharmacol.* 2012; 68(5):505-512.

Comments by author:

"Off-label use is the practice of prescribing a drug outside the terms of its official labeling. Worldwide, about 20% of the commonly prescribed medications are off-label, and the percentage increases in specific patient populations., such as children, pregnant women, and cancer patients.

Off-label use is particularly widespread in oncology for many reasons, including the wide variety of cancer subtypes, the difficulties involved in performing clinical trials, the rapid diffusion of preliminary results, and delays in the approval of new drugs by regulatory organizations/agencies.

Off-label drug utilization is essential in oncology when based on evidence. However, off-label drugs must be prescribed in accordance with existing national laws and only when the potential benefit outweighs the potential toxic effects."

VII.　　DeWitt, M., Gamble, A., Hanson, D., et al. "Repurposing Mebendazole as a Replacement for Vincristine for the Treatment of Brain Tumors." *Mol Med.* 2017; 23:50-56.

Comments by author:

"Our findings documenting a lack of therapeutic efficacy of vincristine in a mouse model for glioma where mebendazole shows significant efficacy, in addition to a lack of evidence for the clinical benefit of vincristine in the treatment of brain tumors, strongly suggest that vincristine should not be used chemotherapeutically in neuro-oncology.

Thus, as mebendazole and vincristine have the same mechanism of action, replacing vincristine with mebendazole may facilitate the elimination of vincristine from neuro-oncological regimens."

VIII.　　Khan, M., Nasti, T., Buchwald, Z., et al. "Repurposing Drugs for Cancer Radiotherapy: Early Success is in Emerging Opportunities." *Cancer J.* 2019; 25(2):106-115.

Comments by author:

"A tremendous opportunity remains to investigate drug combinations in the clinical setting that might increase the benefits of radiation without additional toxicity. We highlight many opportunities to apply repurposing, and survey candidate radiosensitizers that alter DNA repair, decrease hypoxia, block tumor survival signaling, modify tumor metabolism, block growth factor signaling, slow tumor invasiveness, impair angiogenesis, or stimulate anti-tumor immunity.

These candidate drugs, some of which have been previously approved can confer radiation-enhancing effects, and may display low toxicity on their own. Promising agents include such widely used drugs as aspirin, metformin, and statins, offering the potential to improve outcomes, decrease radiation doses, and lower costs."

IX.　　Ozsvari, B., Lamb, R., and Lisanti, M. "Repurposing of FDA-Approved Drugs against Cancer-Focus on Metastasis." *Aging (Albany, NY)* 2016; 8(4):567-568.

Comments by author:

"Aspirin, a widely used anti-inflammatory drug, a potent COX-2 inhibitor, and an anti-aggregant has been recently shown that its regular intake might reduce long-term risk of colorectal, esophageal, gastric, biliary, and breast cancers and the risk of distant metastasis as well.

ADD ASPIRIN, the world's largest ever phase III clinical trial was launched in the UK in October 2015. Oncologists are looking to assess whether regular aspirin use after standard therapy prevents recurrence and prolongs survival in patients with non-metastatic common solid tumors of breast, colorectal, gastroesophageal, and prostate.

Cancer is a leading cause of death worldwide and despite the investment of millions of dollars of large pharmaceutical companies and governments into anti-cancer drug development, the current chemotherapeutic approaches are highly costly while their efficacy is not universally effective in all patients.

These factors are leading to repurposing of well-known FDA approved drugs, which can bypass the early stages of drug development, even Phase-I clinical trials in some cases, thus reducing project costs and time. Taken together, the previously mentioned studies show that FDA approved drugs can be successfully applied in tumor therapies."

The author further states, 'Given that mitochondria have a bacterial origin, antibiotics also target mitochondrial translation and impair mitochondrial function. In our study we have shown a treatment with four or five different classes of FDA approved antibiotics, especially doxycycline can be used to eradicate cancer stem-like cells in several tumor types.'"

X.   McKee, D., Sternberg, A., Stange, U., et al. "Candidate Drugs against SARS-CoV-2 and COVID-19." *Pharmacol Res.* 2020:10-4859.

Comments by author:

"Outbreak and pandemic of coronavirus SARS-CoV-2 in 2019/2020 will challenge global health for the future. Because a vaccine against the virus will not be available in the near future, we herein try to offer a pharmacological strategy to combat the virus.

There exists a number of candidate drugs that may inhibit infection with and replication of SARS-CoV-2. Such drugs comprise inhibitors of TMPRSS2 serine protease and inhibitors of angiotensin-converting enzyme 2 (ACE-2). Blockade of ACE-2, the host cell receptor for the S protein of SARS-CoV-2 and inhibition of TMPRSS2, which is required for S protein priming may prevent cell entry of SARS-CoV-2.

Further, chloroquine and hydroxychloroquine, and off-label antiviral drugs, such as the nucleotide analogue Remdesivir, HIV protease inhibitors lopinavir and ritonavir, broad-spectrum antiviral drugs arbidol and favipiravir as well as antiviral phytochemicals available to date may prevent spread of SARS-CoV-2 and morbidity and mortality of COVID-19 pandemic."

XI.   Sleire, L., Forde, H., Netland, I., et al. "Drug Repurposing in Cancer." *Pharmacol Res.* 2017; 124:74-91.

Comments by author:

"Cancer is a major health issue worldwide, and the global burden of cancer is expected to increase in the coming years. Whereas the limited success with current therapies has driven huge investments into drug development, the average number of FDA approvals per year has declined since the 1990s.

This unmet need for more effective anti-cancer drugs has sparked a growing interest for drug repurposing, i.e., using drugs already approved for other indications to treat cancer. As such, data both from pre-clinical experiments, clinical trials, and observational studies have demonstrated anti-tumor efficacy for compounds within a wide range of drug classes other than cancer.

Whereas some of them induce cancer cell death or suppress various aspects of cancer cell behavior in established tumors, others may prevent cancer development. Here, we provide an overview of promising candidates for drug repurposing in cancer, as well as studies describing the biological mechanisms underlying their anti-neoplastic effects."

XII.   Armando, R., Gomez, D., Gomez, D. "New Drugs are not Enough-Drug Repositioning in Oncology: An Update. *Int J Oncol.* 2020; 56(3):651-684.

Comments by author:

"Developing more effective cancer treatments requires not only the classical design of new molecules, but also intelligent searches for new antitumor medications by repurposing old drugs already approved for other uses.

Such an approach has certain advantages; the development of a new drug is costly and timely, whereas drugs that are already approved have defined safety and pharmacological profiles.

A drug with a long clinical history in humans has properly defined pharmacokinetic and pharmaco-dynamic data, including target identification, toxicity profiles, recommended dosage schemes, and the consistent recognition of adverse effects, often meaning that development for an oncological indication can begin at a later stage, such as phase IIA.

Furthermore, repositioned molecules often are approved quicker with reduced cost. However, there are some hurdles in the path, mainly the interests of companies, and the costly remaining phases of the clinical trials prior to final approval. This review underlines the most promising drugs for repurposing, which are summarized in Table I, and although more research is needed, repositioning could pave the way to new, improved, and more effective treatments for patients with cancer.

Drugs in Table 1 include Artesunate, Auranofin, Albendazole, Flubendazole, Mebendazole, Omeprazole, Chloroquine, and Chlorpromazine."

XIII.   Verbaanderd, C., Rooman, I., Meheus, L., et al. "On-Label or Off-Label? Overcoming Regulatory and Financial Barriers to Bring Repurposed Medicines to Cancer Patients." *Front Pharmacol.* 2020; 10:1664.

Comments by author:

"Repurposing of medicines has gained a lot of interest from the research community in recent years as it could offer safe, timely, and affordable new treatment options for cancer patients with high unmet needs. Increasingly, questions arise on how new uses will be translated into clinical practice, especially in case of marketed medicinal products that are out of basic patent or regulatory protection.

We outlined two routes relevant to the clinical adoption of a repurposed medicine. First, a new indication can be approved, and thus brought on-label, via the marketing authorization procedures established in European and national legislation.

A second option is to prescribe a medicine off-label for the new indication, which is managed at the national level in Europe. While off-label use could provide timely access to treatments with patients with urgent medical needs, it also entails important safety, liability, and financial risks for patients, physicians, and society at large.

In view of that, we recommend finding solutions to facilitate bringing new uses on-label, for example by developing a collaborative framework between not-for-profit and academic organizations, pharmaceutical industry, health technology assessment bodies, payers, and regulators."

XIV. Agrawal, S., Goel, A., Gupta, N. "Emerging Prophylaxis Strategies against COVID-19." *Monaldi Arch Chest Dis.* 2020; 90(1): doi: 10.4081/monaldi.2020.1289.

Comments by author:

"HCQ has the same mechanism of action but a better safety profile than chloroquine and hence makes it a more preferable drug. Both of these drugs are shown to have immunomodulatory effects and can suppress the increase immune factors, which may play a role in reducing the severity of coronavirus disease.

The first ever human trial of chloroquine was conducted by Chinese investigators. The study conducted in more than 100 patients found chloroquine to be superior in reducing symptom duration, exacerbation of pneumonia, radiological improvement, and lead to virus-negative seroconversion.

Hydroxychloroquine along with azithromycin was studied by the French group of investigators. It was an openly bold non-randomized controlled trial. They included 36 patients in the trial and 20 patients were given hydroxychloroquine in dose of 600 mg daily along with azithromycin.

The authors showed significant reduction in viral load on day six of the treatment and much lower average carrying duration of the virus compared to the control group. Currently, many trials are underway to study effects both for prophylaxis and treatment.

Based on these studies the Indian Counsel of research (ICMR) has recommended the use of HCQ for prophylaxis.

A. All healthcare workers those who are involved in the care of suspected or confirmed cases of COVID-19: 400 mg twice a day on day one followed by 400 mg once weekly for the next seven weeks; to be taken with meals.

B. Asymptomatic household contacts of laboratory confirmed cases may be prescribed 400 mg twice a day on day one followed by 400 mg once weekly for the next three weeks; to be taken with meals."

XV. Picot, S., Marty, A., Bienvenu, A., et al. "Coalition: Advocacy for Prospective Clinical Trials to Test the Post-Exposure Potential of Hydroxychloroquine against COVID-19. *One Health.* 2020; April 4:100131.

Comments by author:

"Using post-exposure HCQ is in line with WHO's strategic objectives to limit human-to-human transmission. If we do not seriously consider using this easy and safe option, we are taking the risk of allowing the pandemic to soar further out of control. As recently stated, the urgency of the epidemic necessitates choices about which interventions to employ.

Early HCQ administration to all people at risk of infection from close contact with a positive patient is one of the most reasonable choices. Moreover, it is a choice that could potentially have a considerable impact on the early termination of the COVID-19 pandemic. However, its administration should be done under medical control to avoid potential side effects and to prevent an uncontrolled use leading to supply shortages."

XVI.   Zhou, D., Dai, S., Tong, Q. "COVID-19: A Recommendation to Examine the Effect of Hydroxychloroquine in Preventing Infection and Progression." *J Antimicrob Chemother.* 2020; May 10: doi: 10.1093/JAC/dkaa114.

Comments by author:

"In summary, we propose that HCQ could serve as a better therapeutic approach than CQ for the treatment of SARS-CoV-2 infection. There are three major reasons for this

(1)   HCQ is likely to attenuate the severe progression of COVID-19 through inhibiting the cytokine storm by reducing CD154 expression in T cells;

(2)   HCQ may confer a similar antiviral effect at both pre-and post-infection stages, as found with CQ;

(3)   HCQ has fewer side effects, is safe in pregnancy and is cheaper and more highly available in China. Given the fast-growing number of COVID-19 patients and the urgent need for effective and safe drugs in the clinic, it is more practical to identify reliable candidates by screening currently available drugs.

We herein strongly urge that clinical trials are performed to assess the preventative effects of HCQ on both infection and malignant progression."

XVII.   Shittu, M., Afolami, O. "Improving the Efficacy of Chloroquine and Hydroxychloroquine against SARS-CoV-2 may Require Zinc Additives – A Better Synergy for Future COVID-19 Clinical Trials." *Enfez Med.* 2020; 28(2):192-197.

Comments by author:

"Chloroquine can induce the uptake of zinc into the cytosol of the cell, which is capable of inhibiting RNA dependent RNA polymerase and ultimately halting the replication of coronavirus in the host cell. Currently, there are several clinical trials that are underway in several countries of the world to assess the efficacy of chloroquine as an anti-coronavirus agent.

Since chloroquine has been widely prescribed for use as an anti-malarial its safety is not in doubt. In view of the foregoing, clinical trials predicated upon a synergistic administration of zinc supplement with CQ or HCQ against the novel SARS-CoV-2 virus should be considered so that better COVID-19 clinical trial outcomes can be obtained going forward."

XVIII.   Ferner, R., Aronson, J. Chloroquine and hydroxychloroquine in COVID-19. *BMJ*. 2020;369:m1432

Letters to the Editor:

May 8, 2020

Dr. S. Bhowmick, Clinical Pharmacologist:

"Dear Editor,

As of 8th May , a total of 37,916 (thirty seven thousand nine hundred and sixteen) active Covid 19 cases are present in the country along with a casualty score of over one thousand patients as per the Ministry of Health and Family Welfare, Government of India website (https://www.mohfw.gov.in/ last accessed on 8th May, 2020). The Indian government has taken many proactive steps to halt the rapid spread of the pandemic in this nation of 1.3 billion people.

Measures include implementation of a 40 days complete lockdown of all academic and commercial activities in the country and restricting citizens to their home. (https://www.bbc.com/news/world-asia-india-52277096).

One of the other measures taken by the Indian Council of Medical Research (ICMR), the premier Medical Research body in India which has been the guiding force of the management of Covid 19 pandemic is to issue an advisory on the prophylactic use of Hydroxychloroquine   (HCQ)   for   preventing   Covid   19   infections. (https://www.mohfw.gov.in/pdf/AdvisoryontheuseofHydroxychloroquinasprophy...).

India is the first country to recommend the usage of HCQ as a chemoprophylaxis in Covid 19. As per the advisory, tablet hydroxychloroquine (HCQ) can be given to "high risk population" to prevent the disease occurrence in asymptomatic healthcare workers taking care of suspected or confirmed Covid 19 cases.

A dose of 400 mg Twice daily for day 1 followed by 400 mg once weekly for next 7 weeks has to be taken by these healthcare workers. The second group which can receive HCQ are the asymptomatic household contacts of laboratory confirmed cases. The household contacts are advised to take 400 mg of HCQ twice on day 1 followed by 400 mg weekly for next 3 weeks. ICMR has recommended that this chemoprophylaxis is contraindicated in any children below 15 years of age and in persons with history of retinopathy or with known hypersensitivity of HCQ.

HCQ is an old drug used primarily for the treatment of malaria and in other chronic inflammatory conditions like Rheumatoid arthritis and Systemic lupus erythematosus (SLE).   In   an
in vitro pre-clinical study by Yao et al. (https://doi.org/10.1093/cid/ciaa237), HCQ has exhibited better activity than Chloroquine (CQ) against anti-SARS-CoV-2 in Vero cells derived from the African green monkey kidney.

Some of the clinical trials reported from China and France have inferred that HCQ usage alone or in combination with Azithromycin has been associated with improvement of   virological   clearance   and   improvement   of clinical   symptoms   in   Covid19   patients (https://doi.org/10.1016/j.ijantimicag.2020.105949).

The ICMR advisory was based on the efficacy found in laboratory and in-vivo studies. Following the advisory there was a rush among the common mass to buy this medication resulting in scarcity of drug availability in some parts of the country (https://timesofindia.indiatimes.com/city/kolkata/not-for-public-but-key-...).
However, with timely Government intervention the indiscriminate sale was stopped and situation was brought under control.

As a patient safety professional, the question which comes to my mind is, "Is this data sufficient enough to safely recommend chemoprophylaxis to large number of "high risk" Indians?" We probably need to more evidence for answer this critical question. A systematic review found that although pre-clinical results with HCQ are promising, there is a dearth of evidence to support the clinical efficacy of HCQ in preventing COVID-19. (https://doi.org/10.1111/1756-185X.13842). One of the major limitations of this review was that it did not include any prospectively designed study as none were available.

Recently, ICMR has approved the first observational study to analyze the effectiveness of HCQ prophylaxis in 10,000 (ten thousand) Indian healthcare workers. (https://www.livemint.com/news/india/covid-max-hospital-group-to-study-us...)

Another issue is about the safety aspect of HCQ. According to this editorial (https://doi.org/10.1136/bmj.m1432) "no drug is guaranteed to be safe, and wide use of hydroxychloroquine will expose some patients to rare but potentially fatal harms". Serious adverse effects include retinopathy, chronic cardiomyopathy and carcinogenic potential (https://www.medicines.org.uk/emc/product/1764/smpc).

However, these toxicities have been witnessed with long term usage of HCQ. It is very difficult to predict what kind of toxicities would be experienced at the dosage recommended for short term prophylaxis for Covid 19 and to understand it better, a premier Government Medical college and research institution in Kolkata, India has initiated a Covid 19 chemoprophylaxis registry for healthcare personnel. (http://www.ipgmer.gov.in/chemoprophylaxis.php).

Recently, the Indian government has revised the management strategy of Covid 19 positive cases in lieu of increase demand of hospital beds and has allowed the domiciliary management of patients with mild to moderate symptoms. (https://www.mohfw.gov.in/pdf/GuidelinesforHomeIsolationofverymildpresymp...).

These patients need to be with a caregiver who must be on HCQ prophylaxis. This is a welcome step which would help to optimize the utilization of beds for moderate to sick Covid 19 patients. It would be interesting to note if HCQ reduces the viral transmission amongst the caregivers of these domiciliary Covid 19 patients as this step would be the game changer in Covid numbers in the country. Results from the pharmacovigilance registry and the large observational study would yield real time evidence for prophylaxis use of HCQ in the long run not only for India but for the rest of the world."

May 2, 2020

Dr. Thomas Salvucci, Cardiology:

"Dear Editor,

I am extremely troubled by the contamination of politics into the arena of science in general and medicine specifically.

Everyone of us should be.

COVID-19 has challenged the world by its rapid ascent to pandemic status, initial and to this date unknown mortality risk and severe global economic impact. Naturally, world scientists and political leaders are scrambling to reverse its deleterious course, rapid and widespread as it has been. Time stress often does not bring out the best in us.

Methodical and slow, careful study designs and evaluation of methodology is ideal, but not affordable with this epidemic. People are dying quickly.

Sadly, and I believe I am not the only physician in this camp who tries to analyze and make use of medical research, I am left uncertain as to the study analyses and expert opinions regarding treatment options for COVID-19.

Many commentaries reek political bias. Front and center are the strong political opinions from the world of the president of the United States, Donald Trump. Three years of multi-pronged attempts to oust him from office provides the backdrop for suspicion that anything he may opine or support initiates frantic attempts by his detractors to refute, often at all costs.

Which brings us to this article and the potential benefits of hydroxychloroquine. I emphasize that I do not know the heart, political tilt or intention of this author but the point is suspicion of political bias cannot be helped. Trump is mentioned specifically. My criticism is this: reference to the dangers of hydroxychloroquine.

The two references mentioned, ventricular arrhythmias and hepatic failure are so weak that this article in general cannot be taken seriously.

Corrected QT prolongation isn't always a straightforward measurement and besides, the point of assessing this measurement when using drugs known to prolong it is to discontinue the medication to avoid arrhythmia development. This is standard fare and increases the safe use of such drugs when monitored.

Regarding the reference to hepatic toxicity...I'm shocked such a reference is even mentioned. Even the reference states that severe hepatic toxicity hasn't been reported in its widespread use since 1963.

The conclusion: I am left suspicious that the author is grasping desperately to suggest that proponents of hydroxychloroquine are being reckless and creates yet another criticism of Mr. Trump. For those of us personally and our patients particularly who fall prey to rapidly worsening symptoms from COVID-19, an illness thus far without a definitive cure, denying any reasonable attempt at today's "possible" treatment modalities that statistically are clearly low risk is, in my opinion, reckless and irresponsible.

Ask yourself this question, posed to you on this date, May 2, 2020: if you were COVID-19 positive, febrile and developing worsening dyspnea or already hypoxia, would you consent to therapy with hydroxychloroquine, remdesivir, neither or both?"

April 17, 2020

Dr. Philip L. Davies, General Practitioner:

"Dear Editor

My earlier response to this article [1] was intended to inject urgency into the tackling of this subject matter.

This retort arises from Prof. Ferner's follow up comments where he references his latest article for CEBM [2]

In these two pieces the pages drip with the abundance of biased ink. Indeed, Prof. Ferner is keen to inform that his mind is settled on the matter.

"Drugs that target specific structures in the virus are more likely to work than old drugs that may work in the laboratory but lack data supporting clinical use"[1] ... he goes on to list the diseases in which CQ/HCQ has failed having first shown promise in vitro.

This equates to a clinician telling the chronic smoker to stop trying to quit because he's failed several times already.

Prof Ferner's bias comes bounding forward again in his remarks on Chen et al's small, weak study: it "strengthened our view that HCQ is ineffective in even mild COVID 19."[2]

Indeed, CQ may prove to be ineffective ... but we need to intelligently construct studies capable of delivering a rapid and clear decision on that. Hence my suggestion that we initiate a large cohort study offering CQ as a complete medical countermeasure (prophylaxis and early treatment in lower doses already proven as safe) to all front-line NHS clinical staff. 86% of doctors surveyed (see my earlier response) answered that they are willing to enter this trial.

My final comments concern Prof Ferner's appraisal of the recent study by Mahévas et al: "This is the best study so far published."[2] Prof Ferner supports the study's report; "These results do not support the use of hydroxychloroquine in patients hospitalized for documented SARS CoV-2-positive hypoxic pneumonia."

This is another study that attempts to ascertain if oral HCQ tablets can be of clinical use in patients more than one week into symptomatic disease, hospitalized with bilateral pneumonia and with evidence of established inflammatory reaction (cytokine storm). That's another big ask for any oral medication.

The study is again small (both arms have less than 100 patients). The most significant outcome measured (death) is realized in very small numbers (3 and 4). The confidence levels are extremely wide.

The are several problems with this study. There are marked differences in the two populations. The study honestly attempts to accommodate these confounding factors using a propensity score method (IPTW). Normally this method is valuable but here I can't see that it has been well applied.

It pays to look at the raw data. Bear in mind that Prof Ferner confidently states: "There was no difference in the initial intensity of disease."

Well let's have a look at that:

At baseline (admission), HCQ arm comprises 78.3% men (>20% more of these higher risk patients than control arm with 64.9%); HCQ arm has 21.9% patients with more severe disease in the form of CT showing >50% lung affected). This is >80% more than in control arm (12.1%). HCQ arm has 90.5% patients with CRP > 40mg/l (CRP is a good indicator of impending/current severity). This is 10% higher than control arm (81.9%). HCQ arm had median O2 flow on admission = 3 litres/minute (50% higher than control arm at 2 litres / minute).

So, at baseline, the HCQ arm had significantly more patients with severe disease than control arm. The O2 flow is actually more significant than first sight would suggest. 2 l/m is always the first step in O2 therapy. The data shows us that most patients in the control arm could hold their sats on this first step therapy. This also means they may have been OK on just 1 l/m. We don't know. But we do know that most patients in the HQN could not hold their sats at that first step and needed an increase (3 l/m ... so that's 50-300% more O2 than control arm).

Admittedly there were other confounding factors which compromised the control arm more than HCQ arm (some chronic disease elements). But it's clear to me that disease severity was markedly more established in the HCQ arm.

Another factor to note: the HCQ treatment was not initiated at the moment those baseline values were obtained (on admission). The HCQ was initiated within 48 hours. So let's look again at the timelines. The median duration of symptoms at admission shows that the HCQ arm comprised patients who were further into worsening illness: they were admitted on D8 compared to control, D7. They may not have had HCQ initiated until D10.

Then we look at outcomes: the raw data shows that the disadvantaged HCQ arm actually does better in the two most important outcomes, death and ICU admission. The HCQ delivers 12% less death and ICU admissions than the control arm. Admittedly the numbers are small so the confidence levels are very wide.

So what does that tell us? The answer is not much. But even accepting the poorly aligned baseline for disease severity, the outcomes with their wide 95% confidence levels do deliver a mildly promising indication on the 'swingometer'. They point more towards benefit than harm when using HCQ in this advanced disease state.

As a final comment on significant side effects (increased QT interval) from the use of HCQ. Once again, this trial used a particularly high dose of HCQ (600mg/day...right at ceiling dose for rheumatological use and much higher than the total antimalarial treatment dose). They also added azithromycin (another QT lengthening drug) to 20% of the HCQ patients. It's not surprising at all to find such QT lengthening in a sick, more elderly population taking these medications in particularly high doses)."

Further trials should utilize conservative doses of CQ/HCQ which have been proven safe in many millions of patients.

We don't yet know how this will pan out. We urgently need proper evidence. Statistically robust studies into prophylaxis and early intervention are likely to deliver the most interesting results."

(1)   [1]   Robin   E   Ferner,   Jeffrey   K   Aronson,   'Chloroquine and   hydroxychloroquine   in   COVID-19',   8 April   2020,   BMJ   2020;   369 doi: https://doi.org/10.1136/bmj.m1432 (Published 08 April 2020)

(2)   [2] Robin E Ferner, Jeffrey K Aronson, 'Hydroxychloroquine for COVID-19: what   do   the clinical trials tell us?', 14 April 2020, CEBM; https://www.cebm.net/COVID-19/hydroxychloroquine-for-COVID-19-what-do-th...

XIX.   Rosenberg, E., Dufort, E., Udo, T., et al.   "Association of Treatment with Hydroxychloroquine or Azithromycin with In-Hospital Mortality in Patient's with   COVID-19   in   New   York   State."   *JAMA.*   2020: doi:10.1001/JAMA.2020.8630.

Conflict of interest disclosure; Dr. Dufort reported that her spouse has a Gilead Foundation focus HIV/HCV testing research grant. No other disclosures were reported.

May 11, 2020

Dr. David Chappell, Private Internist and Endocrinologist:

"This study in JAMA and another appearing on May 11, 2020 issue of NEJM (1) both show no clear benefit in treating COVID-19 infected patients with hydroxychloroquine. However, in both studies the treated patients were significantly sicker at baseline than the untreated groups. Both studies were observational; neither had a control group.

Today CNN posted a headline entitled, "Yet another study shows hydroxychloroquine doesn't work against COVID-19." On the contrary, neither study was robust enough to draw definitive conclusions as CNN proposes.

It is unfortunate that the authors of neither study make this clear.

The statement that, "interpretation of these findings may be limited by the observational design" is a cop-out. At the very least the word "may" should be replaced with the word "is." Of note, the editorial by Rubin, et al., in the NEJM May 11 issue was more balanced and left open the possibility that hydroxychloroquine could have had a modest effect to bring the mortality rate of sicker patients down closer to the mortality rate of those less sick. A good clinical study is needed here, not "multiple sensitivity analyses" as done by Rosenberg, et al.

A separate study involving Remdesivir was stopped early by The National Institute of Allergy and Infectious Diseases without achieving statistical significance due to the ethical issues revolving around using a placebo for COVID-19 patients. This occurred despite the fact that many cancer treatment trials carry a higher mortality than does

COVID-19. Now we have another study that fails to meet basic scientific standards and a difficult path forward to overcome this failure.

Scientists and healthcare providers need to guard against the inevitable politicization of scientific data and investigations. False interpretations of scientific data are rampant these days, and the public suffers from this.

I like to ask my patients who have formed their own, often erroneous, medical opinions, "which is more complicated, a nuclear reactor or the physicists who designed it?" Most of us would not presume to offer advice on the design of nuclear reactors, but we sure like to opine on scientific issues surrounding, for example, COVID-19."

May 12, 2020

Dr. Olga Goodman, Rheumatologist and Internist:

"Patients receiving hydroxychloroquine with or without azithromycin were overall sicker on presentation. They were significantly sicker given available information in Table 1 and had multiple other risk factors such as Black or Hispanic were as likely to receive hydroxychloroquine and/or azithromycin (mortality is significantly higher in these groups), and patients receiving hydroxychloroquine plus azithromycin and hydroxychloroquine alone were more likely to be obese and have diabetes, and patients receiving hydroxychloroquine alone had the highest levels of chronic lung disease (25.1%) and cardiovascular conditions (36.5%).

But after receiving treatment much sicker patients had approximately the same mortality rates vs. patients with a milder course of the disease and less risk factors. However, the authors conclude, 'There are no significant benefits.'

Really? No benefits?"

May 12, 2020

Dr. Mubarak Khan states:

"This is a good retrospective observation study of the effects of HCQ and HCQ+AZT in the treatment of COVID-19 infected hospitalized patients but it will be very much premature to conclude these drugs' role in treatment based on short experience and the following questions and concerns.

1. This is an observational study to determine outcomes in the sickest admitted patients.

2. Selection criteria are hospitalized COVID-19 patients. At which stage drugs were administered is not clear in all three groups.

3. Outcome criteria are either death or discharge. What happened to those who got discharged? Was there any hastening in improvement due to these drugs? Was there shortening of duration of illness due to drugs, from Covid positive to negative?

4. Were the drugs tried as prophylaxis? Or only used in hospitalized patients?

5. All patients included are mean age at 70 and with many comorbidities.

6. What dosages were given for HCQ and azithromycin? How many days was treatment given? Were different dosages tried?

7. What type of safety pharmacovigilance was there, beyond noting increased cardiac complications?

8. Were drugs discontinued due to side effects? Did discontinuation lead to any improvements?

9. What side effects were obvious during the treatment periods in patients free from morbidity?

10. When patients succumbed to mechanical ventilation, how and what type of dosages of these drugs were given?

11. Were blood levels of the hydroxychloroquine and azithromycin measured and related to increased complications?"

May 14, 2020

Dr. Flavio Dantas, Retired University Professor:

"Given that early results in France and China suggested that chloroquine and hydroxychloroquine could reduce viral load in COVID-19 patients, it follows that these drugs should primarily be tested in patients soon after their exposure to coronavirus (or in the very initial phase) before getting hospitalized.

This was done in São Paulo (Brazil), after a pandemic was officially declared, with patients from a health care provider dedicated to attending old people (1). Using telemedicine resources, 636 patients with flu-like or COVID-19 symptoms were asked if they consented to use hydroxychloroquine (800 mg first day and 400 mg for 6 days) plus azithromycin (500 mg for 5 days).

Despite the fact that patients treated with hydroxychloroquine and azithromycin had higher prevalence of comorbidities, only 8 (in 412) needed hospitalization (no deaths), whereas in the non-treated patients 12 (out of 224) were hospitalized, and 5 died.

The percentage of hospitalization for patients treated early (<7 days from onset of disease) was 1,17% (for late treatment was 3.2%). The paper was taken out from a preprint site after CONEP (Brazilian Committee of Ethics in Human Research) allegations that patients were enrolled before the study protocol already was approved by CONEP, in the midst of a growing politicization of chloroquine use in Brazil for COVID-19."

REFERENCE

1. Pagliaro, M., Meneguzzo, F. Hydroxychloroquine for the treatment of COVID-19: Evidence, possible mode of action and industrial supply of the drug. *Preprints*. 2020; doi: 10.20944/preprints202004.0381.v1 https://www.preprints.org/manuscript/202004.0381/v1

XX. Sanders, J., Monogue, M., Jodlowski, T., et al., Pharmacologic Treatments for Coronavirus Disease 2019 (COVID-19) A Review. JAMA. 2020; 323(18): 1824-1836

Conflict of Interest Disclosures: Dr Cutrell reported receiving nonfinancial support from Regeneron and Gilead outside the submitted work. No other disclosures were reported.

Dr. Dinesh Ranjan:

"Sanders and colleagues have published a detailed review of pharmacologic treatment options for COVID-19 in JAMA (1). Two drugs, hydroxychloroquine (HCQ) and remdesivir, have garnered most attention by medical journals and public media lately. While the French study touting HCQ with azithromycin had several shortcomings (2), it was hailed by President Trump regardless. The academic medicine, medical journals and main-stream media have condemned HCQ. In contrast however, remdesivir seems to have caught the fancy of the same group who seem to be willing to ignore the shortcomings of remdesivir data.

This double standard is evident in this review. The authors state that they reviewed English language articles catalogued in PubMed. However, they cite a Chinese language paper not catalogued in PubMed, showing no benefit with HCQ (3). They appear to ignore other English language papers supporting HCQ. Finally, the authors conclude that they "do not support adoption" of HCQ/Azithromycin "without additional studies".

In contrast, when discussing remdesivir; the authors recommend that "inclusion of this agent for treatment of COVID-19 may be considered". This recommendation is based upon "anticipated results from RCTs" and "successful case reports" in COVID-19 patients. Recommendations are based on anticipated results? And the successful case reports they state includes a study of 3 (out of 7 hospitalized) patients, without any difference in outcome. The authors, while making a case for its antiviral properties, state that remdesivir was used in clinical trials in Ebola – but they fail to mention that their cited reference did not include humans (4).

They mention other single case reports of remdesivir use in Ebola. Unfortunately, they neglect to mention that the definitive study on Ebola therapeutics: a randomized trial of four therapeutic options, had not supported Remdesivir (5). Surely, a search in PubMed had brought up this NEJM paper? Why was this ignored while the authors were using single case reports to support remdesivir?

That remdesivir has become the favorite in journals and media is obvious (6). And it may yet be the best option for our patients once we have results from trials. We just wish that the reviews and recommendations published in respected journals will use an even-handed approach and not be openly cherry-picking information to support possible preexisting biases."

REFERENCE

1. Sanders JM, Monogue ML, Jodlowski TZ et al. JAMA. 2020 Apr 13. doi: 10.1001/jama.2020.6019.

2. Gautret P, Lagier JC, Parola P et al. . Int J Antimicrob Agents. 2020 Mar 20:105949. doi: 10.1016/j.ijantimicag.2020

3. Chen J,Liu D,Liu L, etal. J Zhejiang Univ (MedSci). Published on line March 6, 2020.doi:10.3785/j

4.   https://www.who.   int/ebola/drc-2018/summaries-of-evidenceexperimental-therapeutics.pdf

5.   Mulangu S, Dodd LE, Davey RT. Randomized, Controlled Trial of Ebola Virus Disease Therapeutics N Engl J Med. 2019 Dec 12;381(24):2293-2303

6.   Grein J, Ohmagari N, Shin D et al. Compassionate Use of Remdesivir for Patients with Severe COVID-19. N Engl J Med. 2020 Apr 10. doi: 10.1056/NEJMoa2007016

XXI.   Mehra, M., Desai, S., Ruschitzka, F., et al., Hydroxychloroquine or Chloroquine with or without a macrolide for treatment of COVID-19: a multinational registry analysis. *The Lancet.* 2020: doi: 10.1016/S0140-6736(20)31180-6

Declaration of interests

MRM reports personal fees from Abbott, Medtronic, Janssen, Mesoblast, Portola, Bayer, Baim Institute for Clinical Research, NupulseCV, FineHeart, Leviticus, Roivant, and Triple Gene.

SSD is the founder of Surgisphere Corporation. FR has been paid for time spent as a committee member for clinical trials, advisory boards, other forms of consulting, and lectures or presentations; these payments were made directly to the University of Zurich and no personal payments were received in relation to these trials or other activities. ANP declares no competing interests.

XXII.   Mehra, M., Desai, S., Ruschitzka, F., et al., Hydroxychloroquine or Chloroquine with or without a macrolide for treatment of COVID-19: a multinational registry analysis. *The Lancet.* 2020: doi: 10.1016/S0140-6736(20)31180-6

A.   *Medpage* Comments [Walker, M. Huge Study Throws Cold Water on Antimalarials for COVID-19. *Medpage Today.* May 22, 2020]

May 22, 2020

Dr. Ellis Lai, Anesthesiology,

"What do you expect from Lancet? It has turned from a respectable medical journal to a leftist political mouthpiece. The public just hasn't realized it yet."

May 23, 2020

Dr. Ron Graf, Endocrinology,

"The article and study conspicuously omitted timing of the drug's administration in relation to the disease phase and patient's state. ANY conclusive study must control against adverse selection bias.

AND, in this case the entire population of the study is an adversely selected in that they are the hospitalized patients being in the advanced state of the disease.

By the fact that Prophylactic and effectiveness at symptom onset is not of interest to these investigators cautions one to trust the results. And, this study would be meaningless to those doctors believing they are seeing positive results from early administration, (especially with zinc). The study, however, will only reinforce the beliefs of those doctors who were already skeptical of HCQ use. Who did the study serve?"

May 22, 2020

Dr. Iraj Akhvan, Internal Medicine,

"Is there any other pharmaceutical left to sponsor this writing? There is no evidence of this being randomized study, this seems to be they picked people who didn't make it out of ICUs (to one account over 90% mortality on intubated patient) and draw the conclusion. Personally have treated patients from 21 to 104 year old as outpatient with HCQ without any complications.

The study should be based on a science not sponsorships, needs to compare, entire populations on treatment with HCQ, in and outpatient, and should be compared with the outcome of other treatments on different categories of treatments. Also taking to consideration all other factors which may have contributed to outcome of this conclusion. It of great importance that the author to disclose the method or methods which were used to collect these data."

May 22, 2020

Dr. Vanita Panjwani, Clinical Pharmacist,

"That study looked at patients who were given hydroxychloroquine to the sickest patients/in the ICU on ventilators, who already are at heightened risks for cardiac side effects as the heart is affected in end stage Covid 19. So it is not correct to completely dismiss an agent that could have potential benefit when used early on the management before the cytokine storm has set in.

Many, many doctors have used HCQ and Zinc at early onset of symptoms for COVID patient and reported good outcomes but unfortunately, they do not make headlines. What is more unfortunate is that patients will be reluctant to participate in a randomized clinical trial after hearing so much negative press that we may never really know via a properly designed scientific trial how the medication could benefit if given at early onset of symptoms, It is very unfortunate to make a conclusion when the drug was inappropriately given to the sickest patients and at much higher doses than are needed for early treatment - that was not it's place in the management of COVID-19"

May 22, 2020

Dr. Robert Campbell,

"There was a 13.2% ventilation/mortality rate in control group...This is far higher than the estimated CFR for COVID-19, which shows that this was again a sick, hospitalized cohort of patients given late treatment with HCQ. The real clinical benefit of HCQ is likely early treatment in an outpatient setting. The Lancet authors acknowledge this limitation stating, 'These data do not apply to the use of any treatment regimen used in the ambulatory, out-of-hospital setting.' Consistently countries that use early HCQ treatment have fewer deaths. HCQ has been politicized more than any drug ever."

May 23, 2020

Dr. Michael Herriges,

"One very telling statement that should have been the headline instead of 'throws cold water' was 'cause and effect cannot be inferred.' Regarding increased risk of arrhythmia. When I see that I question the study even more deeply. In all of my research classes it was beat into our heads that correlation is not causation. This study has some very good information but it was done with seriously ill patients who were already at risk of dying. The fact that the authors admitted they couldn't make the case solid for med induced arrhythmia should have changed the tone of the headline and article.

The tone of the headline comes off sensationalistic instead of rational. Everyone who prescribes medicine knows there are risks. These two are not the only ones that cause arrhythmia and we know that bodies seriously stressed with overwhelming illness are at risk of all sorts of complications. I can't tell the number of times an elderly patient with influenza pneumonia has developed dysrhythmia even without using known arrhythmia risk meds. What about those who have successfully used these early on with great success? Many of them are physicians.

Unfortunately this article implies we need to throw out the baby with the bathwater. These two drugs may work well in early cases in younger patients. Waiting till the patients are knocking on heaven's door to try something then blame the drug for them dying isn't very good science."

May 22, 2020

Dr. Duplantis,

"We are using hydroxychloroquine in Texas in our COVID-19 patients and for prophylaxis with great success and zero side effects! It is obvious to me that this study was tainted and I do not believe it! I find it interesting that many docs in the USA, India, Italy etc. are using it prophylactically and with great success!"

May 22, 2020

Dr. Neal Greenberg, Cardiology,

"The NYU study showed incredible results for Hydroxy plus azithromycin plus zinc. This study didn't look at the zinc issue, so the headline is a bit exaggerated. Mehra's conflicts may be significant. The method for controlling the seriousness of the disease at initiation of the disease should be looked at more carefully."

May 23, 2020

Dr. Brant Mittler, Cardiology,

https://www.icmr.gov.in/pdf/covid/techdoc/V5_Revised_advisory_on_the_use_of_ HCQ_SARS_CoV2_infection.pdf

The Indian Council of Medical Research issued this advisory yesterday continuing to recommend Hydroxychloroquine for prevention as it continues (to) study its use.

Please report to your readers how many US cardiologists received either their basic medical training or cardiology training in India.

India has advanced, sophisticated cardiology programs and a lot of experience in anti-malarial drugs and monitoring.

This online news source should cover India's experience and provide readers a more balanced perspective.

May 28, 2020 Open Letter to Richard Horton (editor of The Lancet) with almost 200 signatures.

Open letter to MR Mehra, SS Desai, F Ruschitzka, and AN Patel, authors of **"Hydroxychloroquine or chloroquine with or without a macrolide for treatment of COVID19: a multinational registry analysis"**. *Lancet*. 2020 May 22:S0140-6736(20)31180-6. doi: 10.1016/S0140-6736(20)31180-6. PMID: 32450107

and to Richard Horton (editor of The Lancet).

Concerns regarding the statistical analysis and data integrity

The retrospective, observational study of 96,032 hospitalized COVID-19 patients from six continents reported substantially increased mortality (~30% excess deaths) and occurrence of cardiac arrhythmias associated with the use of the 4-aminoquinoline drugs hydroxychloroquine and chloroquine. These results have had a considerable impact on public health practice and research.

The WHO has paused recruitment to the hydroxychloroquine arm in their SOLIDARITY trial. The UK regulatory body, MHRA, requested the temporary pausing of recruitment into all hydroxychloroquine trials in the UK (treatment and prevention), and France has changed its national recommendation for the use of hydroxychloroquine in COVID-19 treatment and also halted trials.

The subsequent media headlines have caused considerable concern to participants and patients enrolled in randomized controlled trials (RCTs) seeking to characterize the potential benefits and risks of these drugs in the treatment and prevention of COVID-19 infections. There is uniform agreement that well conducted RCTs are needed to inform policies and practices.

This impact has led many researchers around the world to scrutinize in detail the publication in question. This scrutiny has raised both methodological and data integrity concerns. The main concerns are listed as follows:

1. There was inadequate adjustment for known and measured confounders (disease severity, temporal effects, site effects, dose used).

2. The authors have not adhered to standard practices in the machine learning and statistics community. They have not released their code or data. There is no data/code sharing and availability statement in the paper. The Lancet was among the many signatories on the Wellcome statement on data sharing for COVID-19 studies.

3. There was no ethics review.

4. There was no mention of the countries or hospitals that contributed to the data source and no acknowledgments of their contributions. A request to the authors for information on the contributing centres was denied.

5. Data from Australia are not compatible with government reports (too many cases for just five hospitals, more in-hospital deaths than had occurred in the entire country during the study period). *Surgisphere* (the data company) have since stated this was an error of classification of one hospital from Asia. This indicates the need for further error checking throughout the database.

6. Data from Africa indicate that nearly 25% of all COVID-19 cases and 40% of all deaths in the continent occurred in *Surgisphere*-associated hospitals which had sophisticated electronic patient data recording, and patient monitoring able to detect and record "nonsustained [at least 6 secs] or sustained ventricular tachycardia or ventricular fibrillation". Both the numbers of cases and deaths, and the details provided, seem unlikely.

7. Unusually small reported variation in baseline variables, interventions and outcomes between continents (Table S3).

8. Mean daily doses of hydroxychloroquine that are 100 mg higher than FDA recommendations, whereas 66% of the data are from North American hospitals.

9. Implausible ratios of chloroquine to hydroxychloroquine use in some continents. For example, in Australia 49 received chloroquine and 50 received hydroxychloroquine. However, chloroquine is not readily available in Australia and administration requires authorization from the Therapeutic Goods Administration.

10. The tight 95% confidence intervals reported for the hazard ratios appear inconsistent with the data. For instance, for the Australian data this would imply about double the numbers of recorded deaths as were reported in the paper.

The patient data were obtained through electronic health records, supply chain databases, and financial records. The data are held by the US company *Surgisphere*. In response to a request for the data Professor Mehra replied: "**Our data sharing agreements with the various governments, countries and hospitals do not allow us to share data unfortunately.**"

Given the enormous importance and influence of these results, we believe it is imperative that:

1. The company *Surgisphere* provides details on data provenance. At the very minimum, this means sharing the aggregated patient data at the hospital level (for all covariates and outcomes)

2. Independent validation of the analysis is performed by a group convened by the World Health Organization, or at least one other independent and respected institution. This would entail additional analyses (e.g. determining if there is a dose-effect) to assess the validity of the conclusions

3. There is open access to all the data sharing agreements cited above to ensure that, in each jurisdiction, any mined data was legally and ethically collected and patient privacy aspects respected

June 2, 2020
Dr. Raoul Harf,
"5 weeks to gather data, treat them, submit for publication and edit. 24 hours to ban HCQ by WHO. The question is: who's interest is it?"

June 2, 2020
Dr. Bill Rhoades,

"I wonder if Dr Horton likes to wait till 48 hours after hospitalization before prescribing Tamiflu for his influenza patients?

These are smart people. There's no way they couldn't recognize the flawed protocol of trialing HCQ only on end-stage COVID disease. There must be a hidden agenda for the boffins at WHO & Lancet to be fiddling while millions suffer & economies crumble.

May God have mercy on their souls."

June 1, 2020
Dr. Maria Rivero,

"It appears this study was fabricated. And this made-up study was published by the Lancet and used by the WHO to 1) halt the HCQ arm of a RCT, and 2) advise countries against the use of HCQ. And France, home of Didier Raoult, has banned it!"

June 1, 2020
Dr. Dinesh Ranjan, General Surgery,

"HCQ had two big factors working against it: 1. It is exceedingly cheap (full course <\$5, compared with Remdesivir \$5000+) 2. It was being proposed by Trump"

'You can't waste a crisis on something this cheap'

June 2, 2020
Dr. Bill Rhoades,

"It's also remarkably safe: from WHO monograph on the cardiotoxicity of antimalarials

"Despite hundreds of millions of doses administered in the treatment of malaria, there have been no reports of sudden unexplained death associated with quinine, chloroquine or amodiaquine, although each drug causes QT/QTc interval prolongation."

Compared to Remdesivir:

"25% of patients receiving it have severe side effects, including multiple-organ dysfunction syndrome, septic shock, acute kidney injury. Another 23% demonstrated evidence of liver damage on lab tests". (BioSpace, April 13th Early Data from Gilead's Compassionate Use of Remdesivir for COVID-19 Looks Promising)"

XXIII. Boulware, D., Pullen, M., Bangdiwala, et al., A Randomized Trial of Hydroxychloroquine as Postexposure Prophylaxis for COVID-19. *NEJM.* 2020: doi: 10.1056/MEJMoa2016638

Declaration of Interests:

Supported by David Baszucki and Jan Ellison Baszucki, the Alliance of Minnesota Chinese Organizations, the Minnesota Chinese Chamber of Commerce, and the University of Minnesota. Ms. Pastick and Ms. Okafor are supported by the Doris Duke Charitable Foundation through a grant supporting the Doris Duke International Clinical Research Fellows Program at the University of Minnesota.

Drs. Nicol, Rajasingham, and Pullen are supported by the National Institute of Allergy and Infectious Diseases (K08AI134262, K23AI138851, T32AI055433). Dr. Lofgren is supported by the National Institute of Mental Health (K23MH121220). Dr. Skipper is supported by the Fogarty International Center (D43TW009345). Drs. Lee and McDonald receive salary support from Fonds de Recherche du Québec–Santé.

Dr. Zarychanski receives research support as the Lyonel G. Israels Professor of Hematology at the University of Manitoba. In Quebec, funds were received from the Clinical Practice Assessment Unit of the McGill University Health Centre and the McGill Interdisciplinary Initiative in Infection and Immunity Emergency COVID-19 Research Funding Program.

In Manitoba, research support was received from the Manitoba Medical Service Foundation and Research Manitoba. In Alberta, the trial was funded by the Northern Alberta Clinical Trials and Research Centre COVID-19 Clinical Research Grant. Purolator Canada provided in-kind courier support for the participating Canadian sites. The REDCap software was supported by the National Institutes of Health National Center for Advancing Translational Sciences (grant UL1TR002494).

A.   *Medscape* Comments [Frellick, M. HCQ Fails to Prevent COVID-19 in Randomized Trial. *Medscape*. June 3, 2020]

June 4, 2020
Dr. Ernesto Zilberberg, Psychiatry,

"3 % of participants confirmed by PCR, bias selection of population study (social media recruitment, first responders and healthcare workers who could have been exposed to covid prior to study onset). Higher dose than usual (side effects and loss of double blind), lack of Zinc supplementation, and many other study limitations.

Looks to me like a straw man was built in order to beat it down."

June 3, 2020
Dr. Jeffrey Grolig, Pain Management,

"Interesting that less than 3% of these were actually confirmed by PCR. Also interesting is that less than 0.2% were hospitalized leading one to doubt that these people really had COVID-19. Despite the randomized placebo-blinded label, it is probably worthless in terms of any guidance on the effect of HCQ on prevention. We need valid PCR- validated data, and studies like this do more harm than good."

June 3, 2020
Dr. Loretta Brown, Internal Medicine,

"Not a well thought out clinical trial trying to determine role of HCQ in prevention. First one has to know that the subjects were really exposed to the virus."

June 9, 2020
Dr. Mike Rupe, Emergency Medicine,

"NEJM has been in bed with big pharma for decades. Another bogus study that doesn't fit the mainstream media and their proponents' narrative. Await better trials with significantly less subjective data. A lot of positive literature is already out there regarding prophylaxis."

June 6, 2020
Dr. Jeffrey Grolig, Pain Management,

"The Indian Council of Medical Research just published a case-control study looking at health care workers and their protocol of HCQ prophylaxis: 400 mg per week after a loading dose of 800 mg.

They looked at incidence of infection among health care workers who performed intubations on COVID patients and found almost a 60% risk reduction in those health care workers who took four or more doses. The risk reduction was dose-related with near 80% in six or more doses.

"However, with the intake of four or more maintenance doses of HCQ, the protective effect started emerging," noted Dr. Samiran Panda, director of ICMR- National AIDS Research Institute (NARI) and one of the study authors. "A significant reduction (more than 80%) in the odds of SARS-CoV-2 infection in the HCWs was identified with the intake of six or more doses of HCQ prophylaxis," Dr. Panda added. From IndianExpress, June 4; Preventative Use of HCQ..."

http://www.ijmr.org.in/preprintarticle.asp?id=285520

June 4, 2020
Dr. Olga Goodman, Rheumatology,

"The population treated in lupus and RA are not typically obese or suffer from the Metabolic Syndrome or have the pro-arrhythmic conditions of Obstructive Sleep Apnea"

Not at all. Typically obese, have metabolic syndrome, have higher frequency of rheumatoid lung disease (up to 1/3 of RA patients and even higher in SLE), and have more often have preexisting heart disease, frequently steroid- dependent.

Having RA and SLE is making their "hearts age 10 years older".
But HCQ is extremely safe for them/
Unless someone decided to commit suicide taking 5-10 times higher dose.

For huge local observation data base, there are no single cases of hospital admission in our heavily affected area among patients compliant with HCQ therapy. Unfortunatly some of them stopped it last few weeks after all these "publications" but still appears to be protected from severe disease.

Despite been "immunocompromised, elderly, having preexisting lung and heart issues, on long term steroids, etc.

They still can catch coronavirus but the worst case scenario just reported is as a 'bad cold'."

Regards,

Olga Goodman, MD,

Triple Board Certified in Rheumatology, Internal Medicine, Pediatrics.

June 9, 2020
Dr. Seth Anderson, Dentist,

"I wonder if BIG PHARMA is behind all of these questionable/bogus studies...... Dr. Paul Marik, a pulmonologist at Eastern Virginia Medical School, has published a treatment protocol using Vitamins C, D3, quercetin, famotidine, HCQ with zinc, Ivermectin, remdesivir, and other combinations. Would like to see a follow-up to see how successful it has been."

B.   *Medpage Today* Comments [Walker, M. End of the Road for HCQ in COVID-19? *Medpage Today*. June 6, 2020]

June 6, 2020
Dr. Olga Goodman, Rheumatology,

"Summary: the same mortality rate between treatment and control group.

But...

Investigators gave HCQ dose which considered to be fatal or near fatal, 2400 mg over 1st 24 h. Total dose was 9600 mg/10 days. It's higher that ever used and ~1800 mg/ day required immediate admission to Emergency department. Middle age and elderly patients with advanced stage of Covid, HTD, diabetes, low K and Mg, hypoxia, etc. even more vulnerable to overdose related deaths. At least some treatment group participants were killed by intentional overdose.

After extraction of their deaths, survivors from overdosing actually shows less mortality."

June 8, 2020
Dr. Andrew Johnstone,

"If we 'studied' Tamiflu for people with influenza severe enough to be hospitalized, started it on day five of the illness, and gave 300 mg daily instead of the normal dose, plus gave it with something like amantadine, which might have added toxicity, and the drug caused more harm than good.....would we publish studies saying the drug was useless...??? Or would we perhaps look at the data and pharmacology and decide that unless we give the drug in safe doses, early in the disease process, we are wasting our time and not helping patients...?

Similarly, if we gave patients clavulanic acid for strep infections, but omitted amoxicillin, would we conclude it was useless, or might someone point out that it requires amoxicillin for it to work properly

Try giving hydroxychloroquine in safe doses, with zinc, when the virus hasn't yet overwhelmed the patient, and it seems to work. CLEARLY doing any study early-on like that is a problem, due to the control/placebo arm will not have a high enough incidence of bad outcomes with CoVD19 to separate out 'success' until you have treated many, many patients, and there are so many confounders in studies done on-the-fly and under urgent conditions, and the multiple sites that are inevitable with a disease like this, but eventually such studies may get done.

In the interim, as we try ACE inhibitors, cytokine receptor antibodies, antiviral meds, vitamin D, and all sorts of other things, there is no rational reason NOT to try zinc and hydroxychloroquine in the low, safe, doses many are using. Just because in-patients with severe end-stage disease are not good candidates for plain HCQ doesn't mean wholesale abandonment is rational."

June 8, 2020
Dr. Olga Goodman, Rheumatology,

INTERVIEW EXCLUSIVE: Martin Landray, Regarding Recovery Trial.

http://www.francesoir.fr/politique-monde/interview-exclusive-martin-
landray- recovery-hydroxychloroquine-game-over-uk

FS: From the data you presented, it would appear that they are more elderly patients
with higher level of pre-existing conditions (25% diabetes, 25% heart conditions). Why
?

Comment by OG:

Very sick patients (mortality 24% in control group)- significantly higher than
average hospital mortality across the world

FS: Could you please precise what dosage of HCQ you gave to the patient? and
the results ?

ML: It is 2400 mg in the first 24 hours and 800 mg from day 2 to day 10. It is an
10 day course of treatment in total.

Comment by OG:

2400 mg/24 h is between TD50 and LD50, fatal for up 5-10% of generally
healthy people, for elderly, very sick with multiple comorbidities can cause at
least 25% deaths in the treatment group.

FS: How did you decide on the dosage of HCQ ? ML : The doses were chosen on
the basis of pharmacokinetic modelling and these are in line with the sort of
doses that you used for other diseases such as amoebic dysentery.

Comment #1 by OG.:

It's near fatal dose, No LD5-LD50 dose can be chosen for any reasons.

Comment #2 by OG:

"amoebic dysentery" is not treated by hydroxychloroquine but
hydroxyQUINOLINE.

It appears researches did not realize the difference and chose the dose based on
hydroxyQUINOLINE.

FS: Are there any maximum dosage for HCQ in the UK? ML: I would have to
check but it is much larger than the 2400mg, something like six or 10 times that.

Comments by OG:

Dr Landray states that max HCQ dose is 24 000?
Unbelievable. 1800 mg/24 h requires URGENT admission.
End of the Road for HCQ in COVID-19?
No. It should be "end of the road" for whom who developed and approved this
deadly protocol.

June 8, 2020
Dr. John H. Abeles, Distinguished Cancer Researcher,

> "Perhaps the opinions of a Yale University School of Medicine's professor of epidemiology be set against this study, which once again aims at the wrong - serious, hospitalised - patients:

> https://academic.oup.com/aje/advance-article/doi/10.1093/aje/kwaa093/5847586

> Here's an article on well-conducted study on using HCQ in prophylaxis of Covid19..."
> http://www.ijmr.org.in/preprintarticle.asp?id=285520;type=0

XXIV. Revised advisory on the use of Hydroxychloroquine (HCQ) as prophylaxis for SARS-CoV-2 infection (in supersession of previous rd advisory dated 23rd March, 2020). Indian Council of Medical Research

> "https://www.icmr.gov.in/pdf/covid/techdoc/V5_Revised_advisory_on_the_use_of_HCQ_SARS_CoV2_infection.pdf

APPENDIX G

OPEN LETTER TO DR. ANTHONY FAUCI REGARDING HYDROXYCHLOROQUINE FOR COVID-19

August 11, 2020

Dear Dr. Fauci:

You were placed into the most high-profile role regarding America's response to the Coronavirus pandemic. Americans have relied on your medical expertise concerning the wearing of masks, resuming employment, returning to school, and of course medical treatment.

You are largely unchallenged in terms of your medical opinions. You are the de facto "COVID-19 Czar". This is unusual in the medical profession in which doctors' opinions are challenged by other physicians in the form of exchanges between doctors at hospitals, medical conferences, as well as debate in medical journals. You render your opinions unchallenged, without formal public opposition from physicians who passionately disagree with you. It is incontestable that the public is best served when opinions and policy are based on the prevailing evidence and science, and able to withstand the scrutiny of medical professionals.

As experience accrued in treating COVID-19 infections, physicians worldwide discovered that high-risk patients can be treated successfully as an outpatient, within the first 5 to 7 days of the onset of symptoms, with a "cocktail" consisting of hydroxychloroquine, zinc, and azithromycin (or doxycycline). Multiple scholarly contributions to the literature detail the efficacy of the hydroxychloroquine-based combination treatment. Dr. Harvey Risch, the renowned Yale epidemiologist, published an article in May 2020 in the American Journal of Epidemiology titled "Early Outpatient Treatment of Symptomatic, High-Risk COVID-19 Patients that Should be Ramped-Up Immediately as Key to Pandemic Crisis". He further published an article in Newsweek in July 2020 for the general public expressing the same conclusions and opinions. Dr. Risch is an expert at evaluating research data and study designs, publishing over 300 articles. Dr Risch's assessment is that there is unequivocal evidence for the early and safe use of the "HCQ cocktail." If there are Q-T interval concerns, doxycycline can be substituted for azithromycin as it has activity against RNA viruses without any cardiac effects.

Yet,you continue to reject the use of hydroxychloroquine, except in a hospital setting in the form of clinical trials, repeatedly emphasizing the lack of evidence supporting its use. Hydroxychloroquine, despite 65 years of use for malaria, and over 40 years for lupus and rheumatoid arthritis, with a well-established safety profile, has been deemed by you and the FDA as unsafe for use in the treatment of symptomatic COVID-19 infections. Your opinions have influenced the thinking of physicians and their patients, medical boards, state and federal agencies, pharmacists, hospitals, and just about everyone involved in medical-decision making. Indeed, your opinions impacted the health of Americans, and many aspects of our day-to- day lives including employment and school. Those of us who prescribe hydroxychloroquine, zinc, and azithromycin/doxycycline believe fervently that early outpatient use would save tens of thousands of lives and enable our country to dramatically alter the response to COVID-19. We advocate for an approach that will reduce fear and allow Americans to get their lives back.

We hope that our questions compel you to reconsider your current approach to COVID-19 infection.

QUESTIONS REGARDING EARLY OUTPATIENT TREATMENT

1. There are generally two stages of COVID-19 symptomatic infection; initial flu like symptoms with progression to cytokine storm and respiratory failure, correct?
2. When people are admitted to a hospital, they generally are in worse condition, correct?
3. There are no specific medications currently recommended for early outpatient treatment of symptomatic COVID-19 infection, correct?
4. Remdesivir and Dexamethasone are used for hospitalized patients, correct?
5. There is currently no recommended pharmacologic early outpatient treatment for individuals in the flu stage of the illness, correct?
6. It is true that COVID-19 is much more lethal than the flu for high-risk individuals such as older patients and those with significant comorbidities, correct?

7. Individuals with signs of early COVID-19 infection typically have a runny nose, fever, cough, shortness of breath, loss of smell, etc., and physicians send them home to rest, eat chicken soup etc., but offer no specific, targeted medications, correct?

8. These high-risk individuals are at high risk of death, on the order of 15% or higher, correct?

9. So just so we are clear—the current standard of care now is to send clinically stable symptomatic patients home, "with a wait and see" approach?

10. Are you aware that physicians are successfully using Hydroxychloroquine combined with Zinc and Azithromycin as a "cocktail" for early outpatient treatment of symptomatic, high-risk, individuals?

11. Have you heard of the "Zelenko Protocol," for treating high-risk patients with COVID 19 as an outpatient?

12. Have you read Dr. Risch's article in the American Journal of Epidemiology of the early outpatient treatment of COVID-19?

13. Are you aware that physicians using the medication combination or "cocktail" recommend use **within the first 5 to 7 days** of the onset of symptoms, before the illness impacts the lungs, or cytokine storm evolves?

14. Again, to be clear, your recommendation is no pharmacologic treatment as an outpatient for the flu—like symptoms in patients that are stable, regardless of their risk factors, correct?

15. Would you advocate for early pharmacologic outpatient treatment of symptomatic COVID-19 patients if you were confident that it was beneficial?

16. Are you aware that there are hundreds of physicians in the United States and thousands across the globe who have had **dramatic success** treating high-risk individuals as outpatients with this "cocktail?"

17. Are you aware that there are at least 10 studies demonstrating the efficacy of early outpatient treatment with the Hydroxychloroquine cocktail for high-risk patients—so this is beyond anecdotal, correct?

18. If one of your loved ones had diabetes or asthma, or any potentially complicating comorbidity, and tested positive for COVID-19, would you recommend "wait and see how they do" and go to the hospital if symptoms progress?

19. Even with multiple studies documenting remarkable outpatient efficacy and safety of the Hydroxychloroquine "cocktail," you believe the risks of the medication combination outweigh the benefits?

20. Is it true that with regard to Hydroxychloroquine and treatment of COVID-19 infection, you have said repeatedly that *""The Overwhelming Evidence of Properly Conducted Randomized*

Clinical Trials Indicate No Therapeutic Efficacy of Hydroxychloroquine (HCQ)?"

21. But NONE of the randomized controlled trials to which you refer were done in the first 5 to 7 days after the onset of symptoms-correct?

22. **All** of the randomized controlled trials to which you refer were done on hospitalized patients, correct?

23. Hospitalized patients are typically sicker that outpatients, correct?

24. None of the randomized controlled trials to which you refer used the full cocktail consisting of Hydroxychloroquine, Zinc, and Azithromycin, correct?

25. While the University of Minnesota study is referred to as disproving the cocktail, the meds were not given within the **first 5 to 7 days of illness**, the test group was not **high risk** (death rates were 3%), and no **zinc** was given, correct?

26. Again, for clarity, the trials upon which you base your opinion regarding the efficacy of Hydroxychloroquine, assessed neither the **full cocktail** (to include Zinc + Azithromycin or doxycycline) nor administered treatment **within the first 5 to 7 days of symptoms,** nor focused on the **high-risk group**, correct?

27. Therefore, you have no basis to conclude that the Hydroxychloroquine cocktail when used early in the outpatient setting, within the first 5 to 7 days of symptoms, in high risk patients, is not effective, correct?

28. It is thus false and misleading to say that the effective and safe use of Hydroxychloroquine, Zinc, and Azithromycin has been "debunked," correct? How could it be "debunked" if there is not a single study that contradicts its use?

29. Should it not be an absolute priority for the NIH and CDC to look at ways to treat Americans with symptomatic COVID-19 infections early to prevent disease progression?

30. The SARS-CoV-2/COVID-19 virus is an RNA virus. It is well-established that Zinc interferes with RNA viral replication, correct?

31. Moreover, is it not true that hydroxychloroquine facilitates the entry of zinc into the cell, is a "ionophore", correct?

32. Isn't also it true that Azithromycin has established anti-viral properties?

33. Are you aware of the paper from Baylor by Dr. McCullough et. al. describing established mechanisms by which the components of the "HCQ cocktail" exert anti-viral effects?

34. So- the use of hydroxychloroquine, azithromycin (or doxycycline) and zinc, the "HCQ cocktail," is based on science, correct?

QUESTIONS REGARDING SAFETY

1. The FDA writes the following: "in light of on-going serious cardiac adverse events and their serious side effects, the known and potential benefits of CQ and HCQ no longer outweigh the known and potential risks for authorized use."
    So not only is the FDA saying that Hydroxychloroquine doesn't work, they are also saying that it is a very dangerous drug. Yet, is it not true the drug has been used as an anti-malarial drug for over 65 years?
2. Isn't true that the drug has been used for lupus and rheumatoid arthritis for many years at similar doses?
3. Do you know of even a single study prior to COVID -19 that has provided definitive evidence against the use of the drug based on safety concerns?
4. Are you aware that choloroquine or hydroxychloroquine has many approved uses for hydroxychloroquine including steroid-dependent asthma (1988 study), Advanced pulmonary sarcoidosis (1988 study), sensitizing breast cancer cells for chemotherapy (2012 study), the attenuation of renal ischemia (2018 study), lupus nepritis (2006 study), epithelial ovarian cancer (2020 study, just to name a few)? Where are the cardiotoxicity concerns ever mentioned?
5. Dr. Risch estimates the risk of cardiac death from hydroxychloroquine to be 9/100,000 using the data provided by the FDA. That does not seem to be a high risk, considering the risk of death in an older patient with co-morbidities can be 15% or more. Do you consider 9/100,000 to be a high risk when weighed against the risk of death in older patient with co-morbidities?
6. To put this in perspective, the drug is used for 65 years, without warnings (aside for the need for periodic retinal checks), but the FDA somehow feels the need to send out an alert on June 15, 2020 that the drug is dangerous. Does that make any logical sense to you Dr. Fauci based on "science"?
7. Moreover, consider that the protocols for usage in early treatment are for 5 to 7 days at relatively low doses of hydroxychloroquine similar to what is being given in other diseases (RA, SLE) over many years- does it make any sense to you logically that a 5 to 7 day dose of hydroxychloroquine when not given in high doses could be considered dangerous?
8. You are also aware that articles published in the New England Journal of Medicine and Lancet, one out of Harvard University, regarding the dangers of hydroxychloroquine had to be retracted

based on the fact that the data was fabricated. Are you aware of that?

9. If there was such good data on the risks of hydroxychloroquine, one would not have to use fake data, correct?

10. After all, 65 years is a long-time to determine whether or not a drug is safe, do you agree?

11. In the clinical trials that you have referenced (e.g., the Minnesota and the Brazil studies), there was not a single death attributed directly to hydroxychloroquine, correct?

12. According to Dr. Risch, there is no evidence based on the data to conclude that hydroxychloroquine is a dangerous drug. Are you aware of any published report that rebuts Dr. Risch's findings?

13. Are you aware that the FDA ruling along with your statements have led to Governors in a number of states to restrict the use of hydroxychloroquine?

14. Are you aware that pharmacies are not filling prescriptions for this medication based on your and the FDA's restrictions?

15. Are you aware that doctors are being punished by state medical boards for prescribing the medication based on your comments as well as the FDA's?

16. Are you aware that people who want the medication sometimes need to call physicians in other states pleading for it?

17. And yet you opined in March that while people were dying at the rate of 10,000 patient a week, hydroxychloroquine could only be used in an inpatient setting as part of a clinical trial- correct?

18. So, people who want to be treated in that critical 5-to-7 day period and avoid being hospitalized are basically out of luck in your view, correct?

19. So, again, for clarity, without a shred of evidence that the Hydroxychloroquine/HCQ cocktail is dangerous in the doses currently recommend for **early** outpatient treatment, you and the FDA have made it very difficult if not impossible in some cases to get this treatment, correct?

QUESTIONS REGARDING METHODOLOGY

1. In regards to the use of hydroxychloroquine, you have repeatedly made the same statement: *"The Overwhelming Evidence from Properly Conducted Randomized Clinical Trials Indicate no Therapeutic Efficacy of Hydroxychloroquine."* Is that correct?

2. In Dr. Risch's article regarding the early use of hydroxychloroquine, he disputes your opinion. He scientifically

evaluated the data from the studies to support his opinions. Have you published any articles to support your opinions?

3. You repeatedly state that randomized clinical trials are needed to make conclusions regarding treatments, correct?

4. The FDA has approved many medications (especially in the area of cancer treatment) without randomized clinical trials, correct?

5. Are you aware that Dr. Thomas Frieden, the previous head of the CDC wrote an article in the New England Journal of Medicine in 2017 called "Evidence for Health Decision Making – Beyond Randomized Clinical Trials (RCT)"? Have you read that article?

6. In it Dr. Frieden states that "many data sources can provide valid evidence for clinical and public health action, including "analysis of aggregate clinical or epidemiological data"-do you disagree with that?

7. Dr. Frieden discusses "practiced-based evidence" as being essential in many discoveries, such SIDS (Sudden Infant Death Syndrome)-do you disagree with that?

8. Dr. Frieden writes the following: "Current evidence-grading systems are biased toward randomized clinical trials, which may lead to inadequate consideration of non-RCT data." Dr. Fauci, have you considered all the non-RCT data in coming to your opinions?

9. Dr. Risch, who is a leading world authority in the analysis of aggregate clinical data, has done a rigorous analysis that he published regarding the early treatment of COVID 19 with hydroxychloroquine, zinc, and azithromycin. He cites 5 or 6 studies, and in an updated article there are 5 or 6 more-a total of 10 to 12 clinical studies with formally collected data specifically regarding the early treatment of COVID. Have you analyzed the aggregate data regarding early treatment of high-risk patients with hydroxychloroquine, zinc, and azithromycin?

10. Is there any document that you can produce for the American people of your analysis of the aggregate data that would rebut Dr. Risch's analysis?

11. Yet, despite what Dr. Risch believes is overwhelming evidence in support of the early use of hydroxychloroquine, you dismiss the treatment insisting on randomized controlled trials even in the midst of a pandemic?

12. Would you want a loved one with high-risk comorbidities placed in the control group of a randomized clinical trial when a number of studies demonstrate safety and dramatic efficacy of the early use of the Hydroxychloroquine "cocktail?"

13. Are you aware that the FDA approved a number of cancer chemotherapy drugs without randomized control trials based solely on epidemiological evidence. The trials came later as confirmation. Are you aware of that?

14. You are well aware that there were no randomized clinical trials in the case of penicillin that saved thousands of lives in World War II? Was not this in the best interest of our soldiers?

15. You would agree that many lives were saved with the use of cancer drugs and penicillin that were used before any randomized clinical trials--correct?

16. You have referred to evidence for hydroxychloroquine as "anecdotal"- which is defined as "evidence collected in a casual or informal manner and relying heavily or entirely on personal testimony"- correct?

17. But there are many studies supporting the use of hydroxychloroquine in which evidence was collected formally and not on personal testimony, has there not been?

18. So it would be false to conclude that the evidence supporting the early use of hydroxychloroquine is anecdotal, correct?

COMPARISON BETWEEN U.S. AND OTHER COUNTRIES REGARDING CASE FATALITY RATE

(IT WOULD BE VERY HELPFUL TO HAVE THE GRAPHS COMPARING OUR CASE FATALITY RATES TO OTHER COUNTRIES)

1. Are you aware that countries like Senegal and Nigeria that use Hydroxychloroquine have much lower case-fatality rates than the United States?

2. Have you pondered the relationship between the use of Hydroxychloroquine by a given country and their case mortality rate and why there is a strong correlation between the use of HCQ and the reduction of the case mortality rate.?

3. Have you considered consulting with a country such as India that has had great success treating COVID-19 prophylactically?

4. Why shouldn't our first responders and front-line workers who are at high risk at least have an option of HCQ/zinc prophylaxis?

5. We should all agree that countries with far inferior healthcare delivery systems should not have lower case fatality rates. Reducing our case fatality rate from near 5% to 2.5%, in line with many countries who use HCQ early would have cut our total number of deaths in half, correct?

6. Why not consult with countries who have lower case-fatality rates, even without expensive medicines such as remdesivir and far less advanced intensive care capabilities?

GIVING AMERICANS THE OPTION TO USE
HCQ FOR COVID-19

1. Dr. Harvey Risch, the pre-eminent Epidemiologist from Yale, wrote a Newsweek Article titled: *"The key to defeating COVID-19 already exists. We need to start using it."* Did you read the article?

2. Are you aware that the cost of the Hydroxychloroquine "cocktail" including the Z-pack and zinc is about $50?

3. You are aware the cost of Remdesivir is about $3,200?

4. So that's about 60 doses of HCQ "cocktail," correct?

5. In fact, President Trump had the foresight to amass 60 million doses of hydroxychloroquine, and yet you continue to stand in the way of doctors who want to use that medication for their infected patients, correct?

6. Those are a lot of doses of medication that potentially could be used to treat our poor, especially our minority populations and people of color that have a difficult time accessing healthcare. They die more frequently of COVID-19, do they not?

7. But because of your obstinance blocking the use of HCQ, this stockpile has remained largely unused, correct?

8. Would you acknowledge that your strategy of telling Americans to restrict their behavior, wear masks, and distance, and put their lives on hold indefinitely until there is a vaccine is not working?

9. So, 160,000 deaths later, an economy in shambles, kids out of school, suicides and drug overdoses at a record high, people neglecting and dying from other medical conditions, and America reacting to every outbreak with another lockdown- is it not time to re-think your strategy that is fully dependent on an effective vaccine?

10. Why not consider a strategy that protects the most vulnerable and allows Americans back to living their lives and not wait for a vaccine panacea that may never come?

11. Why not consider the approach that thousands of doctors around the world are using, supported by a number of studies in the literature, with early outpatient treatment of high-risk patients for typically one week with HCQ + Zinc + Azithromycin?

12. You don't see a problem with the fact that the government, due to your position, in some cases interferes with the choice of using HCQ. Should not that be a choice between the doctor and the patient?

13. While some doctors may not want to use the drug, should not doctors who believe that it is indicated be able to offer it to their patients?

14. Are you aware that doctors who are publicly advocating for such a strategy with the early use of the HCQ cocktail are being silenced with removal of content on the internet and even censorship in the medical community?

15. You are aware of the 20 or so physicians who came to the Supreme Court steps advocating for the early use of the Hydroxychloroquine cocktail.
    a.   In fact, you said these were *"a bunch of people spouting out something that isn't true."*
    b.   Dr. Fauci, these are not just "people"- these are doctors who actually treat patients, unlike you, correct?

16. Do you know that the video they made went viral with 17 million views in just a few hours, and was then removed from the internet?

17. Are you aware that their website, American Frontline Doctors, was taken down the next day?

18. Did you see the way that Nigerian immigrant physician, Dr. Stella Immanuel, was mocked in the media for her religious views and called a "witch doctor"?

19. Are you aware that Dr. Simone Gold, the leader of the group, was fired from her job as an Emergency Room physician the following day?

20. Are you aware that physicians advocating for this treatment that has by now probably saved millions of lives around the globe are harassed by local health departments, state agencies and medical boards, and even at their own hospitals? Are you aware of that?

21. Don't you think doctors should have the right to speak out on behalf of their patients without the threat of retribution?

22. Are you aware that videos and other educational information are removed off the internet and labeled, in the words of Mark Zuckerberg, as "misinformation."?

23. Is it not misinformation to characterize Hydroxychloroquine, in the doses used for early outpatient treatment of COVID-19 infections, as a dangerous drug?

24. Is it not misleading for you to repeatedly state to the American public that randomized clinical trials are the sole source of information to confirm the efficacy of a treatment?

25. Was it not misinformation when on CNN you cited the Lancet study based on false data from Surgisphere as evidence of the lack of efficacy of hydroxychloroquine?

26. Is it not misinformation as is repeated in the MSM as a result of your comments that a randomized clinical trial is required by the FDA for a drug approval?

27. Don't you realize how much damage this falsehood perpetuates?

28. How is it not misinformation for you and the FDA to keep telling the American public that hydroxychloroquine is dangerous when you know that there is nothing more than anecdotal evidence of that?

29. Dr. Fauci, if you or a loved one were infected with COVID-19, and had flu-like symptoms, and you knew as you do now that there is a safe and effective cocktail that you could take to prevent worsening and the possibility of hospitalization, can you honestly tell us that you would refuse the medication?

30. Why not give our healthcare workers and first responders, who even with the necessary PPE are contracting the virus at a 3 to 4 times greater rate than the general public, the right to choose along with their doctor if they want use the medicine prophylactically?

31. Why is the government inserting itself in a way that is unprecedented in regards to a historically safe medication and not allowing patients the right to choose along with their doctor?

32. Why not give the American people the right to decide along with their physician whether or not they want outpatient treatment in the first 5 to 7 days of the disease with a cocktail that is safe and costs around $50?

FINAL QUESTIONS

1. Dr. Fauci, please explain how a randomized clinical trial, to which you repeatedly make reference, for testing the HCQ cocktail (hydroxychloroquine, azithromycin and zinc) administered within 5-7 days of the onset of symptoms is even possible now given the declining case numbers in so many states?

2. For example, if the NIH were now to direct a study to begin September 15, where would such a study be done?

3. Please explain how a randomized study on the early treatment (within the first 5 to 7 days of symptoms) of high-risk, symptomatic COVID-19 infections could be done during the influenza season and be valid?

4. Please explain how multiple observational studies arrive at the same outcomes using the same formulation of hydroxychloroquine + Azithromycin + Zinc given in the same time

frame for the same study population (high risk patients) is not evidence that the cocktail works?

5. In fact, how is it not significant evidence, during a pandemic, for hundreds of non-academic private practice physicians to achieve the same outcomes with the early use of the HCQ cocktail?

6. What is your recommendation for the medical management of a 75-year-old diabetic with fever, cough, and loss of smell, but not yet hypoxic, who Emergency Room providers do not feel warrants admission? We know that hundreds of U.S. physicians (and thousands more around the world) would manage this case with the HCQ cocktail with predictable success.

7. If you were in charge in 1940, would you have advised the mass production of penicillin based primarily on lab evidence and one case series on 5 patients in England or would you have stated that a randomized clinical trial was needed?

8. Why would any physician put their medical license, professional reputation, and job on the line to recommend the HCQ cocktail (that does not make them any money) unless they knew the treatment could significantly help their patient?

9. Why would a physician take the medication themselves and prescribe it to family members (for treatment or prophylaxis) unless they felt strongly that the medication was beneficial?

10. How is it informed and ethical medical practice to allow a COVID-19 patient to deteriorate in the early stages of the infection when there is inexpensive, safe, and dramatically effective treatment with the HCQ cocktail, which the science indicates interferes with coronavirus replication?

11. How is your approach to "wait and see" in the early stages of COVID-19 infection, especially in high-risk patients, following the science?

While previous questions are related to hydroxychloroquine-based treatment, we have two questions addressing masks.

1. As you recall, you stated on March 8th, just a few weeks before the devastation in the Northeast, that masks weren't needed. You later said that you made this statement to prevent a hoarding of masks that would disrupt availability to healthcare workers. Why did you not make a recommendation for people to wear any face covering to protect themselves, as we are doing now?

2. Rather, you issued no such warning and people were riding in subways and visiting their relatives in nursing homes without any face covering. Currently, your position is that face coverings are essential. Please explain whether or not you made a mistake in early March, and how would you go about it differently now.

CONCLUSION

Since the start of the pandemic, physicians have used hydroxychloroquine to treat symptomatic COVID-19 infections, as well as for prophylaxis. Initial results were mixed as indications and doses were explored to maximize outcomes and minimize risks. What emerged was that hydroxychloroquine appeared to work best when coupled with azithromycin. In fact, it was the President of the United States who recommended to you publicly at the beginning of the pandemic, in early March, that you should consider **early treatment** with hydroxychloroquine and a "Z-Pack." Additional studies showed that patients did not seem to benefit when COVID-19 infections were treated with hydroxychloroquine late in the course of the illness, typically in a hospital setting, but treatment was consistently effective, even in **high-risk patients,** when hydroxychloroquine was given in a "cocktail" with azithromycin and, critically, **zinc** in the first **5 to 7 days after the onset of symptoms**. The outcomes are, in fact, dramatic.

As clearly presented in the McCullough article from Baylor, and described by Dr. Vladimir Zelenko, the efficacy of the HCQ cocktail is based on the pharmacology of the hydroxychloroquine ionophore acting as the "gun" and zinc as the "bullet," while azithromycin potentiates the anti-viral effect. Undeniably, the hydroxychloroquine combination treatment is supported by science. Yet, you continue to ignore the "science" behind the disease. Viral replication occurs rapidly in the first 5 to 7 days of symptoms, and can be treated at that point with the HCQ cocktail. Rather, your actions have denied patients treatment in that early stage. Without such treatment, some patients, especially those at high risk with co-morbidities, deteriorate and require hospitalization for evolving cytokine storm resulting in pneumonia, respiratory failure, and intubation with 50% mortality. Dismissal of the science results in bad medicine, and the outcome is over 160,000 dead Americans. Countries that have followed the science and treated the disease in the early stages have far better results, a fact that has been concealed from the American Public.

Despite mounting evidence and impassioned pleas from hundreds of frontline physicians, your position was and continues to be that randomized controlled trials (RCTs) have not shown there to be benefit. **However, not a single randomized control trial has tested what is being recommended:** use of the full cocktail (especially zinc), in high-risk patients, initiated within the first 5 to 7 days of the onset of symptoms. Using hydroxychloroquine and azithromycin late in the disease process, with or without zinc, does not produce the same, unequivocally positive results.

Dr. Thomas Frieden, in a 2017 New England Journal of Medicine article regarding randomized clinical trials, emphasized there are situations in which it is entirely appropriate to use other forms of evidence to scientifically validate a treatment. Such is the case during a pandemic that moves like a brush-fire jumping to different parts of the country. Insisting on randomized clinical trials in the midst of a pandemic is simply foolish. Dr. Harvey Risch, a world-renowned Yale epidemiologist, analyzed all the data regarding the use of the hydroxychloroquine/HCQ cocktail and concluded that the evidence of its efficacy when used early in COVID-19 infection is unequivocal.

Curiously, despite a 65+ years safety record, the FDA suddenly deemed hydroxychloroquine a dangerous drug, especially with regard to cardiotoxicity. Dr. Risch analyzed data provided by the FDA and concluded that the risk of a significant cardiac event from hydroxychloroquine is extremely low, especially when compared to the mortality rate of COVID-19 patients with high-risk co-morbidities. How do you reconcile that for forty years rheumatoid arthritis and lupus patients have been treated over long periods, often for years, with hydroxychloroquine and now there are suddenly concerns about a 5 to 7-day course of hydroxychloroquine at similar or slightly increased doses? The FDA statement regarding hydroxychloroquine and cardiac risk is patently false and alarmingly misleading to physicians, pharmacists, patients, and other health professionals. The benefits of the early use of hydroxychloroquine to prevent hospitalization in high-risk patients with COVID-19 infection far outweigh the risks. Physicians are not able to obtain the medication for their patients, and in some cases are restricted by their state from prescribing hydroxychloroquine. The government's obstruction of the early treatment of symptomatic high-risk COVID-19 patients with hydroxychloroquine, a medication used extensively and safely for so long, is unprecedented.

It is essential that you tell the truth to the American public regarding the safety and efficacy of the hydroxychloroquine/HCQ cocktail. The government must protect and facilitate the sacred and revered physician-patient relationship by permitting physicians to treat their patients. Governmental obfuscation and obstruction are as lethal as cytokine storm.

Americans must not continue to die unnecessarily. Adults must resume employment and our youth return to school. Locking down America while awaiting an imperfect vaccine has done far more damage to Americans than the coronavirus. We are confident that thousands of lives would be saved with early treatment of high-risk individuals with a cocktail of hydroxychloroquine, zinc, and azithromycin. Americans must not live in fear. As Dr. Harvey Risch's Newsweek article declares, "The key to defeating COVID-19 already exists. We need to start using it."

Very Respectfully,

George C. Fareed, MD
Brawley, California

Michael M. Jacobs, MD, MPH
Pensacola, Florida

Donald C. Pompan, MD
Salinas, California

APPENDIX H

THE MIRACLE OF THE IMPERIAL VALLEY:
Dr. Tyson's First-Person Account of COVID-19

The Start

We heard about a virus coming out of Wuhan, China, in January of 2020. I had a feeling it was going to make its way to the US due to all the international travel. I told my wife Fabiola; we need to get prepared, and we are going to need a plan. It was long before we started hearing of cases across the US; Washington had the first outbreak and then New York. I remember getting a call from my daughter Mahkenna's music manager Gary Salzman, who she was supposed to fly out and see in late March for her new single.

Gary told me, "I think I have this crap!"

I replied, "How do you feel - Is it bad?"

He said, "It's in my lungs, and I'm having a hard time breathing."

I suggested he go to the ER and get tested to be sure and get available treatment. I had done some research from studies coming out of southern France by Dr. Didier Raoult. A study published by the *Journal of Virology* in 2005 showed Chloroquine was a potent inhibitor of SARS Coronavirus Infection and spread. I told him to get on Hydroxychloroquine, Zinc, and Z-pack.

His response was that he was just at the ER, and they sent him home with no treatment and said he was not even sick enough to get tested. Without that ability to test, treatment as an outpatient was withheld. It wasn't until he became sicker and later ended up in the hospital that they paid any attention to him.

Gary died two weeks later. We were devastated as a family; the music community lost a legend, and we could not even have a funeral. I told myself that I would not allow that to happen with any of my patients. I would find a way to test people and treat people when that day comes.

March

It's now March, and we see the virus all around us. We are scared. My staff was scared, my wife was scared, my parents and in-laws are scared. We have young staff members with newborn kids, others with small kids, and we have small kids and a teenager with Down's syndrome. We had no idea how our lives were about to change.

It's mid-March, and we are seeing sick patients, but we have no tests. We have a screening tool sent out by public health that was not helpful at all to try to determine if patients may or may not have COVID-19. Upper respiratory infections are common in March. What's the difference between COVID-19 symptoms and Influenza? Travel? We are a border town. Many people live in the town of Mexicali (population 1.5M) and work in the Valley (190K).

We are now screening patients outside with a pop-up tent, tables, and some chairs. MAs are scared but strong and take vitals and history from everyone in their cars. They report back to me, and we see them outside in their chairs once the registration process is done. We still had no way to test. I called the hospitals, Public Health, and the Abbott representative to see if we could get the ID kits now that the FDA had approved them because we have the machine already, and the answer was "no" across the board.

There was no way to find out who was positive and who needed treatment. We were now frustrated and scared at the same time. My wife said we should close until we can figure it all out. I was not going to give up. I called all my contacts, and out of the blue, my good friend Terrance found a Lab in Orange County, Equitox, that could get me the serology tests that would show if your IgM or IgG immunity was present.

At last, we had a tool. We also started doing Chest X-rays on all patients with respiratory symptoms. It was not long before we were able to identify the COVID-19 pattern on Chest X-ray and using the IgM, IgG approach. We started treatment on patients. We began with Hydroxychloroquine 400mg by mouth twice a day on the first day, then 200mg three times a day for days 2-5. We would re-evaluate everyone in 2-3 days and see them back at 7 and 14 days to make sure they did better. We also wanted to confirm immunity for patients who then needed to go back to work.

April

By the end of March and April, we were now seeing 200-400 patients a day. We were asked by many essential workers to help keep their services and businesses open. We took care of the many local establishments: Border Patrol, Calipatria and Centinela Corrections Officers, Homeland Security,

Customs, Sheriff's Department, Brawley Beef, RoGar Manufacturing, Imperial Valley Auto, ICOE, and Imperial Valley Superior Court. We also saw many cattle feed and farming seed companies and the various medical and dental offices that needed to stay open.

We knew our system was not perfect, but it was the only one we had. We revised the tents and tables into an insulated carport with mobile clinic functions implemented to have air conditioning for summer, copy machines, registration, air-flow and disinfection on a regular basis.

There was still no way to confirm patients with PCR testing due to a lack of supplies. We didn't even have PPE.

I was called by the Public Health office and asked to stop testing because we were creating too much work for them, and we could not confirm our patients' infections. When I asked where else we could send them for confirmation, I was told the ER. The problem with that was (as my friend Gary told me) they were not sick enough to be tested. I was told by the ER's they only had ten swabs per week for each hospital, and only those sent to the ICU were being tested.

I then got a letter from the ER Medical Director at El Centro Regional Medical Center instructing me to stop prescribing Hydroxychloroquine because it would prohibit the hospitals from getting it for those who needed it. I could not believe what I was hearing. For the first time in my life as a physician, I was being told to stop saving people's lives! My response was clear, "Give me an alternative, and I will use it; until then, I will use whatever I have that has been shown to work. "

I have never understood the pushback in using treatments that were maybe controversial but showed promise over the ridiculous policy of "Home Quarantine for 14 days" without any treatment.

Who does that? Since when is any disease treated by quarantine alone?

We have drugs that work and we have vitamins and supplements that help; why not at least use those? Why confine others at home with known sick people? These are still questions that nobody in the public health department wants to answer. We went to the meetings at public health and asked about the PPE stockpile and were told once again that nothing was available.

During this time, my staff and I were out at the large businesses giving lectures on the virus, how to prevent transmission and that the treatment seemed to be working if they got sick. That seemed to set the standard for our community. Cleaning, social distancing, staying home when not working, and not going to work sick. Early evaluation if symptoms occurred and mandatory seven days off and retesting if the serology test was negative. Mandatory 14 days off if positive.

May

In May, we finally had two labs that were able to get us the PCR nasal swabs. That was good and bad. We were able to finally confirm cases, but the bad was the level of work it took to call all the patients and get the test results out and make the follow-up and treatment calls. I knew all along that the possibility of getting in trouble was there, so we had been keeping a spreadsheet with all the positive patients and the treatment plan and recovery plan. It worked out when we got a call from the State and CDC in June after months of being left alone. We found out that our center was the only place that kept that level of records, and we were chosen to be the Sentinel Site for California and CDC for the Imperial Valley. We were finally validated that everything we did was worth it.

September

We made the news in late September and October when we started publishing our data, and people realized that we had seen more COVID-19 patients face-to-face than probably anyone in the nation, and maybe even worldwide. We did that and have not recorded a single death for anyone that was placed on (our) treatment. We did have to call EMS on two patients that presented to our Urgent Care in respiratory failure and were sent to the hospital before we could start treatment. One of those died, and for the other, we were unable to get follow-up information. As of today, we have over 1900 COVID-19 positive recovered patients – a 100% success rate!

This brought the call to go to Washington, DC.

October

The process in preparing for speaking at the US Supreme Court was intimidating. Those invited were all highly intelligent physicians, scholars, lawyers, and researchers. I felt like I was out of my league. It was intimidating, and once again, I was scared. What will they think? What if I mess up? What if I get laughed at and ridiculed? I still needed to make a statement. I still needed to tell our story.

I still needed to be heard.

Dr. Simone Gold wanted a passionate speech with facts from all of us. After our meetings in DC and the recordings we all did, I felt it was my time. The fear had left me, just like it left me at the clinic in treating all the COVID-19 patients. The staff had been sick but survived. Students were sick and survived. Two of my Nurse Practitioners, both my sons and my manager's mom with MS, all got COVID-19 and survived. That is where my speech came from. It was the buildup and resolution of fear that had us all so scared in the beginning, but now realizing there is treatment.

<u>My Speech</u>

"We can go back to school! We can go back to work! We can go back to life! We can go back to being Americans! We will not let fear take our freedom!!!" I spoke on those steps.

That was a moment I will never forget. It truly was incredible. I have always wanted to do something great for my country, knowing that my grandfathers served in WW2, Vietnam, and Korea. I thought of my grandpa Tyson. My dad served in Vietnam. How scared were they? What must it have been like to have to go into an actual war? This is my war, and it's not over.

We are still fighting the fight, and we will continue to do so. I hoped the video would be a tool that other physicians could see and hear. We need everyone to be able to see the success we had. When it was finally posted on YouTube, it was exciting, it started to go viral, and then something happened.

It was taken down!!

Why? Why would you take down a video with the knowledge, research, links, and website where everyone can see what we are doing?! Why? I don't have any reason. I can't believe that Big Tech and Government controls want to see people die. Why would you take down the message of hope? Why would you take down the message of treatment? Why do you want to continue living in fear when there are clear treatment options now?

There are multiple options. Peter McCullough and his peers published the first peer-reviewed pathway to outpatient treatment in the *American Journal of Medicine,* and that too was recently taken down. We had to get Senate influence to have them re-publish it!!

That should upset people all over the world.

Think about it, the world is looking to us to find a treatment or a cure, and when we do, it gets taken down? Most people would be like – WTF? I was able to channel that anger, I was able to get raw video, and we published it again and again.

We will keep publishing it over and over until it is recognized all over the world that we don't need to be afraid anymore.

People need to know that we will survive this pandemic, just like those of the past. There is treatment available. It works when used early, and it is very effective.

We will get our voices heard because we hear the cry of those in our care. Physicians are people too; we have families and kids. We would never advocate for something we didn't believe.

Scientists are different; they have financial gains and incentives. They have research that needs to be funded, and while they may have the best of intentions, they do not work on the frontlines. They do not care for patients; they do not have to explain the risks and benefits of treatments. They are not there when patients break down and cry when they are told they have a positive test. They don't have to explain to a 9-year-old girl that she will not kill her parents just because she is positive.

Scientists have no skin in the game and no emotional pain when things don't go their way. This virus has killed people!! It will kill more. The question is, how many more will die unnecessarily due to not getting the available treatment?

How many will die in fear, and how many will die alone?

My final point is this: When you get sick, you do not go to the CDC or the NIH or call the FDA to get diagnosed and treated. You go to your doctor! You go to the people who have seen the disease before and know how to treat it. This virus is no different.

-Brian Tyson, MD
Board Certified in Family Medicine
14 Years of ER and Hospital Medicine Experience
All Valley Urgent Care in El Centro, California

APPENDIX I

YOUTUBE CENSORS THE SENATE
& BANS DR. PIERRE KORY

"I will maintain that Ivermectin should be
the standard of care based on these data."
-Pierre Kory, MD.

Dr. Kory's Senate Testimony

The following is adapted from Dr. Pierre Kory's sworn testimony delivered December 8, 2020, to the US Senate Committee on Homeland Security. Minor corrections have been made to grammar and phrasing as necessary. These words were contained in the video that YouTube censored.

The Search for Repurposed Drugs for COVID-19

I am severely troubled by the fact that the NIH, the FDA, and the CDC have not reviewed repurposed drugs. I do not know of any task force that was assigned or compiled to review repurposed drugs in an attempt to treat this disease.

Everything has been about novel and/or expensive and pharmacologically-engineered drugs, those like Remdesivir, monoclonal antibodies, and vaccines. We have had 100 years of medicine development. We are experts in all the medicines we use. I do not know of a task force that has been focused on repurposed drugs. I will tell you that my group and our organization has filled that void. . .

What I want to talk to you about is that we have a solution to this crisis. There is a drug that is proving to be of miraculous impact; when I say miracle, I do not use that term lightly, and I do not want to be sensationalized. This is a scientific recommendation based on mountains of data that has emerged in the last three months. When I am told that we are touting things that are not FDA or NIH recommended, let me be clear. The NIH recommendation to not use it outside clinical trials is from August 27.

We are now in December. This is three or four months later. Mountains of data have emerged from many centers and countries around the world, showing the miraculous effectiveness of Ivermectin. It basically obliterates the transmission of this virus. If you take it, you will not get sick. I want to

399

briefly summarize the data. We have contributed more to the medical knowledge of our specialty, in our careers, than anyone else can claim as a group, and our manuscript posted on the medicine preprint server details all of this evidence. I want to briefly summarize it. We have evidence that Ivermectin is effective not only in prophylaxis, in the prevention, but if you take it, you will not get sick.

Ivermectin is 100% Effective in COVID Prophylaxis

We just came across a trial last night from Argentina by the lead investigator, Dr. Hector Carvallo.   They prophylaxed 800 health care workers; not one got sick. In the 400 they did not prophylax, 58% got sick; 237 of those 400 got sick. If you take it, you will not get sick. It has immense and potent anti-viral activity. We know that from the first study in Monash. It has made the bench to the bedside.

For prophylaxis, we have four large randomized controlled trials totaling over 1500 patients, with each trial showing that as a prophylactic agent, it is immensely effective; you will be protected from getting ill if you take it.

In early outpatient treatment, we have three randomized controlled trials and multiple observational as well as case series showing that if you take it, the need for hospitalization and death will decrease.

The most profound evidence we have is in the hospitalized patients. We have four randomized controlled trials there and multiple observational trials, all showing the same thing, that you will not die or you will die at much, much, much lower rates, statistically significant, large magnitude results if you take Ivermectin. It is proving to be a wonder drug. It has already won the Nobel Prize in Medicine in 2015 for impacts on global health in the eradication of parasitic disease.

It is proving to be an immensely powerful anti-viral and anti-inflammatory agent. It is critical for its use this disease. We stand by our manuscript. It has been submitted for peer review. Please recognize peer review takes time. It takes months; we do not have months. We have 100,000 patients in the hospital right now dying...

Ivermectin Prevents Hospitalizations & Deaths

By the time they get to me in the ICU, they are already dying and almost impossible to recover. Early treatment is the key. We need to offload the hospitals. We are tired. I cannot keep doing this. If you look at my manuscript, and if I have to go back to work next week, any further deaths are going to be needless deaths, and I cannot be traumatized by that.

I cannot keep caring for patients when I know that they could have been saved with earlier treatment. The drug that will treat them and prevent hospitalization is Ivermectin. I am going to be very clear and simple. All I ask is for the NIH to review our data that we have compiled, of all of the emerging data. We have almost 30 studies. Every one is reliably and reproducibly positive showing the dramatic impacts of Ivermectin...

I cannot call on more credibility than we have. We are not just a random doctor who is saying we have a cure. I do not want to say I have a cure. I am just asking you to review our data. We have immense amounts of data that show that Ivermectin must be implemented and implemented now.

Senator, the last thing I want to say is, do you know who is dying here? It is our African-American, Latinos, and elderly. It is some of the most disadvantaged and impoverished members of our society. They are dying at higher rates than anyone else. It is the most severe discrepancy I have seen in my medical career, and we are responsible to protect those disadvantaged members.

We have a special duty to provide countermeasures. The amount of evidence to show Ivermectin is lifesaving and protective is so immense, and the drug is so safe. My colleagues have talked about it. It must be instituted and implemented. I am asking the NIH to review our data and to come up with recommendations for society...

Randomized Controlled Trial Evidence for Ivermectin

Senator Paul, I appreciate your question, and it is critical - the content of your question, which is how we can tell when something is working when many patients get better (anyway)? And there is only one answer to that. And we know what that is. It is one of the central tenets of science, which is that you need a control group. You need to have a group that is comparable to those that you treat, and then you compare them to those that you don't treat.

What I am trying to message today is in our manuscript, we now have eleven randomized controlled trials. Every one of those controlled trials shows that in the Ivermectin-treated group, lives are saved, there is less need for hospitalization, there is less transmission, and less case count. It (Ivermectin) is a fundamentally and powerfully effective therapy against COVID-19. We need the NIH to review these data. We have the data.
Let me say that the amount of patients in those randomized controlled trials, the eleven trials, totals nearly 4,000 with over half treated with Ivermectin.

Let us remind ourselves that the treatment of COVID-19 fundamentally changed after the results of the RECOVERY trial were announced in June. That was a trial of 6,000 patients. Two thousand were treated with steroids. That showed the dramatic and lifesaving effects of corticosteroids. Almost overnight, the treatment of COVID-19 changed as a result of that trial. That was the RECOVERY trial.

The Data for Ivermectin Exceeds RECOVERY Trial Magnitude

I am presenting a paper today with more patients treated with Ivermectin, with larger magnitudes of benefit than in the RECOVERY trial. I will maintain that Ivermectin should be the standard of care based on these data. It is not my opinion. It is the data. If you give anyone else a placebo, based upon the data in our manuscript, I believe that would be malpractice and would lead to a heightened risk of death...

We have four randomized controlled trials in prophylaxis. Each and every one is highly statistically significant. Healthy citizens on Ivermectin do not get COVID...

In the prophylaxis studies alone, which is four, they took COVID-19 patients, who tested positive for COVID-19, they identified their household members and gave them Ivermectin. So they had a whole group of household contacts of COVID-19 patients who took Ivermectin. In the other households, they did not give Ivermectin. Every single randomized controlled trial showed that in the households that were on Ivermectin, drastically reduced rates of transmission. The households did not get sick. You can protect people from this disease with Ivermectin. That's just the prophylaxis trials...

They were drastically statistically significant. And these are from multiple centers and countries around the world. That's just the prophylaxis. We also have trials on early outpatient as well as hospital (treatment). The most dramatic is the hospital. We have four randomized controlled trials in the hospital, all with statistically significant reductions in mortality. Dr. Rajter has a large observational controlled trial from Broward County. In his trial, he also showed the same. The patients who got the Ivermectin died at far lower rates...

The NIH made their last recommendation on August 27, which is either ten years ago or four months ago; I don't know which. On August 27, this was their recommendation, "We recommend against the use of Ivermectin outside of clinical trials."

That recommendation was based upon expert opinion only. There was no data to recommend or recommend against. It was (merely) an expert opinion...

<u>Ivermectin's Unparalleled Safety Profile</u>

3.7 billion doses of Ivermectin have been administered since 1987. It is administered to 63% of Sub-Saharan Africans on a yearly basis. It has an almost unparalleled safety profile with almost no side effects. On a risk/benefit therapeutic analysis, you cannot come up with a credible argument to not give it...

This is not the flu. I have been a doctor for a long time. In one major health care system that I helped work with, they went from 95 ICU beds (in a span of 2.5 weeks) to 350 ICU beds. Gastroenterologists were taking care of dying COVID patients. We do not do that with the flu. We have ICUs dedicated to COVID patients on ventilators. This is not what happens with the flu.

Ivermectin has shown itself to be a highly effective preventative and early treatment agent. It needs to be immediately adopted—systematically, nationally, and globally— period.

***

Ivermectin Goes to Court

This article originally appeared in The Desert Review on January 28, 2021.

Since the NIH heard testimony from Dr. Pierre Kory on January 6, 2021, another 63,822 souls have perished, and based upon the evidence produced by Dr. Andrew Hill of the WHO, some 83% or precisely 52,972 deaths could have been prevented had the NIH instead revised this guidance to recommend or Early Use Authorization.

We are looking at so many preventable deaths that I share Dr. Pierre Kory's disgust. Dr. Kory announced to the Senate on December 8, 2020, that any further deaths are needless because Ivermectin's benefits are now well-known. I keep track of the Kory Count out of reverence to the dead and to keep it known that these deaths were preventable.

The court case where Judith Smentkiewicz's son had to hire an attorney to get an adjunction to force the hospital to provide her Ivermectin underscores the problem our country now faces. My patients and their families all enjoy the protection of Ivermectin because my practice includes education and access.

About 10 percent of other physicians do the same for their patients. The vast majority of doctors do not, and their patients face COVID-19 alone or with research done by family members like Judith Smentkiewicz's son. She was lucky to survive, and one can read her story in "Ivermectin goes to court, and the NIH relaxes its prohibition," published by the *Desert Review* on January 18, 2021.

Her attorney, Ralph Lorigo, saved her life.

It is not every day that an attorney can save a life, but Mr. Lorigo did so when he obtained a court order for the hospital to administer Ivermectin to Ms. Smentkiewicz. She was a single mother who went above and beyond to raise her two children by herself. She worked as a secretary and later cleaned houses four days a week so her children could survive. Her son repaid the favor when the ICU physician told him his mother would probably die. At age 80 and on a ventilator with COVID, her chances were 80% that the virus would take her life. But her son also went above and beyond, and he found an article that suggested that Ivermectin could help her, and the rest is history.

Of course, the naysayers will argue that this was anecdotal at best. And that it did not prove that Ivermectin works. However, the pesky proverbial fly in the ointment is that it happened a second time to Glenna Dickinson, and the same lawyer, Ralph Lorigo, decided to help her family. He went to court and got a second judge to issue a court order to force the hospital to administer the Ivermectin, and she also got better.

So, in whose Brave New World are we now living, where rich, large pharmaceutical companies call the shots, and doctors and regulators can be bought? You and I are expendable resources in a society where the truth and morals no longer matter.

***

YouTube Censors the Senate: The Canary in Our Coal Mine

This article originally appeared in the Desert Review on February 4, 2021.

Senator Ron Johnson wrote an OP-ED in the Wall Street Journal on February 2, 2021, about YouTube removing Dr. Kory's video. Below is an excerpt:

"Google's YouTube has ratcheted up censorship to a new level by removing two videos from a US Senate Committee. They were from a December 8 Committee on Homeland Security and Governmental Affairs hearing on early treatment of Covid-19. One was a 30-minute summary; the other was the opening statement of critical care specialist Pierre Kory.

Dr. Kory is part of a world-renowned group of physicians who developed a ground-breaking use of corticosteroids to treat hospitalized Covid patients. His testimony at a May Senate hearing helped doctors rethink treatment protocols and save lives.

At the December hearing, he presented evidence regarding the use of Ivermectin, a cheap and widely available drug that treats tropical diseases caused by parasites, for prevention and early treatment of Covid-19. He described a just-published study from Argentina in which about 800 health care workers received Ivermectin, and 400 did not. Not one of the 800 contracted the COVID-19; 58% of the 400 did.

Dr. Kory asked the National Institutes of Health to review his group's manuscript outlining dozens of successful trials and to consider updating its August 27 guidance in which he recommended "against the use of Ivermectin for the treatment of COVID-19 except in a clinical trial." On December 10, Sen. Rand Paul and I sent a letter to the NIH requesting that it review Dr. Kory's evidence."
Allow me to add my comment and voice to Senator Johnson's. Since the request was made to the NIH, they, to their credit, invited Dr. Andrew Hill, Dr. Pierre Kory, and Dr. Paul Marik to travel to Bethesda and speak to their committee on COVID-19 treatment on January 6, 2021.

As a result, the NIH broke ranks with the FDA. They removed the restriction against Ivermectin, instead raising their guidance to "neutral" and according it the same status as polyclonal antibodies. This has paved the way for Ivermectin to become widely used in the pandemic by informed patients and informed physicians. However, censorship now blocks this vital and lifesaving information from reaching the public.

When I wrote this book attempting to help my friend survive his brain cancer and drawing upon my 38-years of experience and knowledge as a practicing physician, it never occurred to me that certain powerful interests would not want my message to reach readers. It never occurred to me that censorship still takes place in the United States.

However, with the blatant removal of critical care specialist's Senate testimony, that is exactly what is happening now.

The larger question is, "Why?"

Why should you not be allowed to hear the testimony of scientists who were qualified and invited to speak before the US Senate? Why should cancer patients not be able to read the material in my book? Why do we allow de facto censorship in the United States, and what are the potential future effects of such censorship?

You may believe that YouTube is a kind, generous titan that exists to serve humanity, and its goal is to make certain that you listen to only the best and clearest scientific evidence. If you feel that this type of parental filtering serves your interest, perhaps you would be willing to purchase some ocean-front property in Arizona.

Like me, if you are skeptical, and believe there is a more sinister motive, be alarmed, be vocal, and object to censorship because censorship is merely the canary in the coal mine. If you see them dropping dead all around you, you should take heed.

America needs to awaken and realize that our parental agencies and captains of industry are not behaving in our best interest; instead, they are catering to their own. When the number of preventable US deaths exceeds 200,000, perhaps someone needs to sound the alarm.

Accordingly, I update the "Kory Count' out of respect to the preventable lives lost in the pandemic, those lives that could have been saved with the early outpatient treatment discussed by Dr. Pierre Kory in his Senate testimony that YouTube has now banned.

Dr. Pierre Kory, Dr. Peter McCullough, Dr. Harvey Risch, Dr. George Fareed, Dr. Jean-Jacques Rajter, and other visionaries all testified before Senator Ron Johnson's Homeland Security Committee, and their message must be amplified, not censored. With early outpatient treatment, we can save up to 100,000 lives per month, beginning immediately. Such early outpatient, starting with adding Ivermectin for prevention and treatment, will save countless precious lives, and they may be you, your family, or loved ones.

Tell everyone you know about the canaries in our coal mine. Most importantly, inform those who run the mine that something needs to be done before it is too late.

POSTSCRIPT

It has now been almost six months since the book release. In that time, repurposed drugs have reached the world stage as a potential solution to the COVID-19 pandemic. My friend Evan's tumor continues to shrink, and he is better now than when his cancer was diagnosed more than one year ago – and he attributes this to his use of repurposed drugs.

When I set out to write this book to help Evan beat his diagnosis, I became angry almost immediately because it was so obvious that repurposed drugs could have and should have been made a part of glioblastoma treatment. For that matter, repurposed drugs, in my opinion should be offered in all cases of terminal cancer. They also should have been added long ago as cancer preventative agents.

I sat in disbelief as I watched repurposed drugs get marginalized in this pandemic as half a million Americans perished when repurposed drugs could have saved most. Instead, our public officials delayed and advised against any early outpatient treatment, instead preferring to fashion expensive designer drugs and vaccines while our economy and health crumbled.

Now, more than one year into the pandemic, the truth is leaking out, despite the best efforts by opponents to keep it quiet. We are learning about repurposed drugs, not from our appointed health officials with whom we trusted our lives, but from those intensive care unit doctors who have a conscience – the Dr. Rajters and Dr. Korys of this world – those physicians who continue to place lives above money.

Repurposed drugs have been applied to the coronavirus by some of the most brilliant and academic physicians of our time. Ivermectin has stood out as perhaps the most effective one.

Dr. Kory points out that the current amount of data showing Ivermectin's benefit exceeds the magnitude of the RECOVERY trial data, which showed the benefit of corticosteroids. Although corticosteroid treatment for COVID-19 became the standard of care overnight, no similar change occurred with Ivermectin. Why the double standard?

Merck and the FDA will warn you that Ivermectin still should not be used for coronavirus, despite no data to back up their claim.

Judith Smentkiewicz, Glenna Dickinson, and everyone whose life has been saved from Ivermectin will disagree. So will Dr. Andrew Hill of the WHO, Dr. George Fareed, formerly of Harvard and the NIH, and Dr. Peter McCullough, Vice-Chair of Internal Medicine at Baylor.

In its condemnation of Ivermectin, Merck does not mention that it spent 425 million dollars in purchasing the rights to MK-7110, a potentially expensive and competing drug in Phase III clinical trials that will likely soon receive FDA Emergency Use Authorization to treat COVID-19. Likewise, the FDA does not mention that the US government contributed 356 million dollars to Merck as part of a joint agreement to manufacture and distribute this drug. So long as Big Pharma and our public institutions remain financially entangled, we can never expect cheap repurposed drugs to be judged on a level playing field. We can never expect them to be approved regardless of how well they work against cancer, COVID-19 or any other disease.

Despite the demonization of HCQ, the 1900 patients of Dr. Brian Tyson who survived their infection will also take exception to the FDA's official position that HCQ should not be used to treat COVID-19.

Dr. Pierre Kory's persuasive Senate YouTube testimony went viral, garnering nearly eight million views before it was pulled. Before its censorship, Judith Smentkiewicz's family found it while surfing the internet and researching Ivermectin. As a direct result, Judith, who was on a respirator and dying of COVID in an ICU, got the drug. Within two days she was off of the ventilator, out of the ICU, and breathing on her own. Other families found Dr. Kory's lifesaving video before it was banned. They also fought to get the Ivermectin, and they noticed similar rapid recoveries. Actor Louis Gossett Jr. credits his survival from COVID-19 to finding Dr. Kory's FLCCC website and using Ivermectin.

Dr. Kory does not mince words, "Ivermectin is the solution to the pandemic...The amount of evidence to show Ivermectin is lifesaving and protective is so immense and the drug is so safe. It needs to be immediately adopted—systematically, nationally, and globally— period."

<u>Web Resources on Early Outpatient Treatment for COVID-19</u>

- For more information on Dr. Pierre Kory and Ivermectin, the reader is referred to the FLCCC Alliance website:
  https://covid19criticalcare.com

- For more information about developments with repurposed drugs for cancer and COVID-19, see: www.repurposedpills.com

- For a free patient brochure on early outpatient treatment resources including a list of prescribing physicians:
  https://aapsonline.org/CovidPatientTreatmentGuide.pdf

- For more information about Dr. George Fareed, Dr. Peter McCullough and Dr. Harvey Risch's early sequential multidrug therapy (SMDT), the reader is referred to the following: https://rcm.imrpress.com/EN/10.31083/j.rcm.2020.04.264

ABOUT THE AUTHOR

Dr. Justus Robert Hope, writer's pseudonym, graduated *summa cum laude* from Wabash College where he was named a Lilly Scholar. He attended Baylor College of Medicine, where he was awarded the M.D. degree. He completed a residency in Physical Medicine & Rehabilitation at The University of California Irvine Medical Center.

He is board certified and has taught at the University of California Davis Medical Center in the departments of Family Practice and Physical Medicine & Rehabilitation. He has practiced medicine for over 35 years and maintains a private practice in Northern California. He has authored six books.

CPSIA information can be obtained
at www.ICGtesting.com
Printed in the USA
BVHW051418210921
617191BV00004B/43

9 780998 055428